Reproductive Health and Cancer in Adolescents and Young Adults

Volume 732

For further volumes:
http://www.springer.com/series/5584

Gwendolyn P. Quinn ·
Susan T. Vadaparampil

Editors

Reproductive Health and Cancer in Adolescents and Young Adults

Foreword by Brad Zebrack

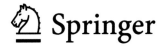 Springer

Editors
Dr. Gwendolyn P. Quinn
Moffitt Cancer Center
Magnolia Drive 12902
33612 Tampa, FL
USA
gwen.quinn@moffitt.org

Dr. Susan T. Vadaparampil
Moffitt Cancer Center
Magnolia Drive 12902
33612 Tampa, FL
USA
susan.vadaparampil@moffitt.org

ISSN 0065-2598
ISBN 978-94-007-2491-4   e-ISBN 978-94-007-2492-1
DOI 10.1007/978-94-007-2492-1
Springer Dordrecht Heidelberg London New York

Library of Congress Control Number: 2011938669

Printed on acid-free paper

Springer is part of Springer Science+Business Media (www.springer.com)

Foreword

Last year marked two major milestones in my life. I turned 50 years old, and I have lived half my life – 25 years – as a cancer survivor.

The invitation to write the forward to this important text on reproductive health for young adults with cancer offered me an opportunity to reflect on my own daughter's birth and my path to parenthood nine years ago.

I recall the day when my wife Joanne and I decided to leave the house for the first time since our daughter Sierra's birth. Living in a self-contained nest, we finally needed food and supplies, and mostly just wanted to get out of the house. So we began to prepare. What might we need when taking a 6-day old infant out into the world? Diaper bag, with all the accoutrements – changing board, spare diapers, wipes. Oh, a bottle in case she gets hungry. Carrier. Stroller. The baby, of course. Oh, maybe we should feed her before we go. Done. OK, now check diaper. Oops! Diaper change. Now dress her. What should she wear on a hot August afternoon in Los Angeles? Redress her. Then dress her back into the first outfit. Find a hat. Blanket?

An hour and a half later we were ready to head to Target. And too tired to go. So we said "forget it; maybe tomorrow."

Fast forward to yesterday. Almost nine years later. Sierra's school is holding its end-of-year Ice Cream Social and street dance. Hundreds of grade school kids and parents are out in the yard, celebrating the anticipation of summer vacation. The once helpless and vulnerable infant who we could not get out of the house on the 6th day of her life is now a thriving 3rd grader, dancing in the street and laughing with her friends. She is beautiful.

These are some of the anxieties and joys of parenthood that I never would have known that I was missing had I not had a child. Yet there was a time when, after unsuccessful attempts at artificial insemination and costly in vitro fertilization, my wife Joanne and I resigned ourselves to a life without children of our own. We each had brothers and sisters with children, and decided that we would play active roles in the lives of our nieces and nephews.

Meanwhile, instead of raising a family during our late 20s and 30s, Joanne and I did a lot together. We hiked and biked and backpacked and travelled. We packed up and moved from California to Michigan for graduate school, then re-packed and returned to California five years later. We got "real" jobs, with benefits! We bought a house. We did what many others our age were doing, except of course raising children. We turned 40 years old. Life was good.

But coming home from work one night and sitting down to dinner, we asked ourselves: Is this all there is? After deciding we would be childless and that we were okay with that decision, we changed our minds. It was time to consider adoption.

Two and half years later, we were at the bedside as our daughter Sierra Grace was born, and thus began the memories and challenges and joys of parenthood that I *now* know and cherish.

I have been a cancer patient but also a clinician who has helped patients and family members deal with the multiple and various challenges that occur throughout phases of cancer diagnosis, treatment, and transitions to off-treatment survival or the end of life. As a researcher and advocate whose work focuses on the quality of life for cancer survivors and their loved ones I feel that this text is an invaluable educational resource that targets unique needs and issues faced by young adults fighting cancer during their reproductive years. The authors provide an excellent review of the impact of cancer on reproductive health and options for maintaining reproductive health throughout a continuum of care. They also address issues and challenges related to family building and parenthood. Most importantly, this book highlights salient challenges, questions, and emotions for clinicians and researchers to consider when working with the young adult cancer population.

Brad Zebrack

Acknowledgements

Writing a book is a lot like having a baby. It begins with the conception of an idea, some hard labor, and the nurturing of the product of that labor for many years to come. Although there are many ways to have a baby or parent a child, there is one constant across them all – it is not done alone. In that regard, we must acknowledge the many individuals who helped bring this book into the world. Starting with Ilse Henson, publishing assistant who saw promise in the idea of a book about reproductive health and cancer and encouraged us to pursue it, created the path for it to happen, and navigated us through the process. Next we had the good fortune of working with authors who were willing to spend long hours drafting chapters, responding to edits, and editing yet again with each step of the review process. We are indebted to this group of skilled experts who shared their knowledge and years of clinical and research experiences in these chapters. We like to think of this group as encompassing the "good genes" that gave rise to the birth of this book. As with a traditional pregnancy, a steady diet of continuous attention, regular appointments, and watching for warning signs are keys to a healthy baby. The constant attention, interest and good work of the following people contributed to the success of this book: Michele Griffin, Alison Nelson, Bethanne Bower, Devin Murphy, and Nicole Hutchins. The extended family of this book, our own families, also donated their efforts by supplying continuous encouragement – we'd like to thank Amanda, Caity, Abby, Blake, Tim, Lisa, Robert, Jennifer, Matt, Joey, Jacob, Maya, Sam, Ali, and Rajesh. Their presence in our lives has allowed us to understand and appreciate the importance of ensuring that all individuals have the opportunity to build families based on their own future desires. We also thank Moffitt Cancer Center for providing the environment and resources to conduct our research. Finally, we are highly appreciative of the cancer survivors who allowed us into their lives by sharing their stories presented in the vignettes that begin each chapter. Your courage and honesty helped to shine a light on the great need for attention to reproductive health issues in the oncology world. We hope we have honored your struggles by creating this book.

This book is intended for current and future health care professionals and researchers who work with adolescent and young adult populations affected by or at risk for cancer. While there are varying definitions of the age range of this population, our goal was to focus on those of "childbearing potential", which typically begins at puberty and extends through the mid-forties. We acknowledge that in this day of reproductive technologies, there are many men, and some women, who become parents beyond this age range. The attention to the broader aspect of reproductive health, outside of childbearing, doesn't begin or end at any age.

Introduction

There are an estimated 70,000 new cancers diagnosed each year among men and women between the age of 15 and 39 and 143,000 in ages 40–45. Recognizing the unique clinical, psychosocial, and quality of life impacts cancer may have based on an earlier than average age of diagnosis, these individuals are often categorized as the Adolescent/Young Adult (AYA) population. The chapters in our text focus either on AYA as a whole or in a few chapters on certain segments of AYA such as pediatric cancer patients or adolescents, or parents of young children.

Infertility and reproductive health issues are an expected consequence of most cancer treatments that include chemotherapy and/or radiotherapy. Although fertility may be regained after some cancer treatments, sustained infertility develops in 50–95% of cancer survivors. Rates of cancer-related infertility in men and women vary and depend on a number of factors, including age, sex, diagnosis, treatment dose/intensity, size/location of radiation field, and the patient's pretreatment fertility status. Women have a 40–80% chance of losing fertility following chemotherapy or radiation during reproductive years and 30–75% of male cancer patients become sterile after cancer treatment. Given the improvements in cancer treatment and survival as well as advances in reproductive medicine that have occurred over the past several decades, the unique reproductive health needs of this group must be considered – beginning at initial diagnosis and continuing through to survivorship care.

There are fertility preservation options available prior to initiation of cancer treatment for AYA populations to assist in preserving or maintaining fertility such as sperm banking, oocyte and embryo cryopreservation and testicular and ovarian tissue freezing. Conversely, reproductive health particularly as it relates to pregnancy and sexually transmitted infection risks are an important consideration. For some cancer patients, there may be a perception that there is little risk of pregnancy due to the cancer treatments and therefore they engage in risky sexual behavior (e.g., unprotected sexual intercourse). The use of contraception for the prevention of pregnancy during treatment is an essential component of quality care. Furthermore, females with certain hormone dependent cancers must consider the type and duration of contraception in relation to their cancer type. Less is known about the need for contraception to prevent a partner from exposure to chemo or radiation during or after treatment.

For patients currently pregnant or who become pregnant after a cancer diagnosis, there are numerous medical and psychosocial considerations. While many survivors' may have healthy pregnancies and offspring, health care professionals and researchers must be aware of the pharmacokinetics of chemotherapeutic agents during pregnancy and lactation, and the effects on placenta, fetus and infant as well as recognizing that additional psychological support may be required in the unique clinical situation of cancer in pregnancy and personalized counseling for contraceptive use during and after treatment. For individuals at high risk of familial cancers, prenatal diagnosis and preimplantation genetic diagnosis should be offered after appropriate genetic consultation and counseling in a regional genetic service.

Early and ongoing consideration about a patient's current and future family building plans and desires is also of critical importance. For those patients who have already experienced loss of fertility through the cancer and/or the associated treatment, counseling about additional family building options such a donor sperm, embryos, gestational carriers, or adoption is warranted. Additionally, for patients who are already parents, there is a tremendous need for support and resources to assist in managing the psychosocial and emotional needs of their children.

The concerns of young cancer survivors in relation to the interplay of body image, relationships, fear of recurrence, and sexuality are often a source of great anxiety which can significantly impact quality of life. New research is aiding in the design of interventions and programs to help AYA survivors prepare for quality survival in relation to the psychosocial "late effects" which may be experienced in ways not seen in the traditional population of older adult cancer survivors.

Despite evidence that patients want information about future fertility, existing research finds large gaps between recommended and actual clinical practice related to discussion of fertility preservation options with cancer patients. There are many barriers at the provider, institutional and policy level that may impact communication and discussion related to fertility preservation and reproductive health issues.

Finally, despite advances in cancer treatment and options to preserve fertility have greatly advanced in the past decade, there are still many considerations related to the ethical and legal issues surrounding these issues such as the disposition of stored gametes and consideration of posthumous reproduction.

Contents

1   **Principles of Cancer Treatment: Impact on Reproduction** . .   **1**
Kenny A. Rodriguez-Wallberg

2   **Fertility Preservation Options for Females** **9**
Amelia P. Bailey and Elizabeth S. Ginsburg

3   **Options for Fertility Preservation in Men and Boys
with Cancer** **29**
Peter J. Stahl, Doron S. Stember, and John P. Mulhall

4   **Contraception and Cancer Treatment in Young Persons** . . .   **41**
Valerie Laurence and Christine Rousset-Jablonski

5   **Sexual Health During Cancer Treatment** **61**
Linda U. Krebs

6   **The Unique Reproductive Concerns of Young Women
with Breast Cancer** **77**
Kathryn J. Ruddy and Ann H. Partridge

7   **Pregnancy and Cancer** **89**
Celso Silva and Farah S. Chung

8   **Preimplantation Genetic Diagnosis for Hereditary Cancers** .   **103**
Sioban B. SenGupta, Susan T. Vadaparampil, and Usha Menon

9   **Non-traditional Family Building Planning** **115**
Judith E. Horowitz

10   **Parenting with Cancer I: Developmental Perspective,
Communication, and Coping** **131**
Kristin S. Russell and Paula K. Rauch

11   **Parenting with Cancer II: Parenting at Different
Stages of Illness** **141**
Kristin S. Russell and Paula K. Rauch

12   **Pediatric Oncology and Reproductive Health** **151**
James L. Klosky, Rebecca H. Foster, and Alexandra M. Nobel

13   **Institutional Approaches to Implementing Fertility
Preservation for Cancer Patients** **165**
Joanne Frankel Kelvin and Joyce Reinecke

14 Patient Provider Communication and Reproductive Health . **175**
Caprice A. Knapp, Gwendolyn P. Quinn, Deborah Rapalo,
and Lindsey Woodworth

15 Fertility Preservation in Cancer Patients:
Ethical Considerations **187**
Bethanne Bower and Gwendolyn P. Quinn

16 The Legal Issue and of Assisted Reproductive Technologies . **197**
Diana Brock

Appendix **211**

Additional Resources **215**

Index **219**

Contributors

Amelia P. Bailey, MD Center for Infertility and Reproductive Surgery, Brigham and Women's Hospital, Boston, MA 02115, USA, apbailey@partners.org

Bethanne Bower, BA Health Outcomes and Behavior Program, Division of Population Sciences, Moffitt Cancer Center, Tampa, Florida, bethannebower@gmail.com

Diana Brock, Esq Adjunct Legal Studies Professor, Hodges University, 2655 Northbrooke Drive, Naples, FL 34119, djzink@gmail.com

Farah S. Chung, MD Department of Obstetrics and Gynecology, University of South Florida, Tampa, FL, USA, fsultanmd@gmail.com

Rebecca H. Foster, PhD Department of Psychology, MS 740, St. Jude Children's Research Hospital, Memphis, TN 38105, USA, Rebecca.Foster@stjude.org

Elizabeth S. Ginsburg, MD In Vitro Fertilization Program Brigham & Women's Hospital, Boston, MA, USA, eginsburg@partners.org

Judith E. Horowitz, PhD Private Practice, 5551 N University Drive, Suite 204, Coral Springs, FL 33067, USA, jhorowitzphd01@aol.com

Joanne Frankel Kelvin, RN, MSN, AOCN Clinical Nurse Specialist, Memorial Sloan-Kettering Cancer Center, New York, NY, USA, kelvinj@mskcc.org

James L. Klosky, PhD Department of Psychology, MS 740, St. Jude Children's Research Hospital, Memphis, TN 38105, USA, james.klosky@stjude.org

Caprice A. Knapp, PhD Department of Health Outcomes and Policy, University of Florida, Gainesville, FL 32608, USA, caprice1@ufl.edu

Linda U. Krebs, PhD, RN, AOCN, FAAN University of Colorado Denver, College of Nursing Campus, Aurora, CO 80045, USA, linda.krebs@ucdenver.edu

Valerie Laurence, MD Department of Medical Oncology, Medical Oncologist, Institut Curie, 75005 Paris, France, valerie.laurence@curie.net

Usha Menon, PhD Gynaecological Cancer Research Centre, Institute for Women's Health, University College London, W1T 7DN London, UK, u.menon@ucl.ac.uk

John P. Mulhall, MD Memorial Sloan-Kettering Cancer Center, New York, NY, USA, mulhalj1@mskcc.org

Alexandra M. Nobel, BA Department of Psychology, MS 740, St. Jude Children's Research Hospital, Memphis, TN 38105, USA, amnobel@gmail.com

Ann H. Partridge, MD, MPH Dana-Farber Cancer Institute, Boston, MA 02215, USA, ann_partridge@dfci.harvard.edu

Gwendolyn P. Quinn, PhD Moffitt Cancer Center, College of Medicine, University of South Florida, Tampa, FL 33612, USA, gwen.quinn@moffitt.org

Deborah Rapalo, MPH Department of Health Outcomes and Policy, University of Florida, Gainesville, FL 32608, USA, rapalo1d@ufl.edu

Paula K. Rauch, MD Marjorie E. Korff, PACT (Parenting At a Challenging Time) Program, Massachusetts General Hospital, Boston, MA, USA; Child Psychiatry Consultation Liaison Service, Massachusetts General Hospital, Boston, MA, USA, prauch@partners.org

Joyce Reinecke, JD Cancer & Fertility Advisor, LIVESTRONG, Lafayette, California 94549, USA, joyce@fertilehope.org

Kenny A. Rodriguez-Wallberg, MD, PhD Division of Obstetrics and Gynecology, Department of Clinical Science, Intervention and Technology, Karolinska Institute, Stockholm, Sweden; Fertility Unit, Division of Obstetrics and Gynecology, Karolinska University Hospital Huddinge, SE-141 86, Stockholm, Sweden, kenny.rodriguez-wallberg@karolinska.se

Christine Rousset-Jablonski, MD Department of Tumor Biology, Gynecologist, Institut Curie, 75005 Paris, France, christine.roussetjablonski@curie.net

Kathryn J. Ruddy, MD, MPH Dana-Farber Cancer Institute, Boston, MA 02215, USA, kathryn_ruddy@dfci.harvard.edu

Kristin S. Russell, MD Child and Adolescent Psychiatry, Marjorie E. Korff, PACT (Parenting At a Challenging Time Program), Massachusetts General Hospital, Boston, MA, USA, ksrussell@partners.org

Sioban B. SenGupta, PhD UCL Centre for PGD, Institute for Women's Health, University College London, WC1E 6HX London, UK, s.sengupta@ucl.ac.uk

Celso Silva, MD Assistant Professor, Director - Center for Fertility Preservation, USF IVF, Division of Reproductive Endocrinology and Infertility, Department of Obstetrics and Gynecology, University of South Florida, Tampa, FL, USA, csilva@health.usf.edu

Peter J. Stahl, MD   James Buchanan Brady Department of Urology, Weill Cornell Medical College, New York, NY, USA, pjs2002@med.cornell.edu

Doron S. Stember, MD   Memorial Sloan-Kettering Cancer Center, New York, NY, USA, doronstember@gmail.com

Susan T. Vadaparampil, PhD, MPH   Health Outcomes and Behavior Program, Department of Oncologic Science, Moffitt Cancer Center and Research Institute, Cancer Prevention and Control, University of South Florida, Tampa, FL 33612, USA, susan.vadaparampil@moffitt.org

Lindsey Woodworth, MA   Department of Health Outcomes and Policy, University of Florida, Gainesville, FL 32608, USA, ljw@ichp.ufl.edu

Principles of Cancer Treatment: Impact on Reproduction

Kenny A. Rodriguez-Wallberg, MD, PhD

A lot of advances have been made in science, technology and reproduction but still we can't say for sure who will or will not be temporarily or permanently sterile from cancer or the treatment. So I think it's best to discuss it will all patients who are of reproductive age. It's not an easy discussion to have. You've just told someone they have cancer and now you tell them they may not be able to have kids. Some people don't care, or at least they think they don't care at the time. Some people are more upset about the news of infertility than they are about the cancer. You can't assume because you look at a patients chart that you know how they feel about fertility. Even if they already have kids or they aren't married or they are struggling financially, it's something that has to be discussed.

I had a testicular cancer patient, Sam, a few years ago with late stage disease. When I talked to him about fertility he got very excited – he said it was the most hopeful thing he'd heard since he came to the hospital. Then I wondered if I had given him false hope, because his odds were not too good, In fact they were pretty dismal. But that guy was bouncing off the wall with joy at the thought of banking sperm, and I thought maybe he would benefit from thinking some happy thoughts for a while. He did bank sperm, and it seemed to lift his spirits but in the end, he didn't survive the cancer.

I had a female patient with a GU cancer who said she wanted no part of a discussion about preserving fertility. She was only 25, but she said she knew she didn't want kids, and had never wanted them. So I stopped trying to talk about it. She did well and she's in graduate school now and just got married. At her last check-up, she told me she wished she had listened to me about the fertility. Now that she's doing well and married she has a new perspective on children and just learned she is infertile. She and her husband are trying to adopt but it's not an easy process for a cancer survivor. That taught me a lesson. I now insist my patients listen to the infertility talk, even if they say they don't want kids I try to explain that a lot of people feel differently when the treatment is over and they go on with their lives. I even tell them about Sam and how much hope that sperm banking gave him in his last days. I think as oncologist we have to not only talk about how to manage the disease, but how to prepare for survivorship. Sometimes we have to talk about end-of-life issues too. None of it is easy, but it's all worth it.
Dr. A, Oncologist

K.A. Rodriguez-Wallberg (✉)
Division of Obstetrics and Gynecology, Department of Clinical Science, Intervention and Technology, Karolinska Institute, Stockholm, Sweden

Fertility Unit, Division of Obstetrics and Gynecology, Karolinska University Hospital Huddinge, SE-141 86, Stockholm, Sweden
e-mail: kenny.rodriguez-wallberg@karolinska.se

Introduction

According to the National Cancer Institute's Surveillance, Epidemiology, and End Results (SEER) database [1], 1,445,000 new cases of invasive cancer (766,860 in men and 678,060 in women) were diagnosed in the US in 2007

G.P. Quinn, S.T. Vadaparampil (eds.), *Reproductive Health and Cancer in Adolescents and Young Adults*, Advances in Experimental Medicine and Biology 732,
DOI 10.1007/978-94-007-2492-1_1, © Springer Science+Business Media B.V. 2012

[1]. Approximately 1,530,000 new cancer cases were expected to be diagnosed in 2010 (789,620 in men and 739,940 in women). Men have an overall 45% risk of developing cancer at some time during their lives, which is higher than in women who present with 37% lifetime cancer risk. Age is the most significant risk factor for cancer in both sexes. However, even younger adults and children may develop cancer, and in people younger than 39 years, the risk is of about 1/72 for men and 1/51 for women. For adults between 40 and 59 years, 1/12 men and 1/11 women will develop cancer.

With modern cancer treatment, nearly two thirds of patients diagnosed with cancer can get cured today. Cancer treatment in young adults and children may have detrimental effects on the reproductive system and negatively affect the quality of life of cancer survivors [2, 3].

As shown in Table 1.1, the most common cancer in females is breast cancer, followed by cancers of the digestive and respiratory systems and genital organs, in particular uterus, ovary and cervix. In males, the most common cancers arise in the genital organs prostate and testicle, followed by cancers of the digestive, respiratory and urinary systems and skin. Haematologycal malignancies and lymphoma are also common cancers in both sexes, particularly presenting at young ages [1].

Principles of Cancer Treatment

Cancer treatment techniques include surgery, radiation therapy, chemotherapy, hormone therapy (in case of hormone sensitive tumors), and biological therapy (including immunotherapy and gene therapy). Surgery and radiation therapy are considered local treatments and chemotherapy and biological therapy are systemic. Hormone therapy is systemic and targeted to specific hormone receptors.

Surgery may impact fertility by removing reproductive organs or damaging structures needed for reproduction. Chemotherapy and radiotherapy have a known toxic effect on the

Table 1.1 Cancer incidence in both sexes expected for year 2010 in the US

Primary site	Estimated new cancer cases for females	Estimated new cancer cases for males
All sites	739,940	789,620
Breast	207,090	1,970
Digestive system	125,790	148,540
Colon	53,430	49,470
Rectum	17,050	22,620
Liver & bile duct	6,690	17,430
Esophagus	3,510	13,130
Stomach	8,270	12,730
Pancreas	21,770	21,370
Respiratory system	110,010	130,600
Lung and bronchus	105,770	116,750
Genital organs	83,750	227,460
Endometrium	43,470	
Ovary	21,880	
Cervix	12,200	
Prostate		217,730
Testis		8,480
Urinary system	41,640	89,620
Urinary bladder	17,770	52,760
Kidney and renal pelvis	22,870	35,370
Endocrine system	35,040	11,890
Thyroid	33,930	10,740
Lymphoma	33,980	40,050
Skin	31,400	42,610
Melanoma	29,260	38,870
Leukemia	18,360	24,690
Myeloma	9,010	11,170
Brain and other nervous	10,040	11,980
Oral cavity and pharynx	11,120	25,420

Adapted from: Cancer Facts & Figures – 2010, American Cancer Society (ACS), Atlanta, Georgia, 2010
Incidence projections are based on rates from the North American Association of Central Cancer Registries (NAACCR) from 1995 to 2006, representing about 89% of the US population
SEER Cancer Statistics Review 1975–2007, National Cancer Institute, updated January 7, 2011 [1]

gonads, ovaries, and testicles, and may induce gonadal failure. The impact of biological therapy on reproduction is largely unknown.

Cancer Surgery

Surgery is the most effective cancer treatment today. Eventually 40–100% of patients may be cured with the highest success when complete removal of the tumor is obtained. Surgery may be also indicated for cancer prophylaxis, such as the case of premalignant disease of the cervix in female patients. In very early stages of cervix cancer, the surgical excision of a significant part of the cervix, known as conization or even a small loop excision, may afford to patients a complete disease-free survival. Surgery of the cervix may induce subfertility by affecting the normal functioning of the cervix and its glandular secretion. These iatrogenically-induced cervical causes of infertility may be treated with success with intrauterine insemination and more advanced techniques of assisted reproduction as In Vitro Fertilization (IVF).

Whenever the complete removal of the tumor aiming to a curative treatment may not be obtained, reduction of tumor size by surgery may improve patient's chances to cure by facilitating the response to adjuvant chemotherapy or radiotherapy in the treatment of cancer tumors.

Surgery may also affect future fertility if there is removal or damage of the reproductive organs. In male patients, surgery for pelvic cancer such as for prostate, bladder or colon cancer may damage nerves and affecting potency or ejaculation. Surgical adjuvant treatment by removing the gonads may be indicated in female and male patients with hormone sensitive tumors.

In case of large tumors, chemotherapy and radiation may be indicated as first line treatment aiming to a reduction of tumor size and control of subclinical metastatic disease before surgical treatment. This is known as neo-adjuvant therapy. Thereafter, surgical treatment is planned to remove residual tumor masses. Neo-adjuvant therapy is usually planned before surgery in female patients with stage III breast cancer and young male cancer patients with bulky testicular cancer.

There has been a gradual development in gynecologic oncologic surgery and urologic oncologic surgery, aiming at preserving reproductive organs in female and male patients, respectively, without compromising survival. Fertility-sparing surgery is an option today for selected patients. The indication for such interventions often includes a well differentiated low-grade tumor in its early stages or with low malignant potential. The surgical fertility-sparing approaches available for women are shown in Table 1.2 [4].

The most established fertility preservation procedure for women in this group is the radical trachelectomy, offered to women with early stage cervical cancer. The surgery aims at removing completely the cervix tumor while preserving the uterus. Although conservative surgery offers the opportunity to preserve the reproductive organs, it offers no guarantee of achieving pregnancy or live-birth. Causes of subfertility may be present in the patients either due to pre-existing conditions or following the surgical treatment (i.e., scar formation) and a number of those patients may further require assisted reproduction treatments. In cases of selected ovarian tumors (i.e. borderline tumors) young female patients may be offered a single oophorectomy aiming at preserving the uterus and the contralateral ovary for future reproduction, (Table 1.2) [4].

In men, testicular cancer is the most prevalent cancer, and it presents often at a young age when fertility concerns may be an issue. For selected patients, unilateral and partial orchidectomies have developed as conservative cancer treatments aiming at preserving hormonal and sperm production and, thus, fertility potential. Experience with this method was first obtained in the treatment of pre-pubertal patients with benign teratomas [5]. The German Testicular Cancer Study Group reported a 98.6% disease-free survival rate at a follow-up of 7 years after conservative surgery of tumors <2 cm with negative biopsy findings of the tumor bed [6].

Radiotherapy in Cancer Treatment

It is known that cancer cells present with defects in their ability to repair sub-lethal DNA, whereas normal cells have the ability to recover. High dose

Table 1.2 Fertility-sparing interventions in female patients (with permission from Rodriguez-Macias Wallberg and colleagues [4])

Diagnosis	Type of surgery	Description	Obstetric outcome	Oncologic outcome
Cervical cancer stage IA1,1A2,1B1	Radical vaginal trachelectomy	Laparoscopic pelvic lymphadenectomy. Vaginal resection of the cervix and surrounding parametria keeping the corpus of the uterus and the ovaries intact	Spontaneous pregnancies described in up to 70%. Risk of second trimester pregnancy loss and preterm delivery	Rates of recurrence and mortality are comparable to those described for similar cases treated by means of radical hysterectomy or radiation therapy
Borderline ovarian tumors FIGO stage I	Unilateral oophorectomy	Removal of the affected ovary only, keeping in place the unaffected one and the uterus	Pregnancies have been reported and favorable obstetric outcome	Oncologic outcome is comparable with the more radical approach of removing both ovaries and the uterus. Recurrence 0–20% vs 12–58% when only cystectomy was performed
Ovarian epithelial cancer stage I, grade 1	Unilateral oophorectomy	Removal of the affected ovary only, keeping in place the unaffected one and the uterus	Pregnancies have been reported and favorable obstetric outcome	7% recurrence of the ovarian malignancy and 5% deaths
Malignant ovarian germ cell tumors/sex cord stromal tumors	Unilateral oophorectomy	Removal of the affected ovary only	Pregnancies have been reported and favorable obstetric outcome	Risk of recurrence similar to historical controls
Endometrial adenocarcinoma Grade 1, stage 1A (without myometrial or cervical invasion)	Hormonal treatment with progestational agents for 6 months	Follow-up with endometrial biopsies every 3 months	Pregnancies have been reported	Recurrence rate 30–40%. Five percent recurrence during progesterone treatment

ionizing radiation is a physical form of cancer treatment that aims at damaging cancer cells by breaking DNA through generation of free radicals from cell water. Damage of cell organelles and membranes kills cancer cells. Radiation therapy is, however, applied locally and although cancer cells are the target, radiation may also induce damage to normal cells in the tissues.

The response to radiation therapy depends on various factors such as the phase of cell cycle the cells are (cells in late G1 and S are more resistant), the degree of cell ability to repair the DNA damage and other factors such as hypoxia (hypoxic cells are more resistant), tumor mass,

and growth fraction. Non-dividing cells are more resistant than dividing cells.

Radiation therapy can be administered as teletherapy, which aims at treating a large volume of tissue. For small volumes of tissue, such as in the case of cervix cancer in the female, radiation therapy can be administered in encapsulated sources of radiation that can be implanted directly into or adjacent to tumor tissue. Radiation therapy is a component of curative therapy for a number of diseases, including breast cancer, Hodgkin's disease, head and neck cancer, prostate cancer, and gynecologic cancers.

Effects of Radiotherapy on Reproduction

The male testis, female ovary, and bone marrow are the most sensitive organs to radiation therapy. The extent of the damage in females and males depends on the dose, fractionation schedule, and irradiation field [7, 8]. Whenever female reproductive organs are involved in the irradiated field, i.e., the ovaries, the uterus and the vagina may be compromised and damaged by direct irradiation. There is also evidence of damage of these organs by scattered radiation. In the female, radiation therapy results in dose-related damage of the gonads by the reduction in the nonrenewable primordial follicle pool. In women, the degree and persistence of the damage is also influenced by age at the time of exposure to radiotherapy due to a greater reserve of primordial follicles in younger women [9]. Table 1.3 presents a compilation of current knowledge on the impact of radiation doses in gonadal function of women and

Table 1.3 Radiation therapy protocols with high or intermediate impact on ovarian and testicular function (Adapted from reference [Rodriguez-Wallberg and Oktay, 10] with permission)

High risk of prolonged azoospermia in males or amenorrhea in females

Total Body Irradiation (TBI) for bone marrow transplant/stem cell transplant

Testicular radiation dose > 2.5 Gy in adult men

Testicular radiation dose $\geq$ 6 Gy in pre-pubertal boys

Pelvic or whole abdominal radiation dose $\geq$ 6 Gy in adult women

Pelvic or whole abdominal radiation dose $\geq$ 10 Gy in post-pubertal girls

Pelvic radiation or whole abdominal dose $\geq$ 15 Gy in pre-pubertal girls

Intermediate risk

Testicular radiation dose 1–6 Gy from scattered pelvic or abdominal radiation

Pelvic or whole abdominal radiation dose 5–10 Gy in post-pubertal girls

Pelvic or whole abdominal radiation dose 10–15 Gy in pre-pubertal girls

Craniospinal radiotherapy dose $\geq$ 25 Gy

men [10]. In female and male pediatric patients, failure in pubertal development may be the first sign of gonadal failure.

In men, radiation therapy damages the gonadal stem cells and the spermatogoniae, which are responsible for the continual differentiation and production of mature spermatozoa. By contrast, the Leydig cells, responsible for the hormonal production of testosterone are more resistant to radiotherapy. However, it is known that Leydig cells of prepubertal boys, which are responsible for the hormonal production of testosterone, have a greater sensitivity to high doses of radiation therapy than those of older males [11]. If Leydig cell function remains after radiation therapy in childhood, patients may present with normal pubertal development in some cases. However, many of those patients will present at adulthood with reduced testicular size, impaired spermatogenesis and infertility, although with well preserved sexual function in most cases.

In adult women and prepubertal girls, use of shielding to reduce scatter radiation to the reproductive organs when possible is the standard medical procedure currently offered to preserve fertility. When shielding of the gonadal area is not possible, the surgical fixation of the ovaries far from the radiation field known as oophoropexy (ovarian transposition) may be considered. It is estimated that this procedure significantly reduces the risk of ovarian failure by about 50% and that those patients may retain some menstrual function and fertility [12]. Scattered radiation and damage of the blood vessels that supply the ovaries are related to the failure of this procedure [12].

Radiotherapy of the uterus in young women and girls has shown to induce tissue fibrosis, restricted uterine capacity, restricted blood flow, and impaired uterine growth during pregnancy, as shown by follow-up of cancer survivors [13, 14]. The uterine damage seems to be more pronounced in the youngest patients at the time of radiotherapy. As a consequence, radiotherapy-treated female patients present with a high risk of unfavorable pregnancy outcomes, such as spontaneous abortion, premature labor, and low birth weight offspring [13, 14].

Irradiation of the vagina is related to fertility and sexual issues due to loss of lubrication, anatomical impairments, and, in some cases, stenosis.

In males, use of shielding to reduce the dose of radiation delivered to the testes when possible is also recommended, and, in most centers, is a standard measure offered currently to adult patients and children.

Total body irradiation (TBI) given in conjunction with myeloablative conditioning prior to bone marrow transplantation is one of the most toxic treatments for the gonads, and is highly related to gonadal failure in both sexes [15, 16].

Cranial Irradiation and Hormonal Dysfunction

Disruption of the hypothalamic-pituitary-gonadal axis is a recognized potential complication of cranial irradiation that can lead to infertility in female and male patients. Follow-up of female patients treated post- and pre-pubertally with cranial irradiation for primary brain tumors has shown a high incidence of primary hypothalamic dysfunction as well as pituitary dysfunction with gonadotropin secretion disturbances. In some cases, precocious puberty may also be induced by cranial irradiation in childhood, which has been attributed to cortical disruption and disinhibition of the hypothalamus.

Chemotherapy

Chemotherapy given as only treatment may be curative for a series of cancer presenting in young adults and children.

Knowledge of the risk of gonadal damage caused by cancer treatment is essential to recognize patients at risk of gonadal failure. Table 1.4 summarizes the gonadotoxic impact of chemotherapy agents on the female ovary and male testis. In a vast majority of cancer treatments, chemotherapy combines several agents and there is a possibility of a synergistic gonadotoxic effect when several agents are given combined, although at lower doses particularly when

Table 1.4 Gonadotoxic impact of chemotherapeutic agents in the female ovary and male testis

High risk of prolonged azoospermia in men or amenorrhea in women

Cyclophosphamide

Ifosfamide

Melphalan

Busulfan

Nitrogen mustard

Procarbazine

Chlorambucil

Intermediate risk

Cisplatin with low cumulative dose

Carboplatin with low cumulative dose

Adriamycin

Low risk

Treatment protocols for Hodgkin lymphoma without alkylating agents

Bleomycin

Actinomycin D

Vincristine

Methotrexate

5-fluorouracil

combining alkylating drugs [16]. In the female, the primordial oocytes, which constitute the female follicle pool, are nonrenewable and reduce through apoptotic loss throughout the female life span, until complete depletion during menopause. Women's undeveloped oocytes and pregranulosa cells of primordial follicles are particularly sensitive to alkylating agents by induced apoptosis, which has been demonstrated in vitro and in vivo when human ovarian tissue has been xenotransplanted in SCID mouse [17, 18]. Ovarian failure is thus common after alkylating treatment [10].

Because of a reduction of the primordial follicle pool with ageing, older women have a higher risk of developing ovarian failure and permanent infertility after a cancer treatment when compared with younger women [8]. Younger patients at the time of cancer treatment may have a higher chance of recovering ovarian function following chemotherapy, and they should be recommended not to delay childbearing for too many years [4]. Although the absence of menstrual cycles, known as amenorrhea, should be considered unfavorable as it may be due to permanent gonadal failure, the presence of cycles should not be interpreted as proof of fertility. In the clinical setting, the gynecological examination by ultrasound, including estimation of small ovarian follicles of approximately 2–7 mm (antral follicle counts, AFC), and the determination of hormones, such as follicle-stimulating hormone (FSH), inhibin, and anti-mullerian hormone (AMH), may help the clinician in evaluating patient's remaining ovarian reserve after a cancer treatment and counseling on her chances to obtain a pregnancy.

Patients should be advised to avoid conception in the 6–12 month period immediately following completion of treatment due to toxicity of cancer treatments on growing oocytes [17]. This is owing to the higher risk of teratogenesis during or immediately following chemotherapy. Recent data support the return of DNA integrity over time after a cancer treatment and most studies conducted in cancer survivors have not shown any significant increase of fetal anomalies in infants that are conceived later [19, 20].

In male patients, prepubertal status does not provide protection from gonadal damage when alkilating agents are given at high doses. Because most chemotherapy agents are given as part of a combination regimen, it has been difficult to quantify the gonadotoxicity of individual drugs [21].

Conclusion

Because of progress in cancer therapy, long-term survival is expected for most of young adults and children of both sexes diagnosed with cancer today. Infertility, as a consequence of cancer treatment, has a recognized negative impact on quality of life of cancer survivors and, therefore, effects of modern cancer therapy on reproductive potential need to be discussed. This chapter outlines general principles of cancer treatment and the impact of the cancer surgery, radiation therapy, and chemotherapy on reproduction.

Provider Recommendations

1. Surgery for cancer is the most effective treatment. Improvements in gynecologic and urologic surgery have improved in the ability to preserve fertility, but some patients may require surgeries that impair fertility.
2. Surgical adjuvant treatment of gonad removal may be indicated in male and female patients with hormone sensitive tumors.
3. Radiotherapy can damage normal tissue cells and may impair male or female fertility by causing damage to reproductive organs. In females, damage to uterine function from radiation may impact ability to maintain a pregnancy.
4. Radiation to the brain can impair fertility by impacting hypothalamic pituitary functioning.
5. Chemotherapy can damage oocytes and sperm as well as the functioning.
6. Patients are advised to avoid conception for at least six months post-chemotherapy treatment.
7. Discussing fertility preservation options with all patients of childbearing age is suggested.

References

1. Altekruse SF, Kosary CL, Krapcho M, Neyman N, Aminou R, Waldron W, Ruhl J, Howlader N, Tatalovich Z, Cho H, Mariotto A, Eisner MP, Lewis DR, Cronin K, Chen HS, Feuer EJ, Stinchcomb DG, Edwards BK (eds) (2010) SEER Cancer Statistics Review, 1975–2007, National Cancer Institute. Bethesda, MD, http://seer.cancer.gov/csr/1975_2007/, based on November 2009 SEER data submission, posted to the SEER web site, 2010
2. Schover LR et al (1999) Having children after cancer. Cancer 86(4):697–709
3. Rosen A, Rodriguez-Wallberg KA, Rosenzweig L (2009) Psychosocial distress in young cancer survivors. Semin Oncol Nurs 25(4)Nov:268–277
4. Wallberg KARM, Keros V, Hovatta O (2009) Clinical aspects of fertility preservation in female patients. Pediatr Blood Cancer 53(2):254–260
5. Sabanegh ES Jr, Ragheb AM (2009) Male fertility after cancer. Urology 73:225–231
6. Heidenreich A et al (2001) Organ sparing surgery for malignant germ cell tumor of the testis. J Urol 166(6):2161–2165

7. Gosden R et al (1997) Impact of congenital or experimental hypogonadotrophism on the radiation sensitivity of the mouse ovary. Hum Reprod 12(11):2483

8. Speiser B, Rubin P, Casarett G (1973) Aspermia following lower truncal irradiation in Hodgkin's disease.
Cancer 32(3):692–698

9. Wallace WHB, Anderson RA, Irvine DS (2005)
Fertility preservation for young patients with cancer:
who is at risk and what can be offered? Lancet Oncol
6(4):209–218

10. Rodriguez-Wallberg KA, Oktay K (2010) Fertility
preservation medicine: options for young adults
and children with cancer. J Pediatr Hematol/Oncol
32(5):390

11. Shalet SM et al (1989) Vulnerability of the human
Leydig cell to radiation damage is dependent upon
age. J Endocrinol 120(1):161–165

12. Lee SJ et al (2006) American Society of Clinical
Oncology recommendations on fertility preservation
in cancer patients. J Clin Oncol 24(18):2917–2931

13. Green DM et al (2009) Ovarian failure and reproductive outcomes after childhood cancer treatment:
results from the Childhood Cancer Survivor Study. J
Clin Oncol 27(14):2374

14. Wo JY, Viswanathan AN (2009) Impact of radiotherapy on fertility, pregnancy, and neonatal outcomes in
female cancer patients. Int J Radiat Oncol Biol Phys
73(5):1304–1312

15. Sklar C (1995) Growth and endocrine disturbances
after bone marrow transplantation in childhood. Acta
Pediatr 84:57–61

16. Thibaud E et al (1998) Ovarian function after
bone marrow transplantation during childhood. Bone
Marrow Transplant 21(3):287–290

17. Meirow D et al (1999) Subclinical depletion of
primordial follicular reserve in mice treated with
cyclophosphamide: clinical importance and proposed
accurate investigative tool. Hum Reprod 14(7):1903

18. Oktem O, Oktay K (2007) A novel ovarian xenografting model to characterize the impact of chemotherapy
agents on human primordial follicle reserve. Cancer
Res 67(21):10159–10162

19. Dodds L, Marrett LD, Tomkins DJ, Green B,
Sherman G (1993) Case-control study of congenital anomalies in children of cancer patients. BMJ
Jul 17;307(6897):164–168. http://www.ncbi.nlm.nih.
gov/pubmed/8343744

20. Langagergaard V, Gislum M, Skriver MV, Nørgård
B, Lash TL, Rothman KJ, Sørensen HT (2006) Birth
outcome in women with breast cancer. Br J Cancer
2006 Jan 16;94(1):142–146

21. Hudson MM (2010) Reproductive outcomes for
survivors of childhood cancer. Obstet Gynecol
116(5):1171–1183

Fertility Preservation Options for Females

Amelia P. Bailey, MD and Elizabeth
S. Ginsburg, MD

My health care team had everything coordinated for me like I was royalty. I had the breast cancer surgery in early March, and two weeks later I was starting my treatment for egg retrieval. I started my chemotherapy, as planned, the next month. I thought doing the egg retrieval right after I finished surgery was going to be too intense, but I was so happy to be doing something that was going to take me one step closer to having the baby I always dreamed of. During the dark days of chemo, I often thought about my frozen eggs and how better things lay ahead for me. I am so thankful that I was in a place that knew how to coordinate all this for me. I read horror stories on line about women who weren't told about infertility or weren't given options or were told it would delay their treatment and there wasn't time. I can't say I'm glad I got cancer, but I am elated with the coordination I had for all aspects of my care.
Courtney, Adult Cancer Patient

Abbreviations

AMH	anti-Mullerian hormone
ART	assisted reproductive technologies
ASRM	American Society for Reproductive Medicine
cGy	centigray
FSH	follicle stimulating hormone
GnRH	gonadotropin-releasing hormone
Gy	Gray
hCG	human chorionic gonadotropin
IVF	in vitro fertilization
IVM	in vitro maturation
OHSS	ovarian hyperstimulation syndrome
PGD	preimplantation genetic diagnosis
SART	The Society for Assisted Reproductive Technologies

A.P. Bailey (✉)
Center for Infertility and Reproductive Surgery, Brigham and Women's Hospital, Boston, MA 02115, USA
e-mail: apbailey@partners.org

Introduction

Nine percent of cancer survivors in the United States are women in their prime childbearing years, ages 20–39 [1]. With recent progress in early detection and diagnosis, as well as in treatment protocols, the number of cancer survivors is increasing. Thus, the prior focus on disease eradication without attention to fertility is outdated and has been replaced with a strong interest by cancer patients to be counseled on fertility preservation alternatives [2, 3]. This patient population now has many options as a result of advances in oncofertility.

Amenorrhea is common after cancer therapy, and its incidence increases after treatment for certain types of cancer (Table 2.1). Amenorrhea may be transient or permanent and acute or chronic in onset. Women may have menstrual cycles immediately after treatment but undergo premature menopause within a few years. Resumption of

G.P. Quinn, S.T. Vadaparampil (eds.), *Reproductive Health and Cancer in Adolescents and Young Adults*, Advances in Experimental Medicine and Biology 732,
DOI 10.1007/978-94-007-2492-1_2, © Springer Science+Business Media B.V. 2012

Table 2.1 Malignancies commonly associated with subsequent decreased female fertility

System	Cancer type	Percent diagnosed at <45 years of age	Treatment that decreases fertility
Reproductive	Breast	12.1	C
	Ovarian/fallopian tube	12	C,S
	Uterine, including gestational trophoblastic disease	7.7	C,R,S
	Cervical	40.3	R,S
	Vaginal	15.5[a]	R,S
	Vulvar	9.4	R,S
Gastrointestinal	Small intestine	7.4[b]	S
	Colon and rectum	5.1[b]	R,S
	Anal	10.5[b]	R,S
Hematologic	Leukemia	20.9[b]	C
	Hodgkin lymphoma	59.6[b]	C,R
	Non-Hodgkin lymphoma	12.3[b]	C,R
	Multiple myeloma	3.8[b]	C
Skin	Melanoma	19[b]	C

[a]SEER Data from 1988 to 2001 and under age 50; [b]men and women included *C* chemotherapy, *R* radiation, *S* surgery
Source: SEER Cancer Statistics, Data from 2004 to 2008 [1]

cyclic menses is often used in the oncology literature as a benchmark for fertility. However, this is not a reliable parameter, as some women with regular menstruation are unable to conceive and others without menses may still have oocytes and be able to reproduce [4, 5]. The presence of menstrual cycles after treatment with chemotherapy and/or radiation or surgery indicates that women have the potential for fertility but by no means indicates that attempted conception would be successful. Pretreatment fertility status also plays a role in prediction of post-treatment reproductive ability.

Ovarian Reserve Testing

Multiple serum markers and imaging modalities are used to assess ovarian reserve, a reflection of the number of oocytes a female has remaining. Ovarian reserve is associated with the likelihood of conceiving a pregnancy either with or without in vitro fertilization (IVF) [6]. Currently, the most reliable method of assessing ovarian reserve is measurement of follicle stimulating hormone (FSH) on menstrual cycle day 2 or 3; an elevated level indicates poor reserve [7]. Anti-Mullerian

hormone (AMH) and inhibin-B are serum tests less commonly used; reduced levels of both indicate decreasing reserve [8, 9]. An advantage of using AMH, especially in cancer patients with treatment timelines, is that it does not vary significantly throughout the menstrual cycle. Thus it can be measured on any day [10]. Ultrasound measurements of ovarian volume, antral follicle count, and ovarian peak systolic velocity can also be used to assess ovarian reserve with low values for each indicating decreased reserve. However, volume and velocity are less reliable than serum markers [10–13].

Fertility preservation is more complicated in women than men [7] because oocytes are not repleted during a woman's life. Starting at 20 weeks gestation, fetal eggs start degenerating; this continues through menopause and does not stop during pregnancy or contraceptive use. Oocytes also progressively decline in quality throughout the reproductive years. These two factors combine to make advancing age predictive of a woman's ability to reproduce. In fact, fertility declines after age 28 at a rate that increases dramatically after age 35 [10]; and the average age of menopause, at which no oocytes remain in the ovaries, is 51 [14]. In contrast, spermatogenesis is ongoing in males until very late in life, allowing men to father children at ages significantly greater than women; and production of sperm by masturbation with subsequent cryopreservation is noninvasive and simple to perform. Despite the complexity of fertility preservation in women, a woman's desire for future fertility should be discussed, and clinicians should not assume that a patient would bring up her concerns. Of course, this conversation should include an age- and health-based estimation of the chance of conception and delivery as well as the likelihood and risks of carrying a pregnancy.

In contrast to the ovaries, the uterus retains its ability to carry a pregnancy to term well after a woman has undergone menopause. In fact, pregnancy and live birth have occurred in mothers in their late 60s. These pregnancies are usually conceived with a donor egg, but the uterine age does not seem to affect implantation rates or pregnancy outcomes [15]. Similarly, the ability of the cervix to maintain a pregnancy does not decrease as a woman approaches menopause. So, a thorough discussion about a patient's future fertility desires is warranted before proceeding with a hysterectomy regardless of her age.

Options for fertility preservation vary based on patient diagnosis, availability of sperm from a partner or donor, time available between diagnosis and start of therapy, the treatments that have already been performed, and the patient's current fertility status and age. The majority of patients are referred to an oncologist and may or may not be counseled on their reproductive options prior to initiation of treatment, yet options for fertility preservation vary widely based on time of presentation. Further, early referral to an oncofertility specialist is paramount as some options may require several weeks. This chapter's purpose is to explain the choices available to attempt maintenance of fertility.

Infertility with Chemotherapy

Chemotherapies vary in their average level of gonadotoxicity, or toxic action on the ovaries (Table 2.2), and the impact may vary from patient to patient. The effects of chemotherapy are dependent primarily on the type of drug but also on patient age, drug dose, dosing interval, type and extent of disease, and administration route (oral versus intravenous). The alkylating agents convey a high risk of ovarian damage by loss of follicles and starting a cascade that leads to hypergonadotrophic hypogonadism and subsequent cessation of menses [4, 16]. This is especially true with cyclophosphamide, which is used to treat breast cancer, leukemia, and lymphoma. These effects on the ovary are both permanent and progressive [17]. In contrast, the antimetabolite chemotherapy agents, such as methotrexate and 5-fluorouracil, act only on metabolically highly active cells and do not appear to have major impacts on ovarian reserve. As women age, ovarian reserve decreases, and risk of gonadotoxicity with a given drug and dose increases. Fewer follicles remain after treatment, thereby increasing the likelihood of infertility and early menopause [18]. There are multiple chemotherapeutic agents with unknown levels of gonadotoxicity, and many of them are part of multi-drug regimens. Even if the gonadotoxicity of the regimen is known, the individual drug's contribution to infertility may be unknown.

In addition, chemotherapy lessens a female's response to ovarian stimulation, so it is important that fertility preservation be performed prior to cancer treatment when possible. Ginsburg et al. found that female cancer patients who had received systemic chemotherapy had a poorer response based on estradiol levels and number of oocytes harvested than women who received local treatment for their cancer. This finding occurred despite the cancer cohort's younger age and higher doses of stimulation medications. Yet there was no difference in the number of embryos obtained between the cases and an infertile cohort [19]. A study on Hodgkin's lymphoma patients showed that those who survived without recurrence ≥3 years and who attempted pregnancy after chemotherapy did not exhibit significant subfertility when compared to sibling and friend controls [20]. Further, 57% of early stage breast cancer survivors who tried to become pregnant

Table 2.2 Risk of permanent amenorrhea, adapted from Lee [4] and www.cancer.gov [158]. Abbreviations are the standard names for each regimen

Degree of risk	Treatment	Common cancer type
High risk (>80%)	Hematopoetic stem cell transplantation with cyclophosphamide/total body irradiation or cyclophosphamide/busulfan	Leukemia Lymphoma
	External beam radiation to a field containing ovaries	Central nervous system, gastrointestinal, or gynecologic cancer; Lymphoma
	CMF, CEF, CAF for 6 cycles in age 40 and older (combinations of cyclophosphamide, methotrexate, fluorouracil, doxorubicin, and epirubicin)	Breast cancer
Intermediate risk (20–80%)	CMF, CEF, CAF for 6 cycles in age 30–39 (combinations of cyclophosphamide, methotrexate, fluorouracil, doxorubicin, and epirubicin)	Breast cancer
	AC for 4 cycles in age 40 and older (doxorubicin and cyclophosphamide)	Breast cancer
	Cisplatin or carboplatin	Ovarian, endometrial, breast, and cervical cancer; leukemia; lymphoma
Lower risk (<20%)	ABVD (doxorubicin, bleomycin, vinblastin, and dacarbazine)	Hodgkin's lymphoma
	CHOP for 4–6 cycles (cyclophosphamide, doxorubicin, vincristine, and prednisone)	Leukemia Lymphoma
	CVP (cyclophosphamide, vincristine, and prednisone)	Lymphoma
	Anthracycline and cytarabine	Acute myelogenous leukemia
	Prednisone, vincristine, and anthracycline with or without cyclophosphamide, imatinib, and/or methotrexate	Acute lymphoblastic leukemia
	CMF, CEF, CAF for 6 cycles in age 29 and younger (combinations of cyclophosphamide, methotrexate, fluorouracil, doxorubicin, and epirubicin)	Breast cancer
	AC for 4 cycles in age 30–39 (doxorubicin and cyclophosphamide)	Breast cancer
Very low or no risk	Vincristine	Leukemia, lymphoma, multiple myeloma
	Methotrexate	Gestational trophoblastic disease
	Fluorouracil	Ovarian, colon/rectal, breast, and stomach cancer
Unknown risk	Taxanes (paclitaxel, docetaxel)	Ovarian and breast cancer
	Oxaliplatin	Colon/rectal cancer
	Irinotecan	Metastatic colon/rectal cancer
	Monoclonal antibodies (trastuzumab, bevacizumab, cetuximab)	Ovarian cancer
	Tyrosine kinase inhibitors (erlotinib, imatinib)	

were successful in a study by Partridge et al. [21]. There are additional studies looking at fertility of childhood cancer survivors.

Infertility with Radiation

The effect of radiation on fertility depends on age, dose, dosing interval, disease, and size and location of the radiation field. Similar to chemotherapy, increasing age at the time of radiation is related to greater gonadotoxicity due to smaller ovarian reserve. Minimal doses and less extensive radiation fields carry a lower risk of infertility [22]. Ovarian failure will occur in over 90% of patients receiving 5 Gray (Gy) of radiation to the pelvis [6]. Standard radiation doses are 40–50 Gy and are even higher with total-body irradiation prior to bone marrow transplantation for recurrent leukemia or lymphoma (Table 2.2) [23, 24]. Even if the beam is not directed toward the pelvis, scatter radiation may still impact a woman's ability to reproduce [25]. Multiple studies show that doses less than 5 Gy do not decrease fertility [26–28].

Radiation affects the uterus in at least three ways. Primarily, damage to the uterine vasculature may cause poor placental-fetal blood flow during future pregnancies resulting in fetal growth restriction [29]. Unfortunately, this does not improve after exogenous hormone administration [30]. Secondly, injury to the endometrium may prevent normal placental attachment, also leading to fetal growth restriction. Lastly, radiation-induced myometrial fibrosis can incite preterm delivery by decreasing uterine volume and distensibility [10]. Thus, all post-radiation pregnancies should be categorized as high-risk. Fortunately, fetuses conceived after completion of radiotherapy do not exhibit an increased incidence of teratogenicity [31–37].

Infertility After Surgery

Standard treatment of gynecologic cancers requires removal of most or all reproductive organs, including the ovaries, fallopian tubes, uterus, and cervix. Thorough pathologic assessment of those organs is important in determining stage and grade of the disease, which guides future treatment. However, some patients remain candidates for fertility-sparing procedures if they have early-stage cancer and are not otherwise infertile.

Fertility-Sparing Surgery

Surgery's role in preserving fertility is case-dependent, and the optimal intervention may not be known until an exploratory operation is performed. The estimated preoperative extent of disease is the primary determining factor when deciding whether to offer fertility-sparing procedures, and standard therapy should always be included as an option [38]. That being said, in appropriate patients with a strong desire to maintain the ability to conceive, there are less extensive procedures that should be offered.

Oophoropexy/Ovarian Transposition

Ovarian transposition and oophoropexy temporarily relocate the ovaries when pelvic radiation is planned; they differ only in their surgical technique, and the terms will be used interchangeably here. This procedure may be helpful not only for gynecologic cancers requiring radiation but also for spinal, colon, rectal, and anal cancers for which radiation is planned due to scatter that affects the ovaries [39]. Ovarian transposition may be performed either at the time of laparotomy or laparoscopically as an isolated outpatient procedure. Performed properly, oophoropexy can reduce ovarian radiation dose by up to 90–95% [10]. Because the ovaries can migrate back to the pelvis, oophoropexy should be conducted immediately before radiation begins [40]. If chemotherapy that is not likely to be highly toxic to the ovaries is planned prior to pelvic irradiation the procedure should be performed before initiation of chemotherapy as patients are immunosuppressed on most chemotherapeutic regimens and, therefore, maynot be able to undergo elective surgery. Ovarian transposition is not indicated with gonadotoxic chemotherapy alone since the ovaries will be adversely affected by the medication regardless of their location.

Ovarian function remains after transposition in 60–89% of cancer patients under 40 years of age [40–43]. Failures likely result from radiation that scatters to the new ovarian location as well as necrosis of the ovary from compromised blood supply due to transposition [44–46]. Necrosis can lead to atresia of follicles and premature menopause [47, 48]. While most women retain enough ovarian tissue for endocrine function, some reports indicate that only 15% of patients are fertile after ovarian transposition [49]. At this time, the procedure remains investigational as a means for fertility preservation.

Spontaneous pregnancies have been reported after oophoropexy, but some patients need either reversal of the procedure or oocyte retrieval with in vitro fertilization because the ovary is no longer in close proximity to the fallopian tube [46, 50]. Oocyte retrieval is more difficult after transposition due to the difficulty in accessing the ovary transvaginally [46]. This situation frequently requires transabdominal aspiration, which can sometimes yield fewer oocytes [10]. However, a recent publication revealed no significant differences between transvaginal and transabdominal aspiration in number of damaged oocytes, fertilization rates, embryo number and quality, and clinical and ongoing pregnancy rates [51].

Additional complications from oophoropexy include pelvic pain from ovarian or fallopian tube infarction or cyst formation. Further, ovarian cancer would be difficult to detect on bimanual examination if the ovaries are no longer located in the pelvis [4]. Gonadal shielding can be performed to reduce the radiation dose to the ovaries if ovarian transposition is contraindicated for any reason, but this is only possible with certain radiation fields and requires expertise in this area [4].

Cancer-Specific Fertility-Sparing Procedures

Fertility-sparing surgery becomes especially important with a gynecologic cancer diagnosis, and the techniques vary depending on which organ is affected. The first goal of any cancer treatment is to remove the tumor burden and see the patient into remission, with a secondary goal of preventing relapse. Fertility-sparing surgery is not intended to displace those objectives but to offer a third elective goal of fertility preservation, and there are many variations in surgical management of cancer that allow retention of the uterus and/or ovaries. Uterine-sparing surgery may be considered on a case by case basis if the patient wishes to carry a future pregnancy herself; ovaries are not necessary for sustaining a pregnancy as all hormones may be exogenously provided to support the endometrium during an embryo replacement cycle. Ovarian-sparing surgery and/or cryopreservation of ovarian tissues, embryos, and oocytes may be offered to appropriate candidates if genetic offspring are desired.

Ovarian Cancer

Tumors of low malignant potential, malignant germ cell tumors, and sex cord-stromal tumors are subtypes of ovarian cancer that are likely to be unilateral and diagnosed at an early stage. Therefore, they are usually amenable to fertility-conserving procedures [38, 52]. Epithelial ovarian cancers at early stages are also amenable to preservation of fertility [38]; unfortunately, only 25% are diagnosed early due to poor screening methods.

Fertility-sparing procedures in the treatment of ovarian cancer include ovarian cystectomy, unilateral salpingo-oophorectomy with or without hysterectomy, and bilateral salpingo-oophorectomy with preservation of the uterus. In the case of cystectomy or unilateral salpingo-oophorectomy, the contralateral ovary would only be biopsied if it appeared grossly involved by tumor [52]. All options should be undertaken concurrently with complete surgical staging including omentectomy, washings to identify cancer cells in the peritoneal cavity, and lymph node dissection in the pelvis and around the aorta. The surgery and treatment is still extensive, but there are multiple reports in the literature of successful pregnancies and live births after conservative management of ovarian cancer [53–57].

Laparoscopic surgery has been considered for these procedures, but does carry an increased risk of cyst rupture which could result in intraperitoneal tumor spread or implantation at trocar sites [58]. If a patient is BRCA1- or 2-positive, and thus at high risk for hereditary breast and ovarian cancer, prophylactic mastectomy and bilateral salpingo-oophorectomy after completion of childbearing should be recommended [38].

Cervical Cancer

Cervical cancer treatment is either surgery or radiotherapy for early disease and chemotherapy for advanced disease. Fortunately, most women present with Stage I cervical cancer. Standard surgery consists of a radical hysterectomy and bilateral pelvic lymphadenectomy. For females who wish to retain the option of having children and have early stage disease, other procedures may be offered that spare the uterus including cold-knife conization (removal of part of the external cervix), simple trachelectomy (removal of the cervix only), radical trachelectomy (removal of the cervix and surrounding tissues), or sparing of the ovaries at the time of radical hysterectomy [4, 38]. Stage IA1 disease encompasses tumors less than 7 mm wide and 3 mm deep and may be treated with a cervical conization provided that margins are negative and the patient receives close follow-up. Stage 1A1 with lymphovascular space invasion and Stage 1A2-IB tumors less than 2 cm in diameter with invasion less than 10 mm may be treated with a vaginal or abdominal radical trachelectomy [59–61], which is usually combined with a laparoscopic lymph node dissection [38] and ovarian transposition if future pelvic radiation is planned.

Women are capable of conceiving after a cold knife conization, but abnormalities of the residual cervix may necessitate use of assisted reproductive technologies (ART). Women are even able to conceive after trachelectomy [62], but ART

is frequently needed in these patients due to absence or constriction of the passageway from the vagina to the uterus. Post-trachelectomy pregnancies also have a much higher rate of second trimester miscarriages and preterm birth [63–65]. To compensate for this, a permanent cerclage is placed after trachelectomy; these women will require future cesarean deliveries [38]. Several successful pregnancies have been reported after radical trachelectomy, but cancer relapses have also occurred in that cohort [65–69]. The trachelectomy recurrence rate to date is similar to standard therapy of radical hysterectomy [70], but further studies are needed.

Endometrial Cancer

Standard therapy for endometrial cancer is hysterectomy with bilateral salpingo-oophorectomy with or without surgical staging depending on the grade and depth of invasion of the tumor. A recent meta-analysis of 218 patients revealed a pregnancy rate of 35.7% after conservative management of endometrial cancer [71]. To maintain fertility in young patients with early lesions (stage IA1 and grade 1), a hysteroscopy and curettage can be offered to remove as much diseased tissue from the uterus as possible [38, 52, 72]. Following this procedure, hormonal therapy is prescribed, and the patient is kept under close surveillance for several years. Progesterone administration is one of the most common therapies used and is available as the progestins megestrol acetate or medroxyprogesterone acetate. However, progestin's efficacy in cancer is less well-documented than in endometrial hyperplasia, which is discussed below [52]. Therefore, hysteroscopy with curettage and a progestin may be best used as a temporizing measure until the patient has completed childbearing.

The precursor to endometrial cancer is complex endometrial hyperplasia with atypia, which is usually diagnosed after an episode of abnormal uterine bleeding. The standard recommended therapy for hyperplasia is hysterectomy with or without removal of both ovaries, but hormonal management is a reasonable conservative alternative. Regression of endometrial hyperplasia has been noted with the progestin protocols mentioned above or an oral contraceptive pill regimen [52].

Assisted Reproductive Technologies

ART should be discussed with every woman until approximately age 43. The likelihood of delivery per initiated IVF cycle using fresh oocytes nationally in women 43 and above is less than 5%. Given that not all oocytes or embryos will survive the cryopreservation process, the risk-cost-benefit ratio likely indicates that women 43 and older are unlikely to have a delivery from oocytes or embryos frozen prior to cancer treatment. Even if the current cancer diagnosis does not usually lead to infertility, a relapse could cause premature menopause; so, fertility preservation methods should be discussed at the time of diagnosis. This section discusses widely used ART (Tables 2.3 and 2.4).

Embryo Cryopreservation

Embryo cryopreservation is the most established fertility preservation method [4, 7]. It has been regularly used since the birth of the first "test tube baby" in 1978 and has progressed to success rates of 30–48% in women under 40 years old [73]. The ovaries are stimulated with FSH injections and luteinizing hormone (LH) for approximately a week and a half. Ultrasounds and blood tests are used throughout this time to monitor development of the ovarian follicles. When the follicles are appropriately sized, an injection of human chorionic gonadotropin (hCG) triggers ovulation, and the eggs are aspirated transvaginally from the follicles just prior to ovulation. This procedure is done in an operating room under intravenous anesthesia. Oocytes are then fertilized and cryopreserved. They can be thawed at a later date and implanted into the uterus of the patient or a gestational carrier who has agreed to carry the pregnancy. Many embryos can be frozen, ideally providing the opportunity for multiple future attempts at pregnancy.

Interestingly, women who have been diagnosed with cancer but have not started chemotherapy or radiation treatment produce as many embryos and oocytes after ovarian stimulation as fertile females undergoing in vitro fertilization for male factor infertility [74]. Unfortunately, only half of patients have counseling on fertility preservation options prior to cancer treatment [75], which is the most appropriate time for discussion and planning to ensure the greatest chance for future success.

Typically embryo cryopreservation requires 2–6 weeks to accomplish dependent upon the phase of the patient's menstrual cycle at presentation to a reproductive specialist. This time constraint leads some physicians to cite delay of treatment as a reason to not pursue fertility-sparing procedures. However, the majority of patients only need 2–3 weeks to preserve embryos or oocytes and even less to cryopreserve ovarian tissue. One report showed no treatment delay in breast cancer patients who chose fertility preservation options over those patients who opted out [76]. Another study showed the average length of fertility preservation treatment was

Table 2.3 Classification of fertility-preserving treatments as widely used or experimental; embryo cryopreservation is the only option considered standard by ASRM [7]

Widely used treatments	Experimental treatments
Oophoropexy/ovarian transposition	Ovarian cortex cryopreservation and transplantation
Gonadal shielding from radiation	In vitro maturation
Conservative surgical or medical management of cancer	Ovarian suppression
Embryo cryopreservation	Uterine transplantation
Oocyte cryopreservation	Generation of gametes from somatic cells
Donor oocyte or embryo	
Gestational carrier	

Table 2.4 Pros, cons, and considerations for each fertility-sparing treatment

Treatments	Pros	Cons	Considerations
Oophoropexy/ovarian Transposition	Can reduce ovarian radiation exposure up to 90–95%.	May require a separate surgery. May cause oocyte atresia or pelvic pain. Ovaries less accessible. Potential for seeding of cancer cells.	Ovaries may migrate back to pelvis. Do not perform if gonadotoxic chemotherapy planned.
Gonadal shielding	Reduces radiation dose to ovaries and uterus.	Not possible in all cases.	Requires a radiation specialist.
Conservative surgery	Usually a smaller procedure and occasionally less invasive.	Chance of recurrence not fully elucidated. May necessitate ART for future pregnancy. Potential for future pregnancy complications.	Only applicable for early stage cancers.
Hormonal treatment	Avoidance of major surgery.	Chance of recurrence not fully elucidated.	Extent of cancer may be undetermined.
Embryo cryopreservation	Only standard option. Highest success rate. Potential for multiple attempts at future pregnancy.	Risk for multifetal pregnancy and OHSS. Significant side effect profile. High hormone levels. Requires at least 2 weeks. Expensive.	Quality of embryos not determined prior to cryopreservation. Requires male partner or sperm donor.
In vitro maturation	Short treatment delay. No sperm needed. No ovarian stimulation.	Lower pregnancy rates than embryo cryopreservation.	Offered in very few centers.
Oocyte cryopreservation	No male partner or sperm donor needed.	Same as with embryo cryopreservation. Lower pregnancy rate than embryo cryopreservation.	Circumvents ethical issues with embryo cryopreservation.
Donor oocyte/donor embryo	Not treatment-or age-dependent. High success rate.	Neither partner's genetic material if donor sperm used.	May fertilize eggs with partner's sperm or donor sperm.
Gestational carrier	No pregnancy-associated risks.	Expensive.	Patient does not carry pregnancy.
Ovarian cortex Cryopreservation and transplantation	No treatment delay. No sperm needed. No ovarian stimulation.	Surgical procedure. Short-term hormonal function only. Oocyte atresia. Potential for transfer of cancer cells.	Only option for prepubertal females. Increases cancer risk in BRCA patients.
Ovarian suppression	Reduced abnormal uterine bleeding.	Significant side effects. Expensive.	Not well-supported with data.
Human uterine transplantation	Patient could carry pregnancy post-hysterectomy.	Lifelong immunosuppressants.	Only one has been performed and did not result in a pregnancy.
Gametes from somatic cells	No treatment delay. No sperm needed. No ovarian stimulation.	Complex ethical issues.	This has not yet resulted in a live human birth.

only 12 days [77]. Also, in certain situations such as breast cancer, there is an approximately 4-week window between surgery and chemotherapy during which fertility-sparing procedures can be performed [78]. Recent reports of brief ovarian stimulation in the follicular or luteal phases of the menstrual cycle with retrieval of immature oocytes and subsequent in vitro maturation allow for shorter periods of stimulation, though a fewer number of mature eggs capable of fertilizing [79]; on average, 6±5 embryos are frozen with traditional stimulation in one study [74] and 3.8±0.8 embryos with brief stimulation using tamoxifen and FSH in another [80].

Innate risks of IVF include pain and infection after oocyte retrieval, medication side effects and allergic reactions, and poor response resulting in few or no eggs or embryos. Another hazard of ovarian stimulation is that it may become uncontrolled and result in ovarian hyperstimulation syndrome (OHSS). This is a potentially serious condition that causes markedly elevated estradiol levels and extravasation of fluid from blood vessels into the peritoneal cavity. Ascites and pleural effusions as well as hemoconcentration and deep venous thrombosis can form, all of which would delay administration of cancer treatment [6, 81].

Elevated estradiol levels lead to a separate concern: the possible progression of hormone-sensitive tumors such as ovarian cancer or estrogen receptor-positive breast cancer. Some studies have shown an increased risk of ovarian cancer after use of clomiphene citrate or gonadotropins [82, 83], but that association has not been observed in more current studies [84]. However, for apprehensive patients, oocyte aspiration can be done without hormonal administration in a process called natural cycle IVF that does not increase estrogen above normal menstrual levels, although it typically results in a low yield of oocytes [80, 85]. Alternative stimulation protocols that utilize letrozole or tamoxifen, which are both used in breast cancer treatment, lower the risk of exposure to estrogen [86]. In small studies these protocols have shown no apparent increase in breast cancer recurrence rates at 2-year follow-up [80, 85, 87] and do not lengthen the time needed to complete a cycle of ovarian stimulation [88]. The impact on cancer treatment of approximately 11 days of elevated hormone levels in a patient preparing for chemotherapy is not currently known [6]. As a precaution, patients should be carefully counseled by a professional exceedingly familiar with the different protocols.

Embryo cryopreservation carries high out-of-pocket costs and requires a male partner or sperm donor. However, it is the most well-established method for fertility preservation and, especially when performed prior to chemotherapy or radiation, offers the best chance for having genetic children in the future. Women may decide in conjunction with their oncologists and reproductive specialists when to implant the embryos, which may occur up to many years later and is a simple procedure requiring no anesthesia. The Society for Assisted Reproductive Technologies (SART) publishes data on success rates from most ART facilities in the United States [73]. This data, although not limited to cancer patients, is useful when counseling women on their options. A frank discussion about disposition of unused embryos should be held as early in the process as possible to facilitate informed decision making.

Given the disadvantages of a time requirement and elevated levels of hormone, oncologists may be deterred from referring patients for fertility preservation discussions; in vitro maturation (IVM) may remove those roadblocks. IVM is a process in which immature oocytes are harvested after a very short course of ovarian stimulation and matured outside of the body. The entire process takes less than a week, and cancer treatment may be started right after the oocyte retrieval [89]. One of the drawbacks of this method is that fewer embryos are generated leading to lower pregnancy rates than with traditional IVF [89]. In fact, with in vitro maturation, only 10–15% of embryos transferred to the uterus implant, and early pregnancy miscarriages are more common [90].

Although data are limited to small case series and reports, there seems to be no increased risk of cancer, birth defects, or genetic abnormalities in the offspring of frozen embryos or oocytes outside of hereditary cancer syndromes [91–99].

With respect to inherited cancer predispositions, preimplantation genetic diagnosis (PGD) provides a possible solution (see Chapter 8), but this method is limited in efficacy since only one cell is analyzed and may be negative while other unsampled cells are positive.

Oocyte Cryopreservation

If there is no male partner or sperm donor or if the patient has objections to freezing embryos, cryopreservation of eggs is another option for fertility preservation. Oocyte cryopreservation has been utilized for decades but has not made advances as rapidly as embryo cryopreservation; its success rate is approximately 8–39% [100–104]. The oocytes are harvested, just as in embryo cryopreservation, with or without hormonal stimulation. Thus, the delay in treatment, risk for OHSS, and exposure to high hormone levels still exist and can be mediated in the same ways with natural cycle IVF or stimulation used in conjunction with letrozole or tamoxifen.

An additional consideration is that eggs may be at higher risk of damage during cryopreservation than embryos causing lower overall pregnancy rates as compared to embryo cryopreservation [105]. A study reviewing 900 babies born as a result of oocyte cryopreservation reported no increased risk of congenital anomalies versus naturally conceived babies [106]. More than half of ART centers offer oocyte cryopreservation [104], and the American Society of Reproductive Medicine (ASRM) supports its use in cancer patients while cautioning that the method is still not considered standard practice [107].

Donor Oocyte/Donor Embryo

If a woman has already undergone cancer treatment that has rendered her unable to conceive using her own eggs or if the number or quality of eggs retrieved is not likely to result in pregnancy, donor eggs may be used to create embryos. Another woman, either known or unknown to the patient, undergoes ovarian stimulation and oocyte retrieval. Those eggs are fertilized with the patient's partner's sperm, and the embryos are implanted in the patient's uterus. Donor eggs may also be fertilized with donor sperm, which can be placed into the patient's uterus. As mentioned above, the patient does not need to have ovaries to carry a pregnancy. She can be given exogenous estradiol and progesterone through the first trimester to maintain the pregnancy until the placenta has grown enough to produce ample estradiol and progesterone itself. SART reports a live birth rate of 55% with fresh donor eggs and 34% with thawed donor eggs [73].

Gestational Carrier

If the patient does not have a uterus but does have ovaries, fresh or frozen embryos may be created with her eggs and implanted into a gestational carrier, alternatively known as a gestational surrogate. This option also works well for women in whom pregnancy is too dangerous. The gestational carrier is thoroughly counseled on all risks of hormonal stimulation and pregnancy. Success rates are the same as with traditional IVF. Gestational carriers are usually unrelated to the patient, but there is no contraindication to the role being filled by a family member. Embryos can also be made using donor eggs and implanted into a gestational surrogate. The cost can range from $15,000 to $35,000 plus additional costs for prenatal care [108]. In traditional surrogacy, in which another woman is inseminated with a female cancer survivor's partner's sperm, the surrogate's uterus and eggs are both utilized, giving her parental rights in the case of a dispute. For this reason, traditional surrogacy is rarely undertaken.

Experimental Fertility-Sparing Technologies

Assisted reproductive technologies are evolving rapidly, and some will become the future of fertility-preserving procedures after thorough clinical trials are conducted. This section explains the promising experimental options and their risks as well as the situations in which one method may be superior (Tables 2.3 and 2.4).

Ovarian Cortex Cryopreservation and Transplantation

Ovarian tissue cryopreservation consists of harvesting ovarian tissue and freezing it. This tissue holds thousands of follicles, which contain immature eggs. The tissue can be removed laparoscopically as an outpatient surgery and reimplanted into the pelvis (orthotopic transplantation) [109–113] or in subcutaneous tissue or muscle (heterotopic transplantation) [114, 115]. Reimplantation may occur years later and allows in vivo maturation of oocytes; however, the best location for placement is currently unknown. This is the best alternative for women who do not have time to undergo ovarian stimulation prior to cancer treatment and is the only choice for prepubertal females. In fact, although there have not been any pregnancies reported from prepubertally harvested ovarian tissue, young children are the ideal candidates given their large number of follicles [116].

Ovarian endocrine function has been noted after transplantation; and a return to premenopausal levels of estradiol, follicle-stimulating hormone, and luteinizing hormone has occurred within 3–7 months [112, 115]. Thus, the reimplanted ovary is capable of supplying hormones to cancer survivors who have undergone premature menopause [109, 112, 113, 115, 117]. Several live births have been noted with orthotopic, but not heterotopic, transplantation [78, 110, 111, 118–121]. However, endocrine function has only been detected for 9 months to 3 years total [122], and some women have required repeat transplantations [123].

This method is still considered investigational and is only offered through clinical trials at a limited number of centers internationally. Neither a sperm donor nor ovarian stimulation is needed, which makes this alternative attractive for single patients or those with hormone-sensitive tumors. Ovarian tissue can be frozen easily [124, 125];

but one concern is that the removed ovary is without a blood supply for about 1 week after it is thawed and reimplanted, as this is the time required for revascularization of the tissue by angiogenesis. During this period, more than 25% of the follicles may become atretic in addition to the loss of follicles that occurs during the freeze-thaw process [88, 126]. Thus, studies are focusing on accelerating the revascularization process, possibly through vascular anastomosis of the transplant, which would immediately restore blood supply [16, 23]. In older women, fewer follicles remain, so a loss of 25% is more significant than in a younger woman and may make this option less beneficial as age increases.

Another concern with ovarian transplantation is the potential to implant tissue carrying hidden cancer cells that survived the freeze and thaw processes, especially in hematologic cancers. To date, there are no reports of tumor recurrence after transplantation of ovarian tissue; but data only exists for few patients over a short time period [4]. Testing of the tissue by histologic, immunohistochemical, genetic, and molecular means can be used to decrease the risk of tumor seeding [16]. None of these methods can guarantee absence of cancer cells in a tissue sample, but quantitative reverse-transcribed polymerase chain reaction shows the most promise [127]. Patients with metastases or high likelihood of ovarian involvement by cancer should not be treated with this option. However, ovarian metastases are rare in most cancers in young women, and the tissue may be implanted subcutaneously if closer surveillance is desired [128]. Women with BRCA mutations are a special population, and reimplantation of ovarian tissue may restore their pre-oophorectomy risk of cancer [6]. Therefore, they should be counseled to seek other options for fertility preservation. Ovarian transplantation is currently investigational, and more studies are needed to answer the above questions.

One way to mitigate concerns about future fertility is to utilize several fertility preservation techniques in the same patient based on personal history and likelihood of success with each method. One case series details removal of ovarian tissue for cryopreservation followed by stimulation of the remaining ovarian tissue and cryopreservation of oocytes with no substantial decrease in average number and quality of oocytes retrieved [129]. Another case series presents eighteen patients who underwent both oocyte and embryo cryopreservation, the former with subsequent in vitro maturation [79]. However, the American Society for Reproductive Medicine states that oocyte and ovarian cryopreservation should only be performed at specialized centers with protocols approved by an Institutional Review Board [7].

Ovarian Suppression

Several studies have shown that suppression of the ovary with either gonadotropin-releasing hormone (GnRH) agonists or antagonists prevents loss of follicles during chemotherapy or radiation, and there are several theories on the mechanism. Most noted is Blumenfeld's, which states that destruction of ovaries by chemotherapy results in elevated FSH, which recruits additional oocytes to mature into a growth state during which they are no longer protected from the chemotherapy's gonadotoxic effects. If the eggs remain quiescent, they might not be targeted by chemotherapy. Blumenfeld postulated that a GnRH agonist would prevent new follicles from being recruited into a vulnerable state [130], yet only animal experiments and non-randomized or small human case series have thus far been offered as evidence [78, 131]. Another small study of GnRH agonist administration to Hodgkin's lymphoma patients failed to show a protective action [132], however these data may be out-dated as treatments have changed over time. There is currently a large, prospective randomized clinical trial investigating the potential fertility benefits of ovarian suppression. A proven advantage, however, of GnRH agonists is the reduction of heavy uterine bleeding associated with decreased platelets during some chemotherapy regimens [133].

Uterine Transplantation

Transplantation of a human uterus has only been performed once, in Saudi Arabia in 2000, and had to be removed 99 days after surgery due to necrosis of the uterus from clotting in the uterine arteries and veins [134]. Despite this apparent failure, great strides have been made in this area over the past several decades due to advances in anti-rejection regimens. Further, the procedure has been successful in animal models with post-transplantation pregnancy demonstrated in mice and dogs and birth by cesarean delivery in sheep [135–139]. Uterine transplantation is investigational in humans at this time, and it would require a patient to be on lifelong immunosuppression medications.

Generation of Gametes from Somatic Cells

Research is currently directed at creating gametes, both egg and sperm, from non-gamete cells in the body. This would allow a patient to have genetic offspring even after oophorectomy. Chromosomal material is transferred from a non-gamete cell into an oocyte whose chromosomal material has been removed [140–144]. Other methods include parthenogenesis in which activation of an oocyte creates an embryo. Kono et al. formed a parthenogenetic mouse from an oocyte composed of two complete sets of the maternal genome, and this mouse maintained the ability to reproduce [145]. Much research is required before this will be considered a viable option, and there are complex ethical issues that arise from this procedure. However, it may ultimately become an established tool in ART.

Special Circumstances

Pregnancies conceived while a patient has cancer should be considered high-risk for several reasons: potential transfer of cancer to the fetus through the placenta, effects of cancer treatment on the fetus, and effects of cancer treatment on the mother. Animal studies and follow-up of pregnant women during atomic fallout exposure in Japan have provided most of our known data on radiation exposure during gestation. The most common side effects are prenatal death, malformations, neurodevelopmental disorders, and childhood cancer [146]. Exposure can be decreased by 30–60% with abdominal shielding [147], and these effects are not usually seen if the radiation exposure to the fetus is less than 10 centigray (cGy) [146]. Small studies have shown no neurodevelopmental effect or increase in malformations or preterm labor in fetuses conceived during chemotherapy [52, 148], but further studies should be performed. If planned, pregnancy should be delayed until cancer treatment is concluded and preferably until the patient is in clinical remission. The optimal delay is unknown, though a minimum of 6 months is estimated based on animal data [52]. Despite these statistics, if the well-known teratogens are avoided, there is not a significantly increased risk of complications during the pregnancy based on small studies [149].

Pregnancies after treatment for cancer are also subject to several risks for both fetus and mother. If long-term damage to the heart or lungs has occurred from radiation or chemotherapy, the mother may be at higher risk of cardiomyopathy, pulmonary fibrosis, or interstitial pneumonitis [150, 151]. Irradiation and trachelectomy can both increase the rate of miscarriage, prematurity, and low birth weight; additionally, the incidence of cervical incompetence is elevated after trachelectomy [33, 67, 95, 152–155].

A child with a cancer diagnosis is another special circumstance that could affect future fertility. This is a unique population, as parents usually have to make the decision about fertility preservation before treatment starts, yet the child will choose how their genetic material is used once they become adults. Options are limited due to the immaturity of the eggs. As mentioned above, ovarian tissue cryopreservation and transplantation is the best option for children despite requiring a laparoscopic procedure under general anesthesia [116]. In the future, it may be possible to harvest primordial follicles from prepubertal children and cryopreserve them for later in vitro maturation and implantation. This process would be highly complicated, though, and will require substantial research before it becomes an established ART method [128].

Conclusions

Cancer survivors may reasonably have concerns about their own longevity after childbearing [4] or the effects of treatment on their future offspring if administered prior to conception or harvesting of oocytes [156]. Despite these concerns, most would prefer to have biological offspring [75], and some choose less effective cancer treatments in order to decrease the potential for infertility [157]. In all situations, though, adoption should be mentioned as part of thorough counseling on ways to become a parent after a cancer diagnosis. Financial limitations are the most common barrier to adoption, with costs in the United States usually exceeding $30,000 [6].

A multi-disciplinary approach provides the most thorough care for a woman recently diagnosed with cancer who is interested or may become interested in retaining fertility. Medical and radiation oncologists, reproductive endocrinologists specializing in oncofertility, and psychosocial support personnel including social workers and psychologists should all be involved from the beginning with inclusion of pediatricians, genetic counselors, and perinatologists as needed. Clear communication among providers is essential.

Fertility-sparing treatment after a cancer diagnosis should be broached with all women of reproductive age who desire to maintain their ability to conceive. Even though there is no guarantee of a successful live birth after any of these methods, it offers a way for a patient to exercise some control of their reproductive life during a frightening time and offers a plan for a normal future. Existing barriers to access include a deficit of information on fertility preservation options, expense due to incomplete insurance coverage, and late referral to reproductive specialists. Once these are overcome, female cancer patients desiring fertility will receive the best and most comprehensive care.

References

1. Surveillance Epidemiology and End Results Cancer Statistics http://seer.cancer.gov. Accessed 2 May 2011
2. Carter J, Sonoda Y, Abu-Rustum N (2007) Reproductive concerns of women treated with radical trachelectomy for cervical cancer. Gynecol Oncol 105:13–16
3. Noyes N, Reh A, Mullin C, Fino ME, Grifo J (2010) Quality-of-life (QOL) assessment at time of fertility preservation (FP) counseling in female cancer patients: results of a university-based registry at two years. J Clin Oncol 28(Supp 15): e1964
4. Lee SJ, Schover LR, Partridge AH, Patrizio P, Wallace WH, Hagerty K, Beck LN, Brennan LV, Oktay K (2006) American Society of Clinical Oncology Recommendations on Fertility Preservation in Cancer Patients. J Clin Oncol 24(18):2917–2931
5. Nakayama K, Ueno NT (2006) American Society of Clinical Oncology recommendations on fertility preservation should be implemented regardless of disease status or previous treatments. J Clin Oncol 24(33):5334–5335
6. Anchan RM, Ginsburg ES (2010) Fertility concerns and preservation in younger women with breast cancer. Crit Rev Oncol Hematol 74:175–192
7. Ethics Committee of the American Society for Reproductive Medicine (2005) Fertility preservation and reproduction in cancer patients. Fertil Steril 83:1622–1628
8. Seifer D, Lambert-Messerlian G, Hogan J, Gardiner A, Blazar A, Berk C (1997) Day 3 serum inhibin-B is predictive of assisted reproductive technologies outcome. Fertil Steril 67:110–114
9. te Velde ER, Pearson PL (2002) The variability of female reproductive ageing. Hum Reprod Update 8:141–154
10. Noyes N, Knopman J, Long K, Coletta JM, Abu-Rustum NR (2011) Fertility considerations in the management of gynecologic malignancies. Gynecol Oncol 120:326–333
11. Ng E, Yeung W, Fong D, Ho P (2003) Effects of age on hormonal and ultrasound markers of ovarian reserve in Chinese women with proven fertility. Hum Reprod 18:2169–2174
12. Syrop C, Dawson J, Husman K, Sparks A, Van Voorhis B (1999) Ovarian volume may predict assisted reproductive outcomes better than follicle stimulating hormone concentration on day 3. Hum Reprod 14:1752–1756
13. Chui D, Pugh N, Walker S, Gregory L, Shaw R (1997) Follicular vascularity – the predictive value of transvaginal power Doppler ultrasonography in an in-vitro fertilization programme: a preliminary study. Hum Reprod 12:191–196
14. WomensHealth.gov: The Federal Government Source for Women's Health Information www.womenshealth.gov/menopause/basics. Accessed 8 June 2011
15. Noyes N, Hampton BS, Berkeley A, Licciardi F, Grifo J, Krey L (2001) Factors useful in predicting success for oocyte donation cycles: a three-year retrospective analysis. Fertil Steril 76:92–97
16. Pendse S, Ginsburg E, Singh AK (2004) Strategies for preservation of ovarian and testicular function after immunosuppression. Am J Kidney Dis 43(5):772–781
17. Blumenfeld Z, Avivi I, Ritter M, Rowe JM (1999) Preservation of fertility and ovarian function and minimizing chemotherapy-induced gonadotoxicity in young women. J Soc Gynecol Investig 6(5): 229–239
18. Rosendahl M, Andersen CY, la Cour Freiesleben N, Juul A, Lossl K, Andersen AN (2010) Dynamics and mechanisms of chemotherapy-induced ovarian follicular depletion in women of fertile age. Fertil Steril 94(1):156–166
19. Ginsburg ES, Yanushpolsky EH, Jackson KV (2001) In vitro fertilization for cancer patients and survivors. Fertil Steril 75(4):705–710
20. Hodgson DC, Pintilie M, Gitterman L, Dewitt B, Buckley CA, Ahmed S, Smith K, Schwartz A, Tsang RW, Crump M, Wells W, Sun A, Gospodarowicz MK (2007) Fertility among female hodgkin lymphoma survivors attempting pregnancy following ABVD chemotherapy. Hematol Oncol 25(1):11–15
21. Partridge AH, Gelber S, Peppercorn J, Ginsburg E, Sampson E, Rosenberg R, Przypyszny M, Winer EP (2008) Fertility and menopausal outcomes in young breast cancer survivors. Clin Breast Cancer 8(1): 65–69
22. Wallace WH, Thomson AB, Kelsey TW (2003) The radiosensitivity of the human oocyte. Hum Reprod 18:117–121
23. Brannstrom M, Diaz-Garcia C (2011) Transplantation of female genital organs. J Obstet Gynaecol Res 37(4):271–291
24. Meirow D (2000) Reproduction post-chemotherapy in young cancer patients. Mol Cell Endocrinol 169:123–131
25. Oktem O, Urman B (2010) Options of fertility preservation in female cancer patients. Obstet Gynecol Surv 65(8):531–542
26. Paris F, Perez GI, Fuks Z, Haimovitz-Friedman A, Nguyen H, Bose M, Ilagan A, Hunt PA, Morgan WF, Tilly JL, Kolesnick R (2002) Sphingosine 1-phosphate preserves fertility in irradiated female mice without propagating genomic damage in offspring. Nat Med 8(9):901–902

27. Wallace WH, Thomson AB, Saran F, Kelsey TW (2005) Predicting age of ovarian failure after radiation to a field that includes the ovaries. Int J Radiat Oncol Biol Phys 62:738–744

28. Wallace WH, Anderson RA, Irvine DS (2005) Fertility preservation for young patients with cancer: who is at risk and what can be offered? Lancet Oncol 6(4):209–218

29. Hawkins MM, Smith RA (1989) Pregnancy outcomes in childhood cancer survivors: probable effects of abdominal irradiation. Int J Cancer 43:399–402

30. Critchley HO, Wallace WH, Shalet SM, Mamtora H, Higginson J, Anderson DC (1992) Abdominal irradiation in childhood; the potential for pregnancy. Br J Obstet Gynaecol 99:392–394

31. Meirow D, Nugent D (2001) The effects of radiotherapy on female reproduction. Hum Reprod Update 7:535–543

32. Nussbaum Blask AR, Nicholson HS, Markle BM, Wechsler-Jentzch K, O'Donnell R, Byrne J (1999) Sonographic detection of uterine and ovarian abnormalities in female survivors of Wilms' tumor treated with radiotherapy. Am J Roentgenol 172:759–763

33. Critchley HO, Bath LE, Wallace WH (2002) Radiation damage to the uterus—review of the effects of treatment of childhood cancer. Hum Fertil 5:61–66

34. Andersen BL, Green DM (2001) Fertility and Sexuality after Cancer Treatment. In: Lenhard RE Jr, Osteen RT, Gansler T (eds) Clinical oncology. American Cancer Society, Atlanta, Georgia

35. Li FP, Fine W, Jaffe N, Holmes GE, Holmes FF (1979) Offspring of patients treated for cancer in childhood. J Natl Cancer Inst 62:1193–1197

36. Hawkins MM, Smith RA, Curtice LJ (1988) Childhood cancer survivors and their offspring studied through a postal survey of general practitioners: preliminary results. J R Coll Gen Pract 38:102–105

37. Byrne J, Rasmussen SA, Steinhorn SC, Connelly RR, Myers MH, Lynch CF, Flannery J, Austin DF, Holmes FF, Holmes GE, Strong LC, Mulvihill JJ (1998) Genetic disease in offspring of long-term survivors of childhood and adolescent cancer. Am J Hum Genet 62(1):45–52

38. Gershenson DM (2005) Fertility-sparing surgery for malignancies in women. J Natl Cancer Inst Monogr 34:43–47

39. Elizur SE, Tulandi T, Meterissian S, Huang JY, Levin D, Tan SL (2009) Fertility preservation for young women with rectal cancer – a combined approach from one referral center. J Gastrointest Surg 13:1111–1115

40. Williams RS, Littell RD, Mendenhall NP (1999) Laparoscopic oophoropexy and ovarian function in the treatment of Hodgkin disease. Cancer 86(10):2138–2142

41. Husseinzadeh N, Nahhas WA, Velkley DE, Whitney CW, Mortel R (1984) The preservation of ovarian function in young women undergoing pelvic radiation therapy. Gynecol Oncol 18(3):373–379

42. Terenziani M, Piva L, Meazza C, Gandola L, Cefalo G, Merola M (2009) Oophoropexy: a relevant role in preservation of ovarian function after pelvic irradiation. Fertil Steril 91(3):935, e15–16

43. Jenninga E, Hilders CG, Louwe LA, Peters AA (2008) Female fertility preservation: practical and ethical considerations of an underused procedure. Cancer 14(5):333–339

44. Clough KB, Goffinet F, Labib A, Renolleau C, Campana F, de la Rochefordiere A, Durand JC (1996) Laparoscopic unilateral ovarian transposition prior to irradiation: Prospective study of 20 cases. Cancer 77:2638–2645

45. Damewood MD, Hesla HS, Lowen M, Schultz MJ (1990) Induction of ovulation and pregnancy following lateral oophoropexy for Hodgkin's disease. Int J Gynaecol Obstet 33:369–371

46. Zinger M, Liu JH, Husseinzadeh N, Thomas MA (2004) Successful surrogate pregnancy after ovarian transposition, pelvic irradiation and hysterectomy. J Reprod Med 49:573–574

47. Blumenfeld Z (2001) Ovarian rescue/protection from chemotherapeutic agents. J Soc Gynecol Invest 8:S60–S64

48. Buekers TE, Anderson B, Sorosky JI, Buller RE (2001) Ovarian function after surgical treatment for cervical cancer. Gynecol Oncol 80:85–88

49. Pfeifer S, Coutifaris C (1999) Reproductive technologies 1998: options available for the cancer patient. Med Pediatr Oncol 33:34–40

50. Morice P, Thiam-Ba R, Castaigne D, Haie-Meder C, Gerbaulet A, Pautier P, Duvillard P, Michel G (1998) Fertility results after ovarian transposition for pelvic malignancies treated by external irradiation or brachytherapy. Hum Reprod 13:660–663

51. Barton SE, Politch JA, Benson CB, Ginsburg ES, Gargiulo AR (2011) Transabdominal follicular aspiration for oocyte retrieval in patients with ovaries inaccessible by transvaginal ultrasound. Fertil Steril 95(5):1773–1776

52. Simon B, Lee SJ, Partridge AH, Runowicz CD (2005) Preserving fertility after cancer. CA Cancer J Clin 55:211–228

53. Gershenson DM (1988) Menstrual and reproductive function after treatment with combination chemotherapy for malignant ovarian germ cell tumors. J Clin Oncol 6:270–275

54. Zanetta G, Bonazzi C, Cantu MG, Bini S, Locatelli A, Bratina G, Mangioni C (2001) Survival and reproductive function after treatment of malignant germ cell ovarian tumors. J Clin Oncol 19:1015–1020

55. Lim-Tam S, Cajigas HE, Scully RE (1988) Ovarian cystectomy for serous borderline tumors: a follow-up study of 35 cases. Obstet Gynecol 72:775–781

56. Zanetta G, Rota S, Chiari S, Bonazzi C, Bratina G, Mangioni C (2001) Behavior of borderline tumors

with particular interest to persistence, recurrence, and progression to invasive carcinoma: a prospective study. J Clin Oncol 19:2658–2664

57. Schilder JM, Thompson AM, DePriest PD, Ueland FR, Cibull ML, Kryscio RJ, Modesitt SC, Lu KH, Geisler JP, Higgins RV, Magtibay PM, Cohn DE, Powell MA, Chu C, Stehman FB, van Nagell J (2002) Outcome of reproductive age women with stage IA or IC invasive epithelial ovarian cancer treated with fertility-sparing therapy. Gynecol Oncol 87:1–7

58. Seracchioli R, Venturoli S, Colombo FM, Govoni F, Missiroli S, Bagnoli A (2001) Fertility and tumor recurrence rate after conservative laparoscopic management of young women with early-stage borderline ovarian tumors. Fertil Steril 76:999–1003

59. Ungar L, Palfalvi L, Hogg R, Sikos P, Boyle DC, Del Priore G, Smith JR (2005) Abdominal radical trachelectomy: A fertility-preserving option for women with early cervical cancer. BJOG 112:366–369

60. Dargent D, Martin X, Sacchetoni A, Mathevet P (2000) Laparoscopic vaginal radical trachelectomy: A treatment to preserve the fertility of cervical carcinoma patients. Cancer 88:1877–1882

61. Plante M, Renaud MC, Francois H, Roy M (2004) Vaginal radical trachelectomy: An oncologically safe fertility-preserving surgery. An updated series of 72 cases and review of the literature. Gynecol Oncol 94:614–623

62. Plante M, Renaud MC, Hoskins IA, Roy M (2005) Vaginal radical trachelectomy: a valuable fertility-preserving option in the management of early-stage cervical cancer. A series of 50 pregnancies and review of the literature. Gynecol Oncol 98:3–10

63. Plante M (2003) Fertility preservation in the management of cervical cancer. CME J Gynecol Oncol 8:97–107

64. Koliopoulos G, Sotiriadis A, Kyrgiou M, Martin-Hirsch P, Makrydimas G, Paraskevaidis E (2004) Conservative surgical methods for FIGO stage IA2 squamous cervical carcinoma and their role in preserving women's fertility. Gynecol Oncol 93:469–473

65. Shepherd JH, Mould T, Oram DH (2001) Radical trachelectomy in early stage carcinoma of the cervix: Outcome as judged by recurrence and fertility rates. BJOG 108:882–885

66. Dargent D (2001) Radical trachelectomy: an operation that preserves the fertility of young women with invasive cervical cancer. Bull Acad Natl Med 185:1295–1304

67. Burnett AF, Roman LD, O'Meara AT, Morrow CP (2003) Radical vaginal trachelectomy and pelvic lymphadenectomy for preservation of fertility in early cervical carcinoma. Gynecol Oncol 88:419–423

68. Roy M, Plante M (1998) Pregnancies after radical vaginal trachelectomy for early-stage cervical cancer. Am J Obstet Gynecol 179:1491–1496

69. Bernardini M, Barrett J, Seaward G, Covens A (2003) Pregnancy outcomes in patients with radical trachelectomy. Am J Obstet Gynecol 189:1378–1382

70. Covens A, Shaw P, Murphy J, DePetrillo D, Lickrish G, Laframboise S, Rosen B (1999) Is radical trachelectomy a safe alternative to radical hysterectomy for patients with stage IA-B carcinoma of the cervix? Cancer 86:2273–2279

71. Erkanli S, Ayhan A (2010) Fertility-sparing therapy in young women with endometrial cancer: 2010 update. Int J Gynecol Cancer 20(7):1170–1187

72. Masciullo V, Amadio G, Lo Russo D, Raimondo I, Giordano A, Scambia G (2010) Controversies in the management of endometrial cancer. Obstet Gynecol Int 2010:638165

73. Society for Assisted Reproductive Technology http://www.sart.org. Accessed 6 May 2011

74. Robertson AD, Missmer SA, Ginsburg ES (2011) Embryo yield after in vitro fertilization in women undergoing embryo banking for fertility preservation before chemotherapy. Fertil Steril 95(2):588–591

75. Schover LR, Rybicki LA, Martin BA, Bringelsen KA (1999) Having children after cancer: A pilot survey of survivors' attitudes and experiences. Cancer 86(4):697–709

76. Baynosa J, Westphal L, Madrigrano A, Wapnir I (2009) Timing of breast cancer treatments with oocyte retrieval and embryo cryopreservation. J Am Coll Surg 209:603–607

77. Noyes N, Labella P, Grifo J, Knopman JM (2010) Oocyte cryopreservation: a feasible fertility preservation option for reproductive age cancer survivors. J Assist Reprod Genet 27:495–499

78. Kim SS, Klemp J, Fabian C (2011) Breast cancer and fertility preservation. Fertil Steril 95(5):1535–1541

79. Maman E, Meirow D, Brengauz M, Raanani H, Dor J, Hourvitz A (2011) Luteal phase oocyte retrieval and in vitro maturation is an optional procedure for urgent fertility preservation. Fertil Steril 95(1):64–67

80. Oktay K, Buyuk E, Libertella N, Akar M, Rosenwaks Z (2005) Fertility preservation in breast cancer patients: A prospective controlled comparison of ovarian stimulation with tamoxifen and letrozole for embryo cryopreservation. J Clin Oncol 23(19):4347–4353

81. Engmann L, DiLuigi A, Schmidt D, Nulsen J, Maier D, Benadiva C (2008) The use of gonadotropin-releasing hormone agonist to induce oocyte maturation after cotreatment with GnRH antagonist in high-risk patients undergoing in vitro fertilization prevents the risk of ovarian hyperstimulation syndrome: a prospective randomized controlled study. Fertil Steril 89(1):84–91

82. Whittemore AS, Harris R, Itnyre J for the Collaborative Ovarian Cancer Group (1992) Characteristics relating to ovarian cancer risk:

collaborative analysis of 12 U.S. case-control studies. II. Invasive epithelial ovarian cancers in white women. Am J Epidemiol 136:1184–1203

83. Rossing MA, Daling JR, Weiss NS, Moore DE, Self SG (1994) Ovarian tumors in a cohort of infertile women. New Engl J Med 331:771–776

84. Brinton LA, Lamb EJ, Moghissi KS, Scoccia B, Althuis MD, Mabie JE, Westhoff CL (2004) Ovarian cancer risk after the use of ovulation-stimulating drugs. Obstet Gynecol 103:1194–1203

85. Oktay K (2005) Further evidence on the safety and success of ovarian stimulation with letrozole and tamoxifen in breast cancer patients undergoing in vitro fertilization to cryopreserve their embryos for fertility preservation. J Clin Oncol 23:3858–3859

86. Oktay K, Hourvitz A, Sahin G, Oktem O, Safro B, Cil A, Bang H (2006) Letrozole reduces estrogen and gonadotropin exposure in women with breast cancer undergoing ovarian stimulation before chemotherapy. J Clin Endocrinol Metab 91:3885–3890

87. Azim AA, Costantini-Ferrando M, Oktay K (2008) Safety of fertility preservation by ovarian stimulation with letrozole and gonadotropins in patients with breast cancer: a prospective controlled study. J Clin Oncol 26:2630–2635

88. Kondapalli L, Hong F, Gracia C (2010) Clinical cases in oncofertility. Cancer Treat Res 156:55–67

89. von Wolff M, Strowitzki T, van der Ven H, Montag M (2006) In vitro maturation is an efficient technique to generate oocytes and should be considered in combination with cryopreservation of ovarian tissue for preservation of fertility in women. J Clin Oncol 24(33):5336–5337

90. Smitz JE, Thompson JG, Gilchrist RB (2011) The promise of in vitro maturation in assisted reproduction and fertility preservation. Semin Reprod Med 29(1):24–37

91. Mosgaard BJ, Lidegaard O, Kjaer SK, Schou G, Andersen AN (1997) Infertility, fertility drugs and invasive ovarian cancer: a case-control study. Fertil Steril 67:1005–1012

92. Rossing MA, Daling JR, Weiss NS, Moore DE, Self SG (1996) Risk of breast cancer in a cohort in infertile women. Gynecol Oncol 60:3–7

93. Hawkins MM (1994) Pregnancy outcome and offspring after childhood cancer. BMJ 309:1034

94. Thomson AB, Campbell AJ, Irvine DC, Anderson RA, Kelnar CJ, Wallace WH (2002) Semen quality and spermatozoal DNA integrity in survivors of childhood cancer: a case-control study. Lancet 360:361–367

95. Green DM, Whitton JA, Stovall M, Mertens AC, Donaldson SS, Ruymann FB, Pendergrass TW, Robison LL (2002) Pregnancy outcome of female survivors of childhood cancer: a report from the Childhood Cancer Survivor Study. Am J Obstet Gynecol 187:1070–1080

96. Sankila R, Olsen JH, Anderson H, Garwicz S, Glattre E, Hertz H, Langmark F, Lanning M, Moller T, Tulinius H (1998) Risk of cancer among offspring of childhood-cancer survivors. Association of the Nordic Cancer Registries and the Nordic Society of Paediatric Haematology. New Engl J Med 338:1339–1344

97. Green DM, Whitton JA, Stovall M, Mertens AC, Donaldson SS, Ruymann FB, Pendergrass TW, Robison LL (2003) Pregnancy outcome of partners of male survivors of childhood cancer: a report from the Childhood Cancer Survivor Study. J Clin Oncol 21:716–721

98. Stovall M, Donaldson SS, Weathers RE, Robison LL, Mertens AC, Winther JF, Olsen JH, Boice JD Jr (2004) Genetic effects of radiotherapy for childhood cancer: gonadal dose reconstruction. Int J Radiat Oncol Biol Phys 60:542–552

99. Boice JD Jr, Tawn EJ, Winther JF, Donaldson SS, Green DM, Mertens AC, Mulvihill JJ, Olsen JH, Robison LL, Stovall M (2003) Genetic effects of radiotherapy for childhood cancer. Health Phys 85:65–80

100. Yang D, Brown SE, Nguyen K, Reddy V, Brubaker C, Winslow KL (2007) Live birth after the transfer of human embryos developed from cryopreserved oocytes harvested before cancer treatment. Fertil Steril 87(6):1469, e1–4

101. Yoon TK, Kim TJ, Park SE, Hong SW, Ko JJ, Chung HM, Cha KY (2003) Live births after vitrification of oocytes in a stimulated in vitro fertilization embryo transfer program. Fertil Steril 79(6):1323–1326

102. Fabbri R, Porcu E, Marsella T, Rocchetta G, Venturoli S, Flamigni C (2001) Human oocyte cryopreservation: new perspectives regarding oocyte survival. Hum Reprod 16(3):411–416

103. Borini A, Sciajno R, Bianchi V, Sereni E, Flamigni C, Coticchio G (2006) Clinical outcome of oocyte cryopreservation after slow cooling with a protocol utilizing a high sucrose concentration. Hum Reprod 21(2):512–517

104. Rudick B, Opper N, Paulson R, Bendikson K, Chung K (2010) The status of oocyte cryopreservation in the United States. Fertil Steril 94(7): 2642–2646

105. Oktay K, Cil AP, Bang H (2006) Efficiency of oocyte cryopreservation: a meta-analysis. Fertil Steril 86(1):70–80

106. Noyes N, Porcu E, Borini A (2009) With more than 900 babies born, live birth outcomes following oocyte cryopreservation do not appear different from those occurring after conventional IVF. Reprod Biomed Online 18:769–776

107. ASRM Practice Committee (2009) ASRM Practice Committee response to Rybak and Lieman: elective self-donation of oocytes. Fertil Steril 92:1513–1514

108. Galbraith M, McLachlan HV, Swales JK (2005) Commercial agencies and surrogate motherhood:

a transaction cost approach. Health Care Anal 13(1):11–31

109. Oktay K, Karlikaya G (2000) Ovarian function after transplantation of frozen, banked autologous ovarian tissue. New Engl J Med 342:1919

110. Donnez J, Dolman MM, Demylle D, Jadoul P, Pirard C, Squifflet J, Martinez-Madrid B, van Langendonckt A (2004) Live birth after orthotopic transplantation of cryopreserved ovarian tissue. Lancet 364:1405–1410

111. Meirow D, Levron J, Eldar-Geva T, Hardan I, Fridman E, Zalel Y, Schiff E, Dor J (2005) Pregnancy after transplantation of cryopreserved ovarian tissue in a patient with ovarian failure after chemotherapy. New Engl J Med 353:318–321

112. Radford JA, Lieberman BA, Brison DR, Smith AR, Critchlow JD, Russell SA, Watson AJ, Clayton JA, Harris M, Gosden RG, Shalet SM (2001) Orthotopic reimplantation of cryopreserved ovarian cortical strips after high-dose chemotherapy for Hodgkin's lymphoma. Lancet 357:1172–1175

113. Tryde Schmidt KL, Yding Andersen C, Starup J, Loft A, Byskov AG, Nyboe Andersen A (2004) Orthotopic autotransplantation of cryopreserved ovarian tissue to a woman cured of cancer-follicular growth, steroid production and oocyte retrieval. Reprod Biomed Online 8:448–453

114. Oktay K, Buyuk E, Rosenwaks Z, Rucinski J (2003) A technique for transplantation of ovarian cortical strips to the forearm. Fertil Steril 80:193–198

115. Oktay K, Economos K, Kan M, Rucinski J, Veeck L, Rosenwaks Z (2001) Endocrine function and oocyte retrieval after autologous transplantation of ovarian cortical strips to the forearm. JAMA 286(12): 1490–1493

116. Wallace WHB, Barr RD (2010) Fertility preservation for girls and young women with cancer: what are the remaining challenges? Hum Reprod Update 16(6):614–616

117. Oktay K, Buyuk E, Veeck L, Zaninovic N, Xu K, Takeuchi T, Opsahl M, Rosenwaks Z (2004) Embryo development after heterotopic transplantation of cryopreserved ovarian tissue. Lancet 363:837–840

118. Demeestere I, Simon P, Buxant F, Robin V, Fernandez SA, Centner J, Delbaere A, Englert Y (2006) Ovarian function and spontaneous pregnancy after combined heterotopic and orthotopic cryopreserved ovarian tissue transplantation in a patient previously treated with bone marrow transplantation: case report. Hum Reprod 21:2010–2014

119. Andersen CY, Rosendahl M, Byskov AG, Loft A, Ottosen C, Dueholm M, Schmidt KL, Andersen AN, Ernst E (2008) Two successful pregnancies following autotransplantation of frozen/thawed ovarian tissue. Hum Reprod 23:2266–2272

120. Silber SJ, DeRosa M, Pineda J, Lenahan K, Grenia D, Gorman K, Gosden RG (2008) A series of monozygotic twins discordant for ovarian failure:

ovary transplantation (cortical vs. microvascular) and cryopreservation. Hum Reprod 23:1531–1537

121. Donnez J, Squifflet J, Jadoul P, Demylle D, Cheron AC, van Langendonckt A, Dolman MM (2011) Pregnancy and live birth after autotransplantation of frozen-thawed ovarian tissue in a patient with metastatic disease undergoing chemotherapy and hematopoietic stem cell transplantation. Fertil Steril 95(5):1787

122. Oktay K, Sonmezer M (2004) Ovarian tissue banking for cancer patients: fertility preservation, not just ovarian preservation. Hum Reprod 19(3): 477–480

123. Kim SS (2006) Fertility preservation in female cancer patients: current developments and future directions. Fertil Steril 85(1):1–11

124. Meirow D, Fasouliotis SJ, Nugent D, Schenker JG, Gosden RG, Rutherford AJ (1999) A laparoscopic technique for obtaining ovarian cortical biopsy specimens for fertility conservation in patients with cancer. Fertil Steril 71:948–951

125. Poirot C, Vacher-Lavenu MC, Helardot P, Guibert J, Brugieres L, Jouannet P (2002) Human ovarian tissue cryopreservation: indications and feasibility. Hum Reprod 17:1447–1452

126. Newton H, Aubard Y, Rutherford A, Sharma V, Gosden R (1996) Low temperature storage and grafting of human ovarian tissue. Hum Reprod 11:1487–1491

127. Dolmans MM, Marinescu C, Saussoy P, Van Langendonckt A, Amorim C, Donnez J (2010) Reimplantation of cryopreserved ovarian tissue from patients with acute lymphoblastic leukemia is potentially unsafe. Blood 116(16):2908–2914

128. Oktay K (2009) Preservation of fertility in patients with cancer. New Engl J Med 360:2680–2683

129. Huober-Zeeb C, Lawrenz B, Popovici RM, Strowitzki T, Germeyer A, Stute P, von Wolff M (2011) Improving fertility preservation in cancer: ovarian tissue cryobanking followed by ovarian stimulation can be efficiently combined. Fertil Steril 95(1):342–344

130. Blumenfeld Z, von Wolff M (2008) GnRH-analogues and oral contraceptives for fertility preservation in women during chemotherapy. Hum Reprod 14:543–552

131. Blumenfeld Z, Avivi I, Linn S, Epelbaum R, Ben-Shahar M, Haim N (1996) Prevention of irreversible chemotherapy-induced ovarian damage in young women with lymphoma by a gonadotrophin-releasing hormone agonist in parallel to chemotherapy. Hum Reprod 11:1620–1626

132. Waxman JH, Ahmed R, Smith D, Wrigley PF, Gregory W, Shalet S, Crowther D, Rees LH, Besser GM, Malpas JS et al (1987) Failure to preserve fertility in patients with Hodgkin's disease. Cancer Chemother Pharmacol 19:159–162

133. Blumenfeld Z (2010) Fertility preservation and GnRH-a for chemotherapy: debate. Arch Gynecol Obstet 282:585–586

134. Fageeh W, Raffa H, Jabbad H, Marzouki A (2002) Transplantation of the human uterus. Int J Gynecol Obstet 76:245–251

135. Eraslan S, Hamernik RJ, Hardy JD (1966) Replantation of uterus and ovaries in dogs, with successful pregnancy. Arch Surg 92:9–12

136. Truta E, Pop I, Popa D, Ionescu M, Truta F (1969) Experimental re- and transplantation of the internal female genital organs. Rom Med Rev 13:53–58

137. Barzilai A, Paldi E, Gal D, Hampel N (1973) Autotransplantation of the uterus and ovaries in dogs. Isr J Med Sci 9:49–52

138. Racho El-Akouri R, Kurlberg G, Dindelegan G, Molne J, Wallin A, Brannstrom M (2002) Heterotopic uterine transplantation by vascular anastomosis in the mouse. J Endocrinol 174:157–166

139. Wranning CA, Marcickiewicz J, Enskog A, Dahm-Kahler P, Hanafy A, Brannstrom M (2010) Fertility after autologous ovine uterine-tubal-ovarian transplantation by vascular anastomosis to the external iliac vessels. Hum Reprod 25:1973–1979

140. Rideout 3rd WM, Eggan K, Jaenisch R (2001) Nuclear cloning and epigenetic reprogramming of the genome. Science 293(5532):1093–1098

141. Hubner K, Fuhrmann G, Christenson LK, Kehler J, Reinbold R, De La Fuente R, Wood J, Strauss JF 3rd, Boiani M, Scholer HR (2003) Derivation of oocytes from mouse embryonic stem cells. Science 300(5623):1251–1256

142. Geijsen N, Horoschak M, Kim K, Gribnau J, Eggan K, Daley GQ (2004) Derivation of embryonic germ cells and male gametes from embryonic stem cells. Nature 427(6970):148–154

143. Friedrich MJ (2005) George Daley, MD, PhD, talks about the clinical promise of stem cell research. JAMA 293(7):787–789

144. Rideout 3rd WM, Hochedlinger K, Kyba M, Daley GQ, Jaenisch R (2002) Correction of a genetic defect by nuclear transplantation and combined cell and gene therapy. Cell 109(1):17–27

145. Kono T, Obata Y, Wu Q, Niwa K, Ono Y, Yamamoto Y, Park ES, Seo JS, Ogawa H (2004) Birth of parthenogenetic mice that can develop to adulthood. Nature 428(6985):860–864

146. de Wildt SN, Taguchi N, Koren G (2009) Unintended pregnancy during radiotherapy for cancer. Nat Clin Pract Oncol 6(3):175–178

147. Mazonakis M, Varveris H, Fasoulaki M, Damilakis J (2003) Radiotherapy of Hodgkin's disease in early pregnancy: embryo dose measurements. Radiother Oncol 66:333–339

148. Nulman I, Laslo D, Fried S, Uleryk E, Lishner M, Koren G (2001) Neurodevelopment of children exposed in utero to treatment of maternal malignancy. Br J Cancer 85:1611–1618

149. Partridge AH, Garber JE (2000) Long-term outcomes of children exposed to antineoplastic agents in utero. Semin Oncol 27:712–726

150. Bar J, Davidi O, Goshen Y, Hod M, Yaniv I, Hirsch R (2003) Pregnancy outcome in women treated with doxorubicin for childhood cancer. Am J Obstet Gynecol 189:853–857

151. Khan A, McNally D, Tutschka PJ, Bilgrami S (1997) Paclitaxel-induced acute bilateral pneumonitis. Ann Pharmacother 31(12):1471–1474

152. Salooja N, Szydlo RM, Socie G, Rio B, Chatterjee R, Ljungman P, Van Lint MT, Powles R, Jackson G, Hinterberger-Fischer M, Kolb HJ, Apperley JF; Late Effects Working Party of the European Group for Blood and Marrow Transplantation (2001) Pregnancy outcomes after peripheral blood or bone marrow transplantation: A retrospective study. Lancet 358:271–276

153. Sanders JE, Hawley J, Levy W, Gooley T, Buckner CD, Deeg HJ, Doney K, Storb R, Sullivan K, Witherspoon R, Appelbaum FR (1996) Pregnancies following high-dose cyclophosphamide with or without high-dose busulfan or total-body irradiation and bone marrow transplantation. Blood 87:3045–3052

154. Crane JM (2003) Pregnancy outcome after loop electrosurgical excision procedure: a systematic review. Obstet Gynecol 102:1058–1062

155. Schlaerth JB, Spirtos NM, Schlaerth AC (2003) Radical trachelectomy and pelvic lymphadenectomy with uterine preservation in the treatment of cervical cancer. Am J Obstet Gynecol 188:29–34

156. Fossa SD, Magelssen H, Melve K, Jacobsen AB, Langmark F, Skjaerven R (2005) Parenthood in survivors after adulthood cancer and perinatal health in their offspring: A preliminary report. J Natl Cancer Inst Monogr 34:77–82

157. Partridge AH, Gelber S, Peppercorn J, Sampson E, Knudsen K, Laufer M, Rosenberg R, Przypyszny M, Rein A, Winer EP (2004) Web-based survey of fertility issues in young women with breast cancer. J Clin Oncol 22:4174–4183

158. American Cancer Society http://www.cancer.gov. Accessed 2 May 2011

Options for Fertility Preservation in Men and Boys with Cancer

Peter J. Stahl, MD, Doron S. Stember, MD, and John P. Mulhall, MD

I was diagnosed with Hodgkin's Lymphoma when I was 15. I guess I was a late bloomer because I'd never really thought about kids or a family. The doctors told my parents there was a good chance I'd never be able to father a child after my treatment. I was only concerned about living, and I didn't want to talk about sperm banking or think about the future. My mom kept bringing it up though – she wouldn't drop it – she kept saying "you'll feel differently one day," or "you'll be sorry when you're older that you didn't think more about it." Truthfully, at the time it was so embarrassing, and the last thing I wanted to do was talk to my mom about sperm banking. I felt lousy I was scared of dying and scared of what the treatments were going to be like, and the biggest thing on my mind was all the baseball practices and games I was going to miss. I yelled at my mom and told her not mention it again – I'd made up my mind I was not going to do the sperm banking.

Now I'm 25 years old and haven't stopped kicking myself. I met the love of my life in college and we married right after graduation. We wanted to start a family right away, and I guess I just forgot that it may be an issue for me. When we couldn't get pregnant, we went to fertility testing and learned that my fertility was very compromised. My wife wondered why I'd never mentioned this possibility to her – she knew I had cancer, but it just didn't sink in to me what my mom and the doctor had been trying to tell me. I regret not listening and not doing the sperm banking. We're going to have to use donor sperm now, and I'm not even sure how I feel about that.

Maybe my mom wasn't the best person to talk to me about it. I might have listened more if the doctor had talked to me alone or maybe if I had talked to some guy a little older than me who'd gone through the same thing. I have no one to blame but myself, and I'm grateful to be alive, but if I had to do it over again, I would have definitely done the sperm banking.
Lionel, Adult Cancer Survivor

Introduction

Fertility is a critical quality of life issue in young men faced with a new diagnosis of malignancy. Fortunately, fertility preservation is possible in the vast majority of cases. Acquisition of sperm for cryopreservation that may be used for future reproduction is the cornerstone of male fertility preservation. The most commonly considered benefit of sperm banking is preservation of the potential for biological paternity. A less commonly considered advantage is maintenance of the opportunity for assisted reproduction with intrauterine insemination (IUI), rather than in vitro fertilization (IVF), by storage of normospermic semen samples in patients at risk for oligospermia. A third benefit of fertility preservation in men is amelioration of anxiety about future infertility. Approximately one third of young men with cancer experience significant

P.J. Stahl (✉)
James Buchanan Brady Department of Urology, Weill Cornell Medical College, New York, NY, USA
e-mail: pjs2002@med.cornell.edu

G.P. Quinn, S.T. Vadaparampil (eds.), *Reproductive Health and Cancer in Adolescents and Young Adults*, Advances in Experimental Medicine and Biology 732,
DOI 10.1007/978-94-007-2492-1_3, © Springer Science+Business Media B.V. 2012

distress concerning their fertility, [1] and two-thirds of cancer patients who cryopreserve sperm feel significantly encouraged by having done so [1, 2].

The benefits of sperm banking must be weighed against the medical and financial costs of sperm acquisition and cryopreservation. In most men, sufficient sperm can be acquired by collection of ejaculated semen, which is inexpensive and has no associated medical risk. However, more invasive procedures, such as electroejaculation (EEJ) and testicular sperm extraction (TESE), may be required in men with ejaculatory dysfunction or azoospermia. These procedures have potential associated medical morbidity, are not universally effective, and are financially expensive. In this chapter, we review the reproductive toxicities of cancer and cancer therapy, and the clinical management of young men whose fertility is threatened by cancer. The optimal utilization of sperm banking and strategies for fertility preservation in men with ejaculatory dysfunction and azoospermia are discussed. Lastly, emerging options for fertility preservation in pre-pubertal boys are reviewed.

Cancer as a Threat to Male Fertility

Sixty-five thousand men of reproductive age (20–44) were diagnosed with cancer in 2009 (www.seer.cancer.gov/statfacts). These men are at significant risk for infertility due to their underlying malignancy and the reproductive toxicities of anti-neoplastic therapy. Concerns about fertility within this population are prevalent. Three-quarters of childless young adults who face a new diagnosis of cancer and 25% of men who already have children consider preservation of the capacity for biological paternity to be a critical quality of life issue [3]. Unfortunately, only 47% of American oncologists routinely refer cancer patients of childbearing age to a reproductive specialist [4].

Timely discussion of fertility preservation is critically important when a young man is diagnosed with cancer. This concept is reflected in statements from both the American Society of Clinical Oncology (ASCO) [5] and the American Society of Reproductive Medicine (ASRM) [5, 6]. The ASCO recommendation dictates that "oncologists discuss at the earliest opportunity the possibility of infertility as a risk of cancer treatment," and that patients interested in fertility preservation should be referred to a fertility specialist as early as possible. The ASCO panel also emphasized that there is no evidence that a history of cancer, cancer therapy, or fertility interventions increase the risk of cancer or congenital malformations in offspring (aside from hereditary genetic syndromes). Guidelines from the ASRM similarly state that "physicians should inform cancer patients about options for fertility preservation and future reproduction prior to treatment." The ASRM panel further stated that concerns regarding the welfare of potential future offspring, including concerns about posthumous parenting, should not impede discussions with cancer patients about options for fertility preservation.

Malignancy as a Risk Factor for Infertility

Cancer itself is associated with infertility, even prior to the initiation of antineoplastic treatment. Although this phenomenon is well-recognized, studies describing the impact of cancer on pretreatment semen analysis parameters are relatively scarce, and some of the data are conflicting. Most of the data suggest that cancer has a significant negative impact on semen quality, which varies according to the cancer diagnosis. In the most contemporary American series to address this issue, Williams and colleagues [7] retrospectively reviewed semen analyses from 409 men who had successfully banked sperm at their institution prior to initiation of cancer treatment [7]. The authors found that men with most types of cancer had pretreatment semen parameters in the National Cooperative Reproductive Medicine Network (NCRMN) fertile range for concentration (mean 47 million sperm per mL) and intermediate range for motility (mean motility score 50%). However, men with testicular cancer had significantly reduced sperm concentrations (mean 33 million sperm per mL, NCRMN intermediate range) compared to men with other malignancies. Moreover, 45% of men with testicular cancer had sperm concentrations in the NCRMN subfertile range (<13.5 million per mL), versus 16% of men with other malignancies and 10% of normal men without cancer who underwent vasectomy. Other studies have found that, in addition to testicular cancer, leukemia and lymphoma are associated with significant reductions in sperm concentrations [8, 9].

It is important to recognize that most studies of pretreatment semen quality in men with cancer have been retrospective and limited by exclusion of men with pretreatment azoospermia. Men with no sperm identified in their ejaculate at the time of sperm banking do not cryopreserve their semen and typically are difficult to retrospectively identify. The limited data that are available suggest that azoospermia affects 10–12% of men of reproductive age with cancer, compared with 1% of the general population. Rates of pretreatment azoospermia seem to vary according to the underlying malignancy, with high rates observed in men with testicular cancer (10–15%) and hematological malignancies (9–13%) and lower rates in other malignancies [8, 10].

Chemotherapy

Regardless of baseline fertility status, cancer treatment places men at increased risk for future infertility. Chemotherapeutic agents have a variable and generally dose-dependent effect on sperm production. Absence of well-designed prospective studies in humans and the common utilization of multi-drug regimens have made it difficult to understand the reproductive sequelae of individual drugs. Various agents, however, can be broadly assigned to risk categories relative to impaired spermatogenesis [5] (Table 3.1).

Alkylating agents cause cellular death by impairing DNA synthesis and RNA transcription. These drugs induce mutations in the rapidly dividing spermatogonial stem cells of the testis and comprise the highest risk group. Patients typically develop severe, and, often permanent, oligozoospermia or azoospermia. Platinum analogs cause DNA crosslink formation and may be equally destructive to spermatogenesis, but 80% of men treated with platinum-based chemotherapy recover some degree of spermatogenesis within 5 years of active treatment. Vinca alkaloids disrupt mitosis by inhibiting microtubule formation. These drugs are associated with significant gonadotoxicity when used in the multi-drug setting, but when used alone cause only a temporary reduction in sperm concentration. Antimetabolites exert anti-neoplastic effects by interfering with DNA synthesis and transcription. In conventional doses, they cause temporary reductions in sperm concentration, but recovery of normal spermatogenesis is the norm. The reproductive sequelae of newer agents, such as monoclonal antibodies, multikinase inhibitors, and taxanes, are not yet known [5, 11].

Radiation Therapy

Radiation therapy (RT) is used to treat many cancers in men of reproductive age, including hematologic malignancies and carcinomas of the testis, penis, prostate, bladder, and rectum. Testicular exposure to RT during treatment for these common malignancies is often significant, despite the use of gonadal shielding. The most common indications for RT in this population are for the retroperitoneal treatment of testicular seminoma; Hodgkins and non-Hodgkins lymphoma; and total body irradiation prior to bone marrow or stem cell transplantation in the setting of advanced hematologic malignancy. Less commonly, men of reproductive age with rectal or prostate carcinoma treated with pelvic RT are exposed to inadvertent testicular irradiation that may be gonadotoxic. In other cases, purposeful testicular RT is delivered for primary testicular processes, such as intratubular germ cell neoplasia. Typical testicular RT exposure in these conditions and the anticipated impact on fertility are summarized in Table 3.2.

The testicular germinal epithelium is exquisitely radiosensitive. Doses as low as 0.1 Gy

Table 3.1 Fertility risk with chemotherapeutic agents

Drug class	Common agents	Common indications	Risk category
Alkylating agents	Ifosfamide	GCT	High risk
	Procarbazine	HL	
	Chlorambucil	NHL	
	Cyclophosphamide	Sarcoma	
	Busulfan carmustine	Glioma	
	Lomustine	Leukemia	
Platinum analogs	Cisplatin	GCT	High risk
		HL	
		NHL	
		Sarcoma	
	Carbolatin		Moderate risk
Vinca alkyloids	Vincristine	HL	Moderate risk
	Vinblastine	NHL	
		Leukemia	
Antimetabolites	Fluorouracil	Colorectal cancer	Moderate risk
	6-Mercaptopurine	Bladder cancer	
	Methotrexate	Leukemia	
	Gemcitabine	HL	
		NHL	
Topoisomerase inhibitors	Etoposide doxorubicin	GCT	Moderate risk
		HL	
		NHL	
		Sarcoma	
		Glioma	
Steroids	Prednisone	HL	Low risk
		NHL	
		Leukemia	
Interferon	Interferon alpha	NHL	Low risk
		Leukemia	
		Kidney cancer	

GCT germ cell tumor, *HL* Hodgkin lymphoma, *NHL* non-Hodgkin lymphoma
Reproductive risks of common chemotherapeutic agents. (adapted from [5])

cause morphological changes in spermatogonia; exposure to 2–3 Gy results in irreversible damage to spermatocytes and an associated sharp decrease in spermatid count; and exposure to greater than 4 Gy typically results in loss of the entire germ cell population. The effects may be transient or irreversible and are typically evident in semen approximately 70 days after RT, which represents the time it takes for sperm to develop and completely transit through the male genital ductal system. From the perspective of semen analysis, oligozoospermia is typically seen with RT doses below 0.8 Gy, transient azoospermia results from 0.8 to 2 Gy, and irreversible azoospermia is a significant risk with doses greater than 2 Gy [11].

Surgery

Cancer surgery may affect fertility in a myriad of ways. It is therefore imperative that surgeons discuss the reproductive implications of surgery with their patients. Men with testicular cancer

Table 3.2 Fertility risk with radiation therapy

Indication for RT	Testicular radiation exposure	Risk category
Intratubular germ cell neoplasia (testicular CIS)	16–20 Gy	High risk
Total body irradiation prior to bone marrow or stem cell transplantation	>6 Gy	High risk
Rectal cancer	0.3–2.1 Gy	Moderate risk
Prostate cancer (external beam radiation therapy)	1.8–2.4 Gy	Moderate risk
Retroperitoneal lymphatic metastases of seminoma	0.3–0.5 Gy	Low risk
Mediastinal or abdominal Hodgkins lymphoma	0.1–0.7 Gy	Low risk

RT radiation therapy, *CIS* carcinoma in situ
Anticipated cumulative radiation exposures and reproductive toxicities of common radiation therapy treatment courses [8, 22, 23]

who undergo retroperitoneal lymphadenectomy (RPLND) are at risk of disruption of the autonomic, sympathetic inputs critical for ejaculation. Though modern nerve sparing techniques have limited the risk substantially, these patients remain at significant risk of postoperative anejaculation or retrograde ejaculation. The autonomic nerves of the pelvis responsible for erection are at risk during extirpative pelvic surgery, such as radical prostatectomy, proctectomy, or cystoprostatectomy. These patients must be counseled about the significant risk of postoperative erectile dysfunction, which threatens their future potential to achieve pregnancy. Furthermore, radical pelvic surgery for the treatment of prostate or bladder cancer includes purposeful and permanent disruption of the male genital ductal system, after which reproduction is only possible with assisted technology.

Acquisition and Cryopreservation of Sperm

For male patients facing a fertility threat, such as impending chemotherapy, an ejaculated semen sample is the preferred method of acquiring sperm for cryopreservation. Ejaculation provides the best quality sperm at the lowest financial cost and avoids invasive procedures. Unfortunately, many patients cannot provide an ejaculated sample because of physical, developmental, or religious reasons. In addition, patients are sometimes able and willing to provide an ejaculated sample, but are found to be azoospermic on microscopic evaluation of the sample. When an ejaculated sample with adequate sperm concentration cannot be obtained, for whatever reason, additional intervention is required to preserve future fertility potential.

Acquisition of Ejaculated Sperm

The vast majority of men and adolescents are able to provide an ejaculated semen sample for cryopreservation. However, these men face a unique set of challenges. The context in which they are asked to provide specimens is fraught with stress. Patients are often facing cancer or other serious medical issues. They, therefore often feel sick, emotionally overwhelmed, are in pain, or are under the influence of narcotics or other medications. They may be hospitalized and, thus, have limited privacy for masturbation. Semen collection is sometimes urgently prescribed prior to starting treatment following a cancer diagnosis and, understandably, patients may be unable to "perform" under severe time pressure. Adolescent boys may never have masturbated or ejaculated. Finally, some of these patients may have religious or personal objections to masturbation that may be difficult or impossible to overcome.

Every attempt should be made to facilitate collection of ejaculated semen. Patients should be provided with a private and relaxing physical environment whenever possible. Sexually stimulating audiovisual materials, such as magazines or videos, should be provided to the patient if appropriate. It is usually important to avoid discussing details of sample collection with adolescent patients in the presence of their families. Separate discussions with the patient and family members help avoid introducing unnecessary embarrassment that might present yet another barrier to successful collection. When applicable, patients should be encouraged to explore religious issues that preclude masturbation with their clergy.

Historically minimal acceptable semen parameters for cryopreservation are no longer applicable in the current era of ICSI. Conception is now possible with only one live sperm, and fertilization and pregnancy rates with ICSI are largely unaffected by semen quality [12]. All samples containing viable sperm, regardless of semen parameters, should therefore be cryopreserved. Collected samples should be microscopically analyzed to determine the concentration, motility, and morphology of sperm prior to cryopreservation. These parameters are useful for determination of the optimal number of semen samples to be banked and may indicate the need for adjunctive techniques during cyropreservation.

Samples are mixed with cryoprotective medium to protect against intracellular and extracellular ice crystal formation that can occur during the cryopreservation freezing process. In samples with poor sperm concentration, motility, or morphology parameters, additional procedures such as swim-up tests or centrifugation help augment concentration and isolate sperm of higher quality. Similar processes are used for sperm acquired via surgical harvesting. Storage facilities typically charge between 50 and several hundred dollars each year for storing samples [13].

The optimal timing of sperm banking is prior to the induction of antineoplastic treatment. As previously discussed, many chemotherapeutic regimens cause immediate and severe impairment of spermatogenesis that may be irreversible. Subsequent invasive attempts at sperm retrieval, such as TESE, are effective in fewer than half of cases in men with post-chemotherapy azoospermia [14]. Furthermore, even in cases when ejaculated or testicular sperm can be acquired, there is theoretical concern that children conceived with sperm that developed during chemotherapy exposure may be at increased risk for congenital anomalies. Though the theoretical risk of congenital anomalies has never been corroborated in humans, chemotherapy does induce genetic defects in sperm. For this reason, no attempts at reproduction or acquisition of sperm should be performed until at least three months following chemotherapy treatment. In practice, most physicians recommend waiting at least six months to a year [15].

Acquisition of Spermatazoa in Azoospermic Patients

Azoospermia is defined as absence of sperm in ejaculated semen and may be due to obstruction (obstructive azoospermia, OA) or testicular failure (nonobstructive azoospermia, NOA). In patients with azoospermia for whom fertility preservation is desired, sperm must be percutaneously or surgically harvested directly from the testis or epididymis. Available procedures for retrieving sperm include microsurgical extraction or percutaneous aspiration of sperm from either the testis or epididymis. Factors to consider in choosing a retrieval technique include the nature of azoospermia (OA versus NOA); surgeon experience and capability; and patient preference.

Patient factors suggestive of OA include a history of prior inguinal hernia surgery; normal size testes and/or non-palpable vasa deferentia on physical examination; and normal serum hormonal profiles. In the normal male, sperm acquire motility and maturity as they transit from the caput to the caudal epididymis. In men with genital ductal obstruction, however, the situation is reversed and the highest quality sperm can be found in the proximal or caudal epididymis.

Retrieval of sperm should thus be directed at the testis or proximal epididymis in these patients. Men with OA are candidates for microsurgical epididymal sperm aspiration (MESA), percutaneous epididymal sperm aspiration (PESA), percutaneous biopsy, testicular fine needle aspiration (TFNA), and testicular sperm extraction (TESE).

MESA is the optimal technique for sperm retrieval in men with OA. MESA is performed as an open surgery with an operating microscope. Direct visualization of the epididymis affords directed puncture of epididymal tubules and micropuncture aspiration typically yields more than 100×10^6 sperm with adequate motility [16]. PESA is an easier procedure to perform, but is less preferable to MESA since it relies on blind targeting of epididymal tissue. Spermatic cord block and local or topical anesthesia is used. Without the benefit of direct visualization or the operating microscope, blood vessels are harder to avoid and bleeding is much harder to control. A 21 gauge butterfly needle is inserted into the caput epididymis and slowly withdrawn until fluid is seen in the tubing.

Sperm may also be retrieved directly from the testis in men with OA. TFNA is the easiest procedure to technically perform, but it yields the lowest number of sperm [17]. Local anesthesia is administered to the scrotal skin, and the spermatic cord is infiltrated with lidocaine. The testis is stabilized between the surgeon's thumb and forefinger, and a small-gauge needle is inserted along the long axis of the testis. The needle is withdrawn slightly and redirected in order to disrupt the testicular architecture. The procedure is repeated until adequate testicular material has been aspirated. Percutaneous biopsy is performed with identical local anesthesia and testicular stabilization, but involves the use of a 15-gauge biopsy gun to obtain cores of testicular tissue rather than a small-gauge needle. Multiple biopsies can be obtained through a single entry site, and this procedure provides higher sperm yield than TFNA.

TESE is an excellent option for sperm acquisition in azoospermia of any etiology, including OA, and is the procedure of choice in men with NOA. NOA should be suspected in azoospermic men with a history of cryptorchidism or gonadotoxin exposure, small soft testicles on physical examination, and elevated serum levels of follicle stimulating hormone (FSH). Although TFNA and percutaneous biopsy are options for retrieval, they are less effective compared to open surgical sperm retrieval and are not recommended in this context.

We advocate performance of TESE with the aid of an operating microscope or loupe magnification, which enables improved visualization of the testicular blood supply and identification of larger, dilated seminiferous tubules that are more likely to contain sperm [18]. The scrotal skin is incised transversely or in the median raphe, and the dartos of the scrotum is divided with cautery. The tunica vaginalis is opened to expose the tunica albuginea of the testis, which is incised in an avascular plane to expose the seminiferous tubules of the testis. The seminiferous tissue is extruded from the testis by gentle compression of the testis. One or multiple biopsies of testicular tissue are sharply excised with scissors and placed in sperm transport medium for subsequent analysis (Fig. 3.1). Hemostasis is obtained with bipolar cautery, and the tunica albuginea is reapproximated with absorbable suture. The procedure may be repeated at multiple sites on one or both testicles to ensure adequate sampling of both

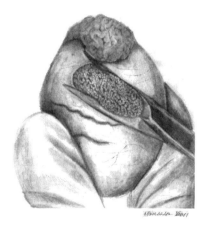

Fig. 3.1 Testicular sperm extraction (TESE) is performed with an open surgical approach with the aid of an operating microscope or loupe magnification. Seminiferous tubular tissue is exposed by incision of the tunica albuginea of the testis and sharply excised

testicles, which is important in cases of NOA in which sperm production may be heterogeneously distributed.

Men with NOA have absolutely minimal reserve of functional germinal epithelium and have a virtually negligible chance for sperm retrieval following chemotherapeutic insult to the gonads. It is particularly important to attempt sperm retrieval in these patients prior to starting chemotherapy. In the largest published series of azoospermic men facing chemotherapy, Schrader and colleagues [19] reported successful retrieval of sperm in 6/14 men with testicular cancer and 8/17 patients with lymphoma. In patients with testicular cancer, radical resection of the tumor-containing testis also provides an opportunity to perform ex vivo sperm retrieval.

Collection of Sperm from Patients Who Cannot Ejaculate

Some young men with cancer who are candidates for fertility preservation may not be able to provide an ejaculated semen sample for sperm banking. This group of patients is diverse and may be broadly divided into men with ejaculatory dysfunction and men who cannot masturbate for social or religious reasons. The cohort of men with ejaculatory dysfunction includes patients with psychogenic anejaculation, spinal cord injuries, peripheral neuropathies, and those who previously underwent retroperitoneal lymphadenectomy for testicular cancer.

Ejaculatory dysfunction may be due to either retrograde ejaculation (RE) or anejaculation. RE is the presumed diagnosis in patients who achieve orgasm without antegrade ejaculation. Initial treatment is pharmacologic induction of antegrade ejaculation with sympathomimetic drugs that increase bladder neck tone during ejaculation. These medications are initiated the night before and the morning of sperm collection. Ephedrine sulfate (25 mg PO BID), imipramine hydrochloride (50 mg PO QD and titrate to 50 mg PO TID), midodin hydrochloride (7.5 mg orally, to max of 20 mg), or pseudoephedrine hydrochloride (90 mg PO QID) have been used successfully in the treatment of RE. If attempts at pharmacologic restoration of antegrade ejaculation are unsuccessful, then sperm may be harvested from the post-ejaculate urine. Alkalinization of urine with 5–10 cc of poly-citra is used with each dose of sympathomimetics [20].

Options for sperm acquisition in anorgasmic patients, anejaculatory patients, and patients who cannot masturbate include penile vibratory stimulation (PVS), EEJ, and surgical sperm retrieval. PVS is minimally invasive and is effective in appropriately selected patients. The frenular surface of the penis is stimulated with a commercially available device, and ejaculation is induced. The procedure may be performed by the physician in his office or by the patient at home. PVS is mediated by a spinal reflex arc that begins with conduction of afferent input from the penis to the sacral spinal cord via the dorsal penile and pudendal nerves. The afferent signal is relayed via spinal interneurons to preganglionic sympathetic nerves that exit the cord at T10-L2. These fibers synapse with postganglionic sympathetic fibers in the paraspinal sympathetic chains, ultimately giving rise to the hypogastric nerves that innervate the ejaculatory apparatus. The reflex arc is subject to inhibitory cortical control, and PVS is, therefore, best suited to patients in whom the reflex arc is intact and in whom cortical inhibition is disrupted, such as patients with spinal cord injury above T10 [20].

EEJ is more invasive than PVS but has the advantage of being effective for anejaculation of any etiology other than complete ejaculatory duct obstruction. The bladder is emptied by urethral catheterization, and a small volume of sperm transport media is injected into the bladder. Ejaculation is induced by direct electric stimulation of the prostate and seminal vesicles, which is delivered with a transrectal probe (Fig. 3.2). Five to 30 volts of energy are delivered cyclically until seminal emission is observed, which may be either pulsatile or occur as a slow drip. Rectal temperature is monitored during the procedure, and peri-procedural anoscopy is performed to confirm that there is no rectal mucosal injury. Urethral catheterization is carried out for collection of any sperm that may have traveled

Fig. 3.2 Electroejaculation (EEJ) is performed by direct stimulation of the prostate and seminal vesicles using a specialized transrectal electrostimulator

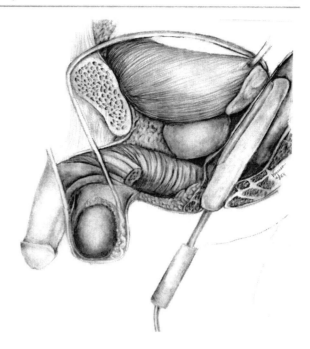

retrograde into the bladder. It is imperative that collected semen is evaluated microscopically at the time of EEJ for the presence of a sufficient number of motile sperm. Inadequate sperm recovery should prompt consideration of immediate TESE, the possibility of which should be discussed and consented preoperatively. In fact, at some centers testicular sperm extraction is preferred over EEJ or PVS for sperm acquisition in patients who cannot ejaculate [20].

Future Directions in Fertility Preservation

As a result of improved diagnostic ability and treatment methodologies in cancer, quality of life issues, such as fertility preservation, are assuming increased importance. It is estimated that more than 75% of males diagnosed with cancer, particularly testis cancer, will have long-term survival. Methods for sperm retrieval in adult males and pubertal boys are identical, although young boys are more likely to have difficulty producing ejaculated semen samples.

Preserving fertility in pre-pubertal boys facing chemotherapy represents an enormously greater challenge, since they do not yet produce functional sperm, and no effective treatment exists. Three strategies are the focus of research and intense interest: autotransplantation of testicular parenchyma, autotransplantation of purified germ cell suspensions, and in vitro maturation of immature germ cells for ICSI [21].

The first approach involves removing testicular tissue prior to chemotherapy and autotransplantation of non-manipulated testicular tissue following treatment. The advantage of this approach is preservation of the microenvironment of spermatagonial stem cells, but reintroduction of occult malignant cells is a major concern. Xenografting of immature testis tissue into immunodeficient mice from non-primate mammals has successfully yielded complete spermatogenesis within the graft, however, suggesting the possibility of sperm retrieval from an animal host to be utilized with ICSI without subjecting the patient to the risk of cancer cells.

Autotransplantation of purified germ cell suspensions, or germ cell transplantation, has been successfully performed in rodent models and non-human primates. The strategy involves retrieving and cryopreserving isolated germ cells before sterilizing treatment for autologous transplantation after the patient recovers. Removing immature germ cells from their usual microenvironment may not prove feasible for fertility but minimizes the risk of reintroduction of malignant cells into the patient.

A final strategy that is being developed involves developing cell-culture systems for spermatogonia. Recent advancements suggest that in vitro spermatogenesis from cryopreserved immature germ cells may be possible in the future [21]. Cryopreservation of immature testicular germ cells or testicular parenchyma should be considered experimental. Although retrieval of testicular tissue is not standard clinical practice, practitioners may consider discussion of the risks and benefits of cryopreservation with prepubertal boys and their parents.

Conclusion

Acquisition of sperm for cryopreservation is feasible in the majority of men with medical conditions that threaten fertility. A major limitation of fertility preservation is lack of patient and physician awareness. Assumptions should never be made about patients' thought processes and desire for future fertility. All patients facing fertility risks deserve a discussion regarding fertility and prompt referral to reproductive specialists when appropriate. Multiple procedures for sperm retrieval are available and can be tailored to individual patients' situations. Preservation of fertility potential remains an elusive goal for prepubertal boys.

Provider Recommendations

1. The presence of cancer may have an impact on semen quality.
2. Cancer treatment impairs spermatogenesis, either temporarily or permanently.
3. Acquisition of sperm for cryopreservation that may be used for future reproduction is the foundation of male fertility preservation.
4. The benefits of sperm banking must be weighed against the medical and financial costs.

5. There are techniques for the acquisition of sperm for banking from males with azoospermia or ejaculatory dysfunction.
6. There are experimental techniques for fertility preservation in prepubertal boys but the effectiveness of these techniques is uncertain.

References

1. Schover LR et al (2002) Oncologists' attitudes and practices regarding banking sperm before cancer treatment. J Clin Oncol 20(7):1890
2. Saito K et al (2005) Sperm cryopreservation before cancer chemotherapy helps in the emotional battle against cancer. Cancer 104(3):521–524
3. Schover LR (2009) Patient attitudes toward fertility preservation. Pediatr Blood Cancer 53(2):281–284
4. Quinn GP et al (2009) Physician referral for fertility preservation in oncology patients: a national study of practice behaviors. J Clin Oncol 27(35):5952
5. Lee SJ et al (2006) American Society of Clinical Oncology recommendations on fertility preservation in cancer patients. J Clin Oncol 24(18):2917
6. (2005) Fertility preservation and reproduction in cancer patients. Fertil Steril 83(6):1622
7. Williams DH et al (2009) Pretreatment semen parameters in men with cancer. J Urol 181(2):736–740
8. Lass A et al (1998) A programme of semen cryopreservation for patients with malignant disease in a tertiary infertility centre: lessons from 8 years' experience. Hum Reprod 13(11):3256
9. Bahadur G et al (2005) Semen quality before and after gonadotoxic treatment. Hum Reprod 20(3):774
10. Ragni G et al (2003) Sperm banking and rate of assisted reproduction treatment: insights from a 15-year cryopreservation program for male cancer patients. Cancer 97(7):1624–1629
11. Brannigan RE (2007) Fertility preservation in adult male cancer patients. Cancer Treatment and Research, 138:28
12. Kuczynski W et al (2001) The outcome of intracytoplasmic injection of fresh and cryopreserved ejaculated spermatozoa–a prospective randomized study. Hum Reprod 16(10):2109
13. Nieschlag E, Behre HM, Nieschlag S (2010) Andrology
14. Chan PTK et al (2001) Testicular sperm extraction combined with intracytoplasmic sperm injection in the treatment of men with persistent azoospermia postchemotherapy. Cancer 92(6):1632–1637
15. Wyrobek AJ, Schmid TE, Marchetti F (2005) Relative susceptibilities of male germ cells to genetic defects induced by cancer chemotherapies. JNCI Cancer Spectrum 2005(34):31
16. Sheynkin YR et al (1998) Controlled comparison of percutaneous and microsurgical sperm retrieval

in men with obstructive azoospermia. Hum Reprod 13(11):3086

17. Friedler S et al (1997) Testicular sperm retrieval by percutaneous fine needle sperm aspiration compared with testicular sperm extraction by open biopsy in men with non-obstructive azoospermia. Hum Reprod 12(7):1488

18. Schlegel PN (1999) Testicular sperm extraction: microdissection improves sperm yield with minimal tissue excision. Hum Reprod 14(1):131

19. Schrader M et al (2003) Onco-tese: Testicular sperm extraction in azoospermic cancer patients before chemotherapy: New guidelines? Urology 61(2): 421–425

20. Ohl DA et al (2009) Anejaculation: an electrifying approach. Semin Reprod Med 27:179–185

21. Wyns C et al (2010) Options for fertility preservation in prepubertal boys. Hum Reprod 16(3):312

22. King CR, Maxim PG, Hsu A, Kapp DS (2009) Incidental testicular irradiation from prostate IMRT: it all adds up. Int J Radiat Oncol Biol Phys 2010 77(2):484–489

23. Manzonakis M, Damilakis J, Varveris H, Gourtsouiannis N (2006) Radiation dose to testes and risk of infertility from radiotherapy for rectal cancer. Oncol Rep 15(3):729–733

Contraception and Cancer Treatment in Young Persons

Valerie Laurence, MD and Christine Rousset-Jablonski, MD

I always thought my patients were too sick to even think about sex. I had a twenty-one year old male patient who was so weak from chemo he had to use a wheelchair. Halfway into his treatment he told me his girlfriend was pregnant and he couldn't understand how. I'd talked to him and his parents about the need to sperm bank and so he thought he didn't need to use protection. It was a difficult situation because he also managed to get chlamydia in the process.
Dr. B, Oncologist

Introduction

Cancer in adolescence and young adulthood is relatively uncommon. However, after a decreasing incidence in early childhood until 9 years of age, it steadily increases through adolescence and young adulthood, with an annual incidence of 203 per million for the 15–19 year-old, 352 per million for the 20–24 year-old and 547 per million for the 25–29 year-old in the United States between 1975 and 2000 [1]. The most frequent cancers in AYAs are Hodgkin's disease, germ cell tumors, leukemia, cancers of the central nervous system, non-Hodgkin's lymphoma, non-rhabdomyosarcoma soft-tissue sarcomas, Ewing's tumors, osteosarcoma, thyroid cancers, and melanomas [1–3]. Survival rates have improved over the past decades with the use of combined surgery, radiation, and dose-intensive combination chemotherapy.

A range of factors influences the degree, nature of fertility defects in children, and adolescents undergoing treatment for cancer including age, tumor site, treatment modality, and sex. The most important study, which investigated 2,283 adult survivors of childhood and adolescent cancer in five centers, showed a relative risk of fertility of 0.93 for females and 0.76 for males [4]. Alkylating agents and subdiaphragmatic radiation were deemed most likely to impair fertility. Cancer therapy may induce amenorrhea, the onset and duration of which depends on the age of the patient, type, intensity and duration of treatments, and premature menopause [4, 5]. Norwegian data showed that in the 10 years after a cancer diagnosis women are about half as likely as women without cancer to become pregnant [6].

Although many AYAs undergoing treatment for cancer remain fertile, in females their window of fertility may be shortened. Adolescence and young adulthood is a time when personal experimentation, development of new relationships, exploring sexual awareness, and sexual activity are essential tasks. Except for the most extremely ill, AYAs with chronic conditions have the same sexual, marital, and romantic aspirations as healthy AYAs. It can be assumed

V. Laurence (✉)
Department of Medical Oncology, Medical Oncologist,
Institut Curie, 75005 Paris, France
e-mail: valerie.laurence@curie.net

G.P. Quinn, S.T. Vadaparampil (eds.), *Reproductive Health and Cancer in Adolescents and Young Adults*, Advances in Experimental Medicine and Biology 732,
DOI 10.1007/978-94-007-2492-1_4, © Springer Science+Business Media B.V. 2012

that for those AYA with normal pubertal development and peer relationships, they will have sexual behaviors similar to their peers [7–9]. Advances in therapeutic modalities for adolescents with cancer (including solid tumors as well as hematological malignancies) means that they can aspire to the same sexual and reproductive health activities as other healthy adolescents and young adults. Furthermore, AYAs with cancer and those who have had cancer face developmental issues in terms of independence and separation from their parents, health concerns, and questions about their fertility potential. These complex issues may encumber their sexual education and their perception of information on sexual health and contraception. Their particular needs as AYAs with cancer, emerging sexual identities and practice have been poorly addressed by health professionals [10].

Given that young people with cancer and those who survived childhood cancer are likely to have the same sexual behavior as their healthy peers, they share with them the same need for effective contraception and information about sex to avoid unwanted pregnancies and prevent sexually transmitted infections (STIs). Many cytotoxic drugs, as well as radiotherapy, are teratogenic and mutagenic and conception during chemotherapy may result in abortion of the embryo, or in gross congenital abnormalities of the fetus, thus emphasizing the need for effective contraception in sexually active young people undergoing treatment for cancer [11].

Recommendations from the World Health Organization (WHO) offer that "in general, adolescents are eligible to use any method of contraception and must have access to a variety of contraceptive choices." Age alone does not constitute a medical reason for denying any method of contraceptives to adolescents. Social and behavioral issues should be important considerations in the choice of contraceptive methods by adolescents. Adolescents, married or unmarried, may be less tolerant of side effects of contraceptives and therefore have high discontinuation rates. Method choice may be influenced by factors such as sporadic patterns of intercourse and the need to conceal sexual activity and contraceptive use.

Expanding the number of method choices offered can lead to improved satisfaction, increased acceptance, and increased prevalence of contraceptive use. Proper education and counseling both before and at the time of method selection can help adolescents address their specific problems and make informed and voluntary decisions. Every effort should be made to prevent service and method costs from limiting the options available [12]. Therefore, contraception for AYAs undergoing cancer treatment raise several medical and educational issues, different from those of cancer survivors [13].

Contraceptive Methods and Their Use in Young People with Cancer

Several contraceptive options are available and can be classified as behavioral methods, nonbarrier methods with estrogen-containing methods and progestin-only methods, barrier methods, intrauterine devices (IUDs), and surgical sterilization (which we will not discussed here). They are summarized in Table 4.1.

Table 4.1 Contraceptive methods

Abstinence
Behavioral method
– No methods
– Withdrawal
– Periodic abstinence
Oral contraception
– Oral combined pill (OCP)
– Progestin-only pill (POP)
– Emergency contraception ("morning-after pill")
– Oral progestogens
Injectable contraceptives (Depo-Provera®)
Implant contraceptives (Norplant®, Jadelle®, Implanon®)
Intra-uterine devices (IUDs)
– Copper IUD
– Levonorgestrel IUS
Barrier methods
– Female barrier methods (diaphragm, cervical cap, vaginal sponge, female condom, vaginal spermicides)
– Male condoms

Behavioral Methods

Abstinence

Abstinence or postponement of sexual activity is the most effective method of preventing pregnancy and STIs [14, 15]. For some AYAs with cancer, abstinence is common, normal, and acceptable. However, abstinence-only programs are not as effective as those in which other contraceptive options are offered at the same time [16].

It should be recognized that AYAs with cancer may have a sense of not having enough time to postpone a sexual relationship with their partner. It is difficult to add the loss of a potential sexual life to the many other restrictions these patients face, and it may be important for a teen or young adult facing death to have experienced a sexually fulfilling relationship before dying [17]. It is therefore difficult to recommend abstinence as a contraceptive method for these very special patients, unless they are strongly motivated and willing to use it.

No Method

It has been reported that as many as 25–50% of sexually active adolescents in the United States do not use contraception at first intercourse. As far as teenagers are concerned, it is far more convenient not to use any method of contraception. However, such an approach to sexual activity leads to a very high risk of acquiring STIs, HIV transmission, and getting pregnant (85% in the first year) [18]. Without clear guidance from health professionals, young women with complex medical history or medical conditions may not feel comfortable asking a health professional for birth control counseling, and therefore may limit themselves to behavioral or barrier methods [19, 20]. Young people with cancer are strongly advised to use an effective method of contraception at all times.

Withdrawal

Withdrawal remains a common method used by AYAs, especially within the first year of becoming sexually active. Effectiveness of withdrawal (or coitus *interruptus*) depends on the man's ability to withdraw the penis before ejaculation. First-year failure rates approach 24–27% with typical use, and there is a risk of STIs and HIV [13, 18]. Although it is a free and convenient method, withdrawal is not recommended as an effective contraceptive method.

Periodic Abstinence

Periodic abstinence relies on abstaining from sexual intercourse during the fertile window during which sexual intercourse can result in pregnancy. This "fertile window" consists of the 5 days before ovulation and the day of ovulation, itself and can be identified by observing changes in cervical secretions, monitoring increases in basal body temperature, or using calendar calculations [21–23]. However, even normal healthy women with usually regular menstrual cycles have highly unpredictable fertile windows based on clinical guidelines, resulting in a typical failure rate as high as 25% within 12 months of initiating use [24, 25]. In addition, these methods do not prevent STIs and HIV. Not only is this an unreliable method for many young women who have irregular cycles, but it is a much more inadvisable contraceptive method for those with cancer, whose cycles may be more irregular with chemotherapy, and who may suffer from febrile infections, thus making basal temperature monitoring impossible.

Non-barrier Methods

Combined Hormonal Contraceptives: Oral Combined Pill (OCP), Vaginal Ring, and Transdermal Patch

The combined oral contraceptive pill (OCP) contains both synthetic estrogens and progestin, and prevents ovulation by inhibiting gonadotropin-releasing hormone. Additionally, progestin-induced changes, such as increased cervical mucus viscosity, endometrial atrophy, and changes in tubal transport mechanism provide secondary contraceptive mechanisms. There are many brands used throughout the world, containing 15, 20, 30, 35 or 50 μg of ethinyl estradiol as the estrogen. A new contraception containing estradiol valerate combined with the progestin dienogest is available in some countries. Estradiol-containing OCP might have less impact on various metabolic and homeostatic parameters than ethynil-estradiol-containing contraception [26, 27]. Several generations of progestins are used: first generation – ethynodiol diacetate, norethindrone acetate, norethindrone; second generation – norgestrel, levonorgestrel; or third generation – desogestrel, norgestimate, gestodene. Several new progestins are designed to minimize side effects related to androgenic, estrogenic, or glucocorticoid receptor interactions. Drospirenone, developed as combination oral pills with ethinyl estradiol. Dienogest has been combined both with ethynil estradiol and, more recently, with estradiol valerate. Nomegestrol acetate has been used as a progestin-only method and more recently combined with estradiol [28]. OCPs containing third generation progestin or new progestins are more expensive and may therefore be more difficult to obtain. OCPs are either monophasics, which contain a constant amount of hormones, or multiphasics (biphasic or triphasics), which vary the amount of progestin, and sometimes estrogen, over the course of a 21-day cycle.

Historically, combined hormonal contraceptives have been packaged and used in a regimen of 21 hormonally active days followed by seven hormone-free days (21/7). In the past several years, there has been increased interest in and use of combined hormonal contraception in extended regimens in which hormones are taken for longer than 21 continuous days and the hormone-free interval either shortened or eliminated. An important indication for using these newer extended regimens is the treatment of menstrual disorders, such as dysmenorrhea, menorrhagia, and endometriosis. The most commonly prescribed extended regimen is 84 continuous hormone days followed by 7 hormone-free days. Many other regimens are used include hormone-free intervals shorter than 7 days and continuous regimens that eliminate the hormone-free interval completely [29].

The OCP is the most widely used contraceptive method with a rate of use approaching 50% in teenagers [16]. OCPs, especially those with low dose estrogen, are effective only if used consistently and correctly. The typical failure rate of OCPs in adults is 3% [30], and in adolescents 5–15% [15, 16]. Adolescents are less compliant than adults, with over half of them stopping the pill during the first year of use [31].

Vaginal ring and transdermal patch are also combined contraceptives. The ring releases continuous low doses of ethinyl estradiol and etonogestrel. The patch is a rectangular (4 × 5 cm) adhesive polyester patch that delivers continuous low doses of ethynilestradiol and norelgestromin. The patch is worn on the arm, thigh, abdomen, torso, or buttocks, changed every week for 3 consecutive weeks, and followed by a patch-free week. Like OCPs, the ring and the patch inhibit ovulation, induce regular scheduled periods, and have a low one-year method failure rate of about 1% [32, 33]. In comparison to OCPs, the ring and the patch offer women greater convenience since they do not require daily administration. With monthly administration, the ring has seemingly superior advantage over the patch. The patch can be concealed with appropriate site selection; however, partners or parents might see the method when clothes are removed. Despite apprehension concerning these two methods regarding vaginal insertion, sexual partner perceptions for the vaginal ring, ease of remembering, visibility issues, and perceived health risk concerning the patch, they have a good acceptability [34]. Overall approval of the ring might even be higher than that of OCPs [35]. However, despite transdermal administration of both hormones, they have the same metabolic and vascular contra-indications as OCPs.

Medical eligibility criteria have been published for the use of contraceptive methods by the WHO [12]. The conditions affecting eligibility for the use of each contraceptive method were classified under one of the following four categories:

1. A condition for which there is no restriction for the use of the contraceptive method.
2. A condition for which advantages of using the method generally outweighs the theoretical or proven risks.

3. A condition for which theoretical or proven risks usually outweigh the advantages of using the method.
4. A condition for which represents an unacceptable health risk if the contraceptive method is used.

The malignancies in which the use of OCPs is absolutely contraindicated is in breast cancer and liver malignant tumors. The WHO medical eligibility criteria apply to AYAs as well. Nevertheless, OCP prescription for young people with cancer involves far more specific issues than the issues common to their healthy peers. For young people receiving chemotherapy and/or radiotherapy, complicating factors include:

Thrombocytopenia

Chemotherapy may induce thrombocytopenia, the nadir, duration, and time of onset of which depends on the drug regimen and protocol, with the critical issue being the control of menstrual flow. Patients with a predictable short course of thrombocytopenia usually do well on cyclic monophasic OCPs. Combined OCP is useful for cycle regulation and inhibition of the growth and development of the endometrium. There is some evidence that OCP significantly reduces mean menstrual blood loss in women with normal periods and those with menorrhagia. On the other hand, the efficacy of OCP in reducing the menstrual loss in women with bleeding disorders has not been well established [36].

For the OCPs provided in 28-day packs, omission of placebo pills will avoid bleeding, and patients may take continuous monophasic pills without bleeding [16]. Extended cycles of combined hormonal contraceptives are now more frequently used in classical daily practice for patients who desire to avoid bleedings on specific events, to have less frequent menses, and to treat common gynecologic conditions like menorrhagia, dysmenorrheal, and endometriosis. The most commonly prescribed extended regimen seems to be 84 continuous hormone days followed by 7 hormone-free days, most often with a monophasic oral contraceptive containing 30 μg of ethinyl estradiol [29]. These extended regimens are usually well tolerated, but may induce breakthrough bleeding and spotting. Instituting a 3-day hormone-free interval is often efficient to control these bleedings [37]. For patients in whom severe and/or prolonged thrombocytopenia can be expected, cyclic OCP use should not be recommended. Continuous monophasic OCPs could be suitable, given good compliance and the absence of gastrointestinal (GI) side effects (cf below).

Gastro-Intestinal Tract Side Effects

Chemotherapy-induced vomiting and mucositis may significantly reduce absorption of OCPs. Changes in bacterial flora may occur following chemotherapy-induced diarrhea. Infection or repeated courses of antibiotics in febrile neutropenic patients may result in changes in gastro-hepatic circulation with decreased effectiveness of OCPs [38]. Vaginal ring and transdermal patch are good options in these situations. For AYAs undergoing highly emetogenic and aggressive chemotherapy with anticipated severe GI side effects, OCPs cannot be recommended. In contrast, vaginal ring and transdermal patch are good options.

Drug Interactions

Cancer patients who frequently receive polypharmacy and OCPs have many known drug interactions. Use of antibiotics is a category 1 condition in the WHO recommendations, with no restrictions for OCPs, except for rifampicin and rifabutin. Antacids (magnesium and aluminium types) block absorption of OCPs and should be avoided for at least 3 h after ingesting the pills. Many analgesics, anticonvulsants, and antifungals interfere with microsomal enzymes, thereby reducing efficacy of OCPs, vaginal ring, and transdermal patch. Equally, OCPs may decrease clearance of benzodiazepines, tricyclic antidepressants, prednisolone, cyclosporin, and other medications. Hence, use of OCPs in these patients requires careful monitoring [12, 15, 39]. OCPs should be avoided in patients with allogenic bone marrow transplant for whom prednisolone and cyclosporins are necessary to prevent graft-versus-host disease and graft reject.

Thrombosis

OCPs, vaginal ring, and transdermal patch are contraindicated in women with deep vein thrombosis or pulmonary embolism [12, 40]. However, young women with a history of thromboembolic events related to known foreign bodies (such as central lines) that have been removed are allowed to take OCPs [39]. In summary, prescription and use of combined hormonal contraceptives in AYAs with cancer should be discussed and assessed on an individual basis, with careful evaluation of specific issues of relevance to each patient.

Progestin-Only Pills (POP)

The POP mini-pill contains no estrogen. Traditional POPs work through secondary contraceptive methods (thick and less penetrable cervical mucus, endometrial involution, and tubal motility changes) without reliable ovulation inhibition (ovulation is inhibited in under 40% of cycles with traditional POPs) [41]. In contrast to traditional POPs, the desogestrel-only pill Cerazette®, consistently inhibits ovulation [41, 42]. It is an acceptable contraceptive option for AYAs if estrogen is contraindicated or not tolerated. Traditional POPs require rigorous compliance with dependence on users to take the pill on a rigid schedule (with need for a back-up method if the pill-taking is more than 3 h late). Ovulation inhibition with desogestrel-only pill is maintained after 12 h delays in tablet intake and return of ovulation takes at least 7 days. These properties distinguish desogestrel-only pill from all other POPs [42]. Although some POPs have been associated with lower contraceptive effectiveness than OCPs, the desogestrel-only POP has shown similar contraceptive effectiveness. The most commonly reported complaints in women using all POPs are bleeding problems

[43]. It should be avoided in patients with a history of ectopic pregnancy, who are poorly compliant, or taking rifampicin, griseofulvin, and certain anticonvulsants (phenytoin, carbamazepine, barbiturates, primidone, topiramate, and oxcarbazepine). POPs raise the same issues in patients undergoing chemotherapy as those already listed for OCP.

The progestogens used on a continuous basis can be used to suppress the uterine endometrium to avoid dysfunctional and breakthrough bleeding in AYAs undergoing chemotherapy for hematological malignancies (for example chlormadinone acetate or nomegestrol daily during all the treatment). Cyclical progestogens are widely used in the treatment of dysfunctional uterine bleeding but are effective only when administered in a 21-day course starting from day 5 of the cycle. In women with a bleeding disorder, progestogen treatment may be useful in high doses alone or in combination with desmopressin or factor concentrate to arrest acute menorrhagia. Cyclical progestogens from day 5–26 of the cycle can be used as a second-line treatment for patients not responding to extended OCPs regimen or when they are contraindicated. Because of their side effects and the long duration of treatment for each cycle, the compliance with this regimen is usually not good [36, 44]. Consequently, POPs should not be recommended as a first choice contraceptive method for AYAs undergoing chemotherapy. However, progestogens might be useful to avoid dysfunctional bleeding in adolescents and young women undergoing chemotherapy.

Emergency Contraception

Hormonal emergency contraception (EC), also called the "morning-after pill," has been available for over 20 years and is a useful backup method when the usual contraceptive methods fail or unplanned and unprotected sexual activity takes place [16, 45]. Different drug regimens are available: (1) the levonorgestrel-only EC (Levonorgestrel 1.5 mg as a single dose or two tablets of levonorgestrel 750 μg, administered 12 h apart within 72 h of unprotected intercourse). The WHO trial established levonorgestrel-only EC as the gold standard in hormonal emergency contraception [46] and more than 80 countries have now approved this regimen. Levonorgestrel has no medical contraindications, except current ongoing pregnancy [39, 47]. (2) A new emergency contraception using a Selective Progesterone Receptor Modulator has recently emerged. A single dose of 30 mg Ulipristal acetate provides women and health care providers with an effective alternative for EC that can be used up to 5 days after unprotected sexual intercourse [48]. This new EC is already available in some countries by prescription only (i.e., in France, Ella-One®). (3) The combination regimen of progestin–estrogen (dubbed as the Yuzpe regimen), consisting of two doses of 100 μg of ethinyl estradiol and 0.50 mg of levonorgestrel taken approximately 12 h apart, is now rarely used.

Availability of hormonal EC is variable around the world. In France, the levonorgestrel-only EC is available for sale for women aged less than 18 years at pharmacies and can be given by nurses freely in schools. In the United States, EC is available from a pharmacist without a prescription for women eighteen years or older. For girls under 18, EC is available exclusively by prescription in most states, but some states have made it available by pharmacists without prescription (Hawaii, Alaska, California, Massachusetts, New Hampshire, New Mexico, Vermont, and Washington). Young girls are capable of using EC correctly and safely. Access to EC is not associated with increased rates of unprotected intercourse, with compromised contraceptive or sexual behavior, or with higher rates of pregnancy or STIs [49, 50]. Thus, restricting access to EC clinics seems unreasonable [50].

Since AYAs with cancer run the same risk of unplanned and unwanted pregnancy as healthy ones, discussion of EC should be part of counseling to increase awareness of this method.

The copper intrauterine device (IUD) is a highly effective form of EC with treatment failure rates at less than 1%. It can be inserted up to 5 days after the earliest estimated date of ovulation (i.e., up to day 19 in a woman with a 28-day cycle) [51].

The high risk of STIs in this age group, as well as the risk of thrombocytopenia and neutropenia in young patients undergoing treatment for cancer, renders it unsuitable as an emergency contraceptive method.

Injectable Contraceptives: Depo-Provera

Depot medroxyprogesterone acetate (DMPA, Depo-Provera®) is the most widely used injectable method, is very effective, reversible, and does not interfere with sexual intercourse. It provides contraceptive efficacy for 12 weeks without the need for daily compliance. When given at a dose of 150 mg by deep intramuscular injection every 12 weeks, studies have shown failure rates ranging from 0 to 0.7 pregnancies per 100 women years [52]. Its mechanisms of action include persistent suppression of ovulation and ovarian production of oestradiol, through inhibition of the secretion of gonadotrophins, as well as alteration of the yield, composition, and physical characteristics of cervical mucus. It induces the formation of a thin and quiescent endometrium with decreased glandular activity. These effects are collectively responsible for the high level of clinical efficacy. The most common side effect is menstrual irregularities and most users eventually become amenorrhoeic. Amenorrhea occurs in 8% of women after their first injection and in 45% during 10–12 months of use [53]. However, despite its efficacy and acceptability, the use of Depo-Provera® raises two major concerns in young women with cancer. Firstly, in patients undergoing chemotherapy with the potential for thrombocytopenia and neutropenia, a deep intramuscular injection in the deltoid or the gluteal muscle may be a source of hematoma formation and/or infection. The other area of concern is the potential decrease of bone density with prolonged use of DMPA [54–58] and the potential increase of fracture risk [59]. Adolescence is a crucial time for bone growth, with bone mass accumulating rapidly, with most of the bone mass in the spine and hip being accumulated by the age of 18 years [60]. It has been recommended that DMPA should be avoided in teenagers at risk for osteoporosis such as those with chronic renal failure

[15]. Furthermore, it has been shown that children and adolescents undergoing chemotherapy have an increased risk of bone mineral density loss [61, 62]. Lastly, DMPA offers no protection against STIs. It would therefore seem prudent to avoid the use of Depo-Provera® in adolescent girls undergoing chemotherapy.

Implant Contraceptives: Norplant®, Jadelle® (levonorgestrel), Implanon® (Etonegestrel)

Norplant I® was the first implantable contraceptive for women to be developed made of six silastic rods containing levonorgestrel; it provides effective contraception for 5 years. Previously commonly used in the AYAs because of the long-term contraception provided and a high 12-month continuation rate, the difficulty in removing the six rods limited the use of this method [16], and it was withdrawn from the market in many countries. The Jadelle® implant (Norplant II) consists of two silastic rods containing levonorgestrel. Implanon® is made of one rod of vinyl ethylene acetate polymer with etonegestrel and provides effective contraception for 3 years, with an easy insertion and removal. These implants provide reversible contraception and need to be placed subdermally, usually in the upper arm [63, 64]. They do not provide any protection against STIs and HIV transmission. Side effects include irregular menstrual bleeding, amenorrhea, weight gain, headaches, and mood changes. Menstrual irregularities are common and may deter young women from using this method or result in a request for removal after insertion [65]. This method is convenient and relatively popular with AYAs in that it sidesteps the issue of compliance, it is reliable (failure rate of 0.2 pregnancies per 100 woman-years), and works for a long time. However, this method may create difficulties for young women mostly because of the cost, fear of the subcutaneous insertion, side effects of menstrual irregularities, acne, and weight gain [55, 66–68]. Patient satisfaction with implants varies and is most directly related to the quality of pre-insertion counseling. Little is known regarding the long-term side effects of Implanon® in teenagers.

For patients undergoing chemotherapy and expecting severe and/or prolonged thrombocytopenia, there is an issue with irregular menstrual bleeding induced by implants. Furthermore, subdermal insertion of a contraceptive device is an invasive procedure contraindicated in potentially thrombocytopenic patients. Data are lacking about the tolerance and potential sepsis in immunocompromised patients. It is not recommended to initiate the use of contraceptive implants in young women undergoing chemotherapy. The situation might be different for newly diagnosed patients already using an implant and in whom chemotherapy regimen induces a short and moderate thrombocytopenia. In such cases, removal of the implant might not be necessary, especially if such patients chose to use implants because of failure or side effects of other contraceptive methods.

Common Contraindications to Hormonal Contraception in AYAs with Cancer

The only absolute contraindication for the use of hormonal contraceptives in female cancer patients is the presence or suspicion of breast cancer and malignant liver tumors. The use of OCPs, vaginal ring, transdermal patch, POPs, progestogens, Depo Provera®, and progestin subdermal implants falls under category 4 of the WHO medical eligibility criteria [12, 69]. Breast cancer is rare, but not unknown in very young women. 1% of breast carcinomas occur between 20 and 29 years [70] whilst invasive breast cancer accounts for 0.5% in 15–19 years olds and 4.1% in 20–24 years olds of all female cancers [2].

Ovarian tumors rank fourth amongst female cancers in the age group between 15 and 24 years, although subtypes change with age: germ-cell tumors are the most frequently occurring among 15–19 years olds whilst "non-germ cell" cancers account for 70% of ovarian tumors amongst 20–24 years old [2]. Although extensive surgery with bilateral oophorectomy and hysterectomy is part of the strategy for treatment of ovarian epithelial cancer, conservative unilateral oophorectomy can be discussed in early stage I disease as well as for all germ cell tumors in young women where conservation of fertility is desired. Estrogen (ER) and progestogen receptors (PR) have been described in ovarian epithelial cancer tissue, with 67% of tumors positive for ER and 47% positive for PR: however, data regarding the potential role of receptor status in ovarian cancer as a predictor of activity of hormonal therapy is inconclusive [71]. No evidence exists regarding the effects of OCPs on recurrence rates in women with conservative treatment for ovarian epithelial cancer. However, it is probably safer to use contraceptive methods other than OCPs and long-acting progestogens in young women who have undergone conservative surgery for non germ-cell tumors when the hormonal receptor status is unknown. Although there have been concerns regarding the use of OCPs in melanoma patients, they do not appear to be contraindicated in these patients [72].

Intrauterine Devices

The IUDs, used by millions of women all over the world, are very effective contraceptive methods. Copper IUDs have failure rates of less than one per 100 women years. The intrauterine system releasing 20 μg of levonorgestrel daily (LNG-IUS) is as efficient as the copper IUDs with >250 mm^2 copper surface area. Traditionally, IUDs were not recommended as first choice contraceptive methods for adolescents [15, 18, 31, 69]. Higher rates of expulsion and removals due to bleeding and pain have been described in nulliparous women [73]. Some evidence suggests IUD size and shape play a role in performance. However, all existing copper IUDs are suitable and are now widely used in nulliparous women. They are interesting alternatives in case of contraindication to hormonal contraceptives. In case of thrombocytemia induced by chemotherapy, copper IUDs should be avoided given the risk of menorraghia and heavy bleeding. The LNG-IUS is approved as treatment for heavy menstrual bleeding in more than 80 countries [51], and could be an option in these cases. Data on their use in women with bleeding disorders or receiving anticoagulant therapy suggests that LNG-IUS is a viable and safe option for the management of

menorrhagia in these women [74]. Acceptability is high in nulliparous women when compared either to parous LNG-IUS users or to nulliparous users of combined oral contraceptive pills [75].

Undoubtedly, copper IUD use is associated with an increased incidence of dysmenorrhoea and menorrhagia as well as pelvic inflammatory disease in women exposed to sexually transmitted pathogens. The presence of an LNG-IUS does not increase the risk of pelvic inflammatory disease in either parous or nulliparous women and it may be protective against infection [75]. Young women often participate in "serial monogamy," or have multiple partners, putting them at increased risk of STIs. The presence of cervical ectropion, common during adolescence, also predisposes AYAs to acquisition of STIs [31]. Thus, copper IUDs or LNG-IUS can be used, with caution, in AYAs.

The LNG-IUS falls under category 4 of the WHO medical eligibility criteria in case of breast cancer in the last 5 years [12]. Given adequate and appropriate counseling, STI screening, and medical care, the copper IUDs can provide effective long-term contraception for adolescents. However, the risk of neutropenia and thrombocytopenia in AYA cancer patients undergoing chemotherapy strongly suggest avoidance of this method. In case of heavy bleeding due to thrombocytemia. LNG-IUS can be an alternative.

Barrier Methods

Female Barrier Methods (Diaphragm, Cervical/Vault Cap, Vaginal Contraceptive Sponge, Female Condom, Vaginal Spermicides)
Diaphragms and Cervical Caps
Diaphragms are shallow, flexible, thin latex or silicone rubber hemispheres reinforced by a flexible flat or coiled metal spring, available in a variety of sizes, which are placed high in the vagina to cover the cervix. They are used with spermicidal jelly or cream, can be inserted at any time convenient before sexual intercourse, and must be left in place for at least 6 h after intercourse. Additional spermicidal jelly or cream must be inserted if

intercourse takes place more than 3 h after insertion of the device and for each repeat coital act. First-year probability of failure is 13–17% for typical use and 4–8% for perfect use [76]. They require proper fitting by a knowledgeable health professional, who must initially perform a pelvic examination to fit the device, a situation not many adolescents would be willing to tolerate. Besides, many adolescents may be unwilling or unable to deal intimately with their own bodies or prepare so carefully for each act of sexual intercourse [15]. Of notable importance (although without an evidence base) in these patients is the need for a change in size of the diaphragm if there is change of more than 3 kg in weight. However, for highly motivated AYAs with cancer, this can be an effective method.

The cervical cap is a thimble-shaped dome of rubber that is used with spermicides and applied over the cervix. Cervical cap also needs proper fitting by clinicians, and fitting the cap to the cervix is more difficult than fitting a diaphragm. It can be inserted immediately before or up to 30 min before intercourse and must remain in place at least 8 h before removal, but may be left in place for up to 48 h. Subsequent coital acts require additional spermicidal jelly or pessary to be added to the vaginal side of the cap. Its insertion and removal tends to be more difficult than for the diaphragm while failure rates are similar [15, 18, 69, 77].

Cervical cap and diaphragm usage increases the risk of toxic shock syndrome, urinary tract infection, bacterial vaginosis, and vaginal candidiasis. They reduce STIs in varying ranges (50–100% for trichomonas, gonorrhoea, and Chlamydia), but their role in preventing HIV infection is not clear [78].

Vaginal Sponge

This is a sustained-release spermicidal system which absorbs semen and prohibits entrance of sperm through the cervical ostium. It is generally available over the counter, can be inserted anytime up to 24 h before intercourse, and has a contraceptive action lasting 24 h. Some studies indicate that sponges are less effective than condoms or diaphragms [79]. First-year probabilities of failure are 17% for typical use and 11–12% for perfect use [76]. While in nulliparous women the first-year failure rate may be similar to that of the diaphragm, failure rates seem to be higher in parous women (19–21% versus 9–10% in nulliparous women) [76, 80]. As for diaphragm and cervical caps, AYAs need to be given detailed instructions on sponge use. Development of toxic shock syndrome is not a concern as the nonoxynol-9 contained in the sponge is known to reduce staphylococcal replication and toxin production. While sponges may reduce STI concern has been expressed about the possibility of enhancing HIV transmission because of vaginal mucosal injury [81].

Female Condom

Polyurethane female condom is a soft sheath which is fitted into the vagina before coitus. It is pre-lubricated on its inside with silicone and has two rings, the internal one at the closed end which covers the cervix and the external one at the open end which partially covers the perineum [82]. It is poorly utilized due to difficulty with insertion, discomfort, and suboptimal functional performance during intercourse. Latex female condom has been introduced as an updated version using synthetic latex for greater affordability. It has been developed in an effort to overcome these obstacles [83]. It has a thin, pliable plastic pouch that conforms to the shape of the vagina, and has a flexible soft outer ring that is intended to protect the external genitalia. Contraceptive failure rates for polyurethane female condom range from 15 to 21%, and tends to result from user failure [82]. The US FDA approved female condom in 1993 as the first barrier contraceptive for women that offered protection against STIs. Indeed, this condom may offer a significant protection from STIs [84, 85].

Female condoms have some disadvantages: it is costly, aesthetically displeasing, and associated with a high rate of problems such as misdirection of the penis during intercourse and slippage of the condom [82]. Latex female condom seems to lead to less failure, to have fewer adverse events, and to be more acceptable than the polyurethane one. However, discontinuation rates are high [86].

Non-prescription Spermicides

Spermicides are valuable adjuncts to the pregnancy and STI-preventive functions of condoms, diaphragms, and caps, and do not need to be prescribed by a health professional. They are widely available (foam, cream, jelly, film, suppository or tablet) and may be used alone or with diaphragms, cervical caps, sponges, or condoms. Typical failure rates in the first year of use range between 21 and 30% [87, 88]. They have to be inserted 10–30 min before intercourse, and reliable protection lasts 1 h. However, leakage from the vagina is inevitable and this common problem of "messiness" described by users as well as vulval, penile, or vaginal irritation resulting from the detergent action on cell membranes makes their use less acceptable. Some recent spermicides also have a microbicide effect or may reinforce normal vaginal acidity to inactivate both sperm and acid-sensitive sexually transmitted pathogens [89–91]. Their efficacy is comparable to that of a common spermicide with diaphragm [91]. Female barrier methods have not received a widespread acceptance by AYAs: they are coital-related methods, interfere with the spontaneity of sex, and young women describe preparation and insertion as messy and inconvenient. Used alone, they have a questionable efficacy in STI prevention and can not be relied upon as an effective method of birth control. Furthermore, the concerns about the increased risk of toxic shock syndrome, urinary tract infection, lower genital tract infection, and the high failure rate suggest that they should not be recommended in potentially immunosuppressed AYAs with cancer.

Male Barrier Methods (Condoms)

Male condoms are non-prescription, single-use contraceptives that serve as a mechanical barrier to sperm, bacteria, and viruses. Classical condoms are made of latex. Non-latex male condoms made of polyurethane film or synthetic elastomers (polyisoprene) were developed in the early 1990s as alternative male barrier methods for individuals with allergies, sensitivities, or preferences that prevented the consistent use of condoms made of latex. For the user, it decreases

infection acquired through exposure to viral and bacterial agents from cervical, vaginal, vulval or rectal secretions or lesions. For partners of condom users, contact with seminal fluid, infectious urethral discharge, or penile shaft or glans penis infectious lesions are prevented. However, transmission of infectious agents from lesions on the areas of the skin not covered by the male condom is still possible, although latex condoms have been shown to prevent the transmission of a whole range of pathogens [92]. Improved education about condoms and fear of STIs, especially HIV, has led to an increased utilization of condoms by AYAs over the past decade. The failure rate for the condom is highest in the first years of use (cumulative failure rate of 7.8% within the first 2 years of use and 4.5% within the next 3 years (third to fifth year of use) [93]. Women aged less than 30 are at higher risk of condom failure, when compared with women age 30 and older (relative risk (95%CI) = 1.55 (1.11–2.16) [25]. There is a large gap between the probabilities of failure with typical use (17% during the first 12 months) and perfect use (2%), underlining the importance of education about condom use [25, 94]. Condom failure may result from inconsistent use or from incorrect use, with the consequence in condom slippage or breakage. Breakage rates during vaginal intercourse in developed countries range from 0 to 6.7%. Although the nonlatex condoms (polyurethane or synthetic elastomers) are associated with higher rates of clinical breakage, these new condoms still provide an acceptable alternative for those with allergies, sensitivities, or preferences that might prevent the consistent use of latex condoms. No difference in terms of pregnancy rates (typical use efficacy) between polyurethane, synthetic isomers, and their latex counterparts was found [95].

Condoms do not require parental or healthcare professional involvement and allow confidentiality for adolescents. They are readily accessible (from shops or from a machine), cost-effective, and portable, and allow male participation in contraceptive planning. However, for maximum efficacy, adolescents need to be instructed in the correct and consistent use of condoms. There is no medical contraindication to the use of male condoms. They prevent STIs and potential HPV transmission, avoid contact with seminal fluid and vaginal secretions, and are effective if properly used. They may be recommended for use to AYAs with cancer after adequate instructions in their use.

Advantages of Barrier Methods
Avoiding Exposure to Cytotoxics in Genital Secretions

During chemotherapy, one might expect cytotoxic drugs to be excreted in vaginal secretions or seminal fluid of the patient. In rats, cyclophosphamide penetrates the male reproductive tract and can be transmitted to the female partner and affect progeny [96]. The occurrence of vulvovaginitis has been reported in the wife of a patient with Hodgkin's disease and treated with vinblastine, occurring if sexual intercourse happened during the first three or four days after patient taking vinblastine, and prevented by the use of condom [97]. We are not aware of any studies of levels of cytotoxic drugs in human prostatic secretions, seminal fluid, or vaginal secretions. However, considering these two reports, the use of barrier methods, especially male condoms, need to be discussed before commencement of cytotoxic treatment to avoid contact with seminal fluid or vaginal secretion.

Preventing Transmission of Sexually Transmitted Infections

The occurrence of rapidly changing relationships amongst adolescents, the high probability of multiple sequential sexual partners, and to some extent their greater physiological susceptibility leads to an increased risk of acquiring STIs. Occurrence of bacterial STIs can have serious implications in potentially neutropenic patients.

The most common STI in young women is human papilloma virus (HPV) infection, with a prevalence of approximately 30–50% in sexually active young women [98], and a cumulative incidence during the 3 years following first intercourse of approximately 50% [99]. The frequency of infection persistency is positively correlated with age, and HPV infections are more likely to be transient in AYAs than in older women [100]. However, adolescents who have persistent infection with "high-risk" HPV types have an increased risk of developing high-grade squamous intraepithelial lesions (SIL) [98, 101, 102]. HPV infection may be asymptomatic or have a wide clinical spectrum from benign to precancerous lesions. The clinical sequelae of HPV-infections are linked with the type of HPV. Low-risk types are usually associated with anogenital condylomata and high-risk types with low-grade or high-grade intraepithelial lesions and invasive anogenital cancers. Adolescents are more vulnerable biologically to HPV infections, with postulated mechanisms including inadequate production of cervical mucus, relatively large area of cervical ectopy, increased sensitivity to minor traumas during sexual intercourse, and incompletely developed immune response [98].

It has been well-established that women who have undergone renal, liver, or lung transplantation with chronic immunosuppression are at increased risk for HPV-related genital and oral disease, including cancer [103–105]. Cell-mediated immunity plays a central role in HPV infection control, and this risk for HPV disease in chronically immunosuppressed women are thought to be due to prolonged persistence of virus due to impaired clearance of the immune system [106–108]. Children and adolescents undergoing hematopoietic stem cell transplant (HCST) experience extreme immunosuppression as a result of pretransplant conditioning. Although most patients will have complete immune reconstitution by 2 years post-transplant, the duration and severity of immunodeficiency depends on several factors including type of the stem cells and their pre-transplant manipulation, graft vs. host disease (GVHD), and the age of the transplant recipient. This delay in immune recovery increases the likelihood of infectious complications from bacteria, fungi, and viruses, such as HPV [109]. Women who underwent bone marrow transplant are at significantly increased risk for cervical dysplasia and second cancers, including cervical cancers [110].

Female cancer patients treated with therapies toxic to mucosal surfaces, such as anthracyclines and radiotherapy, may be more prone to HPV infection simply on the basis of impaired genital tract epithelial cell function, as well as survivors with chronic GVHD involving the genital tract mucosa. Women who have received pelvic irradiation are significantly more likely to experience HPV-related cervical and vaginal dysplasia, and carcinomas of the genital tract [111, 112].

Both quadrivalent and bivalent vaccines are highly effective in preventing persistent infection with high-risk HPV-16 and -18 types, and in preventing HPV cervical cancer precursor lesions [113, 114]. Routine HPV vaccination is currently recommended by the Advisory Committee on Immunization Practices for adolescent girls aged 11 and 12 years. Recent data showed a vaccination coverage among adolescents aged 13–17 years in 2009 of 44.3% for 1 dose or more, and 26.7% for 3 doses, widely variable among states, and a good acceptance of adolescent girls parents [115].

Although the immunogenicity of the HPV vaccine has not yet been established among immunocompromised individuals, the Children's Oncology Group's Long-Term Follow-Up Guidelines for Survivors of Childhood, Adolescent and Young Adult Cancer Version 3.0, has recommended HPV vaccination for all eligible females surviving childhood cancer [116].

HPV vaccination must not prevent male condom use. Given that HPV is transmissible through non-penetrative sexual contact with both male and female partners and that imperfect condom use does occur, protection by condom against HPV transmission is not as high as for other STIs. However, there is an inverse and temporal association between the frequency of condom use by male partners and the risk of HPV infection in young women. Women whose partners use condoms for all instances of vaginal intercourse are significantly less likely to acquire HPV than are women whose partners used condoms less than 5% of the time [117]. Condom use offers similar protection against both high-risk and low-risk types of HPV [117]. Male condom use has to be promoted in AYAs undergoing chemotherapy, as it is the most protective method against bacterial and viral pathogens, and the only

protection against HIV. The dilemma associated with condom use is its poorer rate of contraceptive efficacy compared with other methods. Ideally, to protect these patients against pregnancy and STIs, dual protection would be the best option, i.e., condom plus another method with a lower failure rate for pregnancy. An alternative approach would be condom use with the ability to use emergency contraception in the event of condom accident.

Education and Information for Staff and Parents

Fertility is a major concern to AYA with cancer as well as AYA survivors of childhood cancer and their families. It is now openly discussed between patients, families, oncology teams, and assisted-conception units. However, the prevalence of infertility is far less than 50% in cancer survivors, whilst teenage pregnancy is a not an unusual problem, especially in the United States [4]. Most of the time, adolescent patients and their families do get the "risk of infertility" message provided by the health providers. However, they are not aware that, if the AYA is sexually active, he/she is more likely to need protection against pregnancy, as well as against STIs. Furthermore, young cancer patients may not take note of the sexual education provided by school, community centers, or any other sources, due to the belief that they do not need it.

A multitude of medical and psychosocial factors has to be taken into consideration when choosing a contraceptive method for an AYA cancer patient during or following cancer treatment. Each decision has to be made on an individual basis, in partnership with the young person.

How practice can be improved to share the information about sexual health and contraceptive issues with these patients is a pertinent and very important topic. No literature is available on this specific topic in this population and it should be noted that the organization of healthcare and the family planning services vary from country to country with different socio-cultural backgrounds. Nevertheless, some suggestions can be made:

Table 4.2 Advantages/disadvantages and recommendations of the different contraceptive methods in AYAs with cancer

Methods	Advantages	Disadvantages	Recommendations
No method	Convenient, free	No STIs/HIV prevention No pregnancy prevention	Not to be recommended
Abstinence	Best form of pregnancy and STIs prevention, free, no medical CI	Patients with life-threatening conditions not willing to miss a sexual life	Difficult to recommend
Withdrawal	Free, convenient	No STIs/HIV prevention High failure rates	Not to be recommended
Periodic abstinence	Free	No STIs/HIV prevention Inadequate during adolescence	Not to be recommended
OCPs	Low failure rates Most used contraceptive method in teenagers Involving physician and education No breakthrough bleeding if continuous in potentially thrombocytopenic patients	No STIs/HIV prevention Poor compliance in teenagers girls Issues of thrombocytopenia, nausea/vomiting, mucositis, drug interactions	To be discussed on individual basis Ideally combined with male condoms
Progestin-only pill	Suitable if estrogen CI	Same issues as OCP Needs rigorous compliance Increased failure rates	Not to be recommended
Progestogens	Useful to avoid dysfunctional bleeding	No STIs/HIV prevention Poor compliance in teenagers girls	Not to be recommended as a first choice contraceptive method
Hormonal emergency contraception ("morning-after pill")	Post coital method Solution if unprotected or unwanted intercourse	No STIs/HIV prevention Cost Not same easy access in each country	To be discussed as part of the counselling
Injectable contraceptives (Depo-Provera®)	Highly effective No problems of compliance	No STIs/HIV prevention Intramuscular injection in potentially thrombocytopenic and neutropenic patients Decrease in bone mineral density	Not to be recommended if chemotherapy
Subdermal implants	Highly effective Long lasting (3–5 years), reversible No problems of compliance	No STIs/HIV prevention Irregular bleedings in potentially thrombo-cytopenic patients Insertion and foreign body in immunocompromised patients	Not to be recommended if chemotherapy To discuss removal or not if already inserted at time of diagnosis
Copper intra-uterine device	Very effective	No STIs/HIV prevention Unsuitable for adolescent girls Unsuitable for thrombocytopenic and immunocompromised patients	Not to be recommended

Table 4.2 (continued)

Methods	Advantages	Disadvantages	Recommendations
Levonorgestrel intra-uterine device	Very effective Useful to avoid dysfunctional bleeding	No STIs/HIV prevention Unsuitable for adolescent girls Unsuitable for immunocompromised patients	Not to be recommended
Female barrier methods	No medical CI Spermicides/sponges/ female condoms easily available	STIs/HIV prevention uncertain High failures rates Teenagers not prepared to deal so intimately with their own bodies	Not to be recommended
Male condom	Easily available No medical CI STIs/HIV prevention Protection against exposure to seminal/vaginal secretions	Poorer rate of contraceptive efficacy in teenagers	Recommended +/- spermicides Ideally, dual method (condom + another method)

CI Contraindication, OCP Oral combined pill, STIs Sexually transmitted infections

- Provision of adequate and relevant information on specific issues to the staff taking care of these patients.
- Establishment of close working relationships within a multidisciplinary setting between AYA oncology and family planning services staff.
- Provision of practical information about family planning clinics (address, timetables, phone number, web site if available), as well as the leaflets used in family planning clinics about contraceptive methods, sexual health, and STIs, available in the oncology units and out patients clinics taking care of these patients. This can be difficult and has to be discussed in an environment where the units and clinics are shared by children and adolescents, parents of young adolescents can be reluctant to discuss such topics openly, and older adolescents and young adults may have long-term partners, or even children.
- These issues need to be kept in mind when dealing with AYAs who need to be made aware of the staff's willingness to discuss the issues with them whilst respecting their need for confidentiality. Inclusion of parents/guardians in such discussions has to be determined on an individual basis in conjunction with the adolescent. It may be pertinent to remind staff that in many countries, contraception can be given to young persons under 18 without parents/guardians being informed.

Contraception guidance may need to be provided at different times of the patient's cancer journey. Even if there is no need for effective contraception at the time of diagnosis, this may change as the situation improves or after treatment. AYA cancer patients may become sexually active in the months following completion of therapies and professionals have to be aware of these changes in the follow-up clinics. An additional problem may be determining the duration of medical contraindication of pregnancy. This decision depends mainly on the cancer prognosis and the risk of relapse. It is an individual decision to be discussed with the patient in case of pregnancy desire. No specific guidelines are available [11, 118].

Provider Recommendations

1. Contraceptive issues need to be highlighted with AYAs with cancer. This demands awareness and education of oncology teams, and collaboration with family planning units.
2. Multiple issues must be considered when choosing a contraceptive method for AYA cancer patients.

3. Table 4.2 summarizes the advantages and disadvantages of each method in these patients. Decisions should be made on the basis of the age of the patient, disease, type of treatment, and specific requirements of the individual.

4. Along with respect for confidentiality and a non judgemental approach, the cornerstones of the discussion process should include education about sexual health, STIs, and pregnancy prevention.

5. Use of the male condom is strongly recommended as it is the best protection against viral (especially HPV) and bacterial pathogens, the only protection against HIV, and a protection against seminal and vaginal secretions which potentially contain cytotoxic drugs.

6. Dual method with condom plus another method with a better contraceptive effect would be ideal and should be discussed whenever medically possible.

References

1. Bleyer A, Viny A, Barr R (2006) Cancer in 15- to 29-year-olds by primary site. Oncologist 11(6):590–601

2. Wu XC, Chen VW, Steele B, Roffers S, Klotz JB, Correa CN, Carozza SE (2003) Cancer incidence in adolescents and young adults in the United States, 1992–1997. J Adolesc Health 32(6): 405–415

3. Chapter: Smith MA, Gloecler-Ries LA (2002) Childhood cancer: incidence, survival and mortality. In: Pizzo PA, Poplack DG (eds) Principles and practice of pediatric oncology. Williams and Wilkins, Philadelphia, Lippincot pp 1–12.

4. Byrne J, Mulvihill JJ, Myers MH, Connelly RR, Naughton MD, Krauss MR, Steinhorn SC, Hassinger DD, Austin DF, Bragg K et al (1987) Effects of treatment on fertility in long-term survivors of childhood or adolescent cancer. N Engl J Med 317(21):1315–1321

5. Wallace WH, Anderson RA, Irvine DS (2005) Fertility preservation for young patients with cancer: who is at risk and what can be offered? Lancet Oncol 6(4):209–218

6. Cvancarova M, Samuelsen SO, Magelssen H, Fossa SD (2009) Reproduction rates after cancer treatment: experience from the Norwegian radium hospital. J Clin Oncol 27(3):334–343

7. Coupey SM, Alderman EM (1992) Sexual behavior and related health care for adolescents with chronic medical illness. Adolesc Med 3(2):317–330

8. Suris JC, Resnick MD, Cassuto N, Blum RW (1996) Sexual behavior of adolescents with chronic disease and disability. J Adolesc Health 19(2):124–131

9. Blum RW (1997) Sexual health contraceptive needs of adolescents with chronic conditions. Arch Pediatr Adolesc Med 151(3):290–297

10. Morgan S, Davies S, Palmer S, Plaster M (2010) Sex, drugs, and rock 'n' roll: caring for adolescents and young adults with cancer. J Clin Oncol 28(32):4825–4830

11. Gbolade BA (2000) Teenage pregnancy rates and the age and sex of general practitioners. Record linkage analysis could have been used. BMJ 321(7257):381–382; author reply 382–383

12. World Health Organization (2009) Improving access to quality care in family planning: medical eligibility criteria for contraceptive use, 4th edn. WHO, Geneva, Switzerland

13. Schwarz EB, Hess R, Trussell J (2009) Contraception for cancer survivors. J Gen Intern Med 24(Suppl 2):S401–S406

14. Jemmott JB 3rd, Jemmott LS, Fong GT (1998) Abstinence and safer sex HIV risk-reduction interventions for African American adolescents: a randomized controlled trial. JAMA 279(19): 1529–1536

15. Greydanus DE, Patel DR, Rimsza ME (2001) Contraception in the adolescent: an update. Pediatrics 107(3):562–573

16. Lara-Torre E (2009) Update in adolescent contraception. Obstet Gynecol Clin North Am 36(1): 119–128

17. Grinyer A (2002) Sexuality and fertility: confronting the "taboo". In: Clarke D (ed) Cancer in young adults: through parent's eyes. Open University Press, Buckingham-Philadelphia, pp 61–75

18. Rieder J, Coupey SM (1999) The use of nonhormonal methods of contraception in adolescents. Pediatr Clin North Am 46(4):671–694

19. Schwarz EB, Sobota M, Charron-Prochownik D (2010) Perceived access to contraception among adolescents with diabetes: barriers to preventing pregnancy complications. Diab Educ 36(3): 489–494

20. Schwarz EB, Manzi S (2008) Risk of unintended pregnancy among women with systemic lupus erythematosus. Arthritis Rheum 59(6):863–866

21. Wilcox AJ, Weinberg CR, Baird DD (1995) Timing of sexual intercourse in relation to ovulation. Effects on the probability of conception, survival of the pregnancy, and sex of the baby. N Engl J Med 333(23):1517–1521

22. Dunson DB, Baird DD, Wilcox AJ, Weinberg CR (1999) Day-specific probabilities of clinical pregnancy based on two studies with imperfect measures of ovulation. Hum Reprod 14(7): 1835–1839

23. Wilcox AJ, Weinberg CR, Baird DD (1998) Postovulatory ageing of the human oocyte and embryo failure. Hum Reprod 13(2):394–397

24. Wilcox AJ, Dunson D, Baird DD (2000) The timing of the "fertile window" in the menstrual cycle: day specific estimates from a prospective study. BMJ 321(7271):1259–1262

25. Kost K, Singh S, Vaughan B, Trussell J, Bankole A (2008) Estimates of contraceptive failure from the 2002 National Survey of Family Growth. Contraception 77(1):10–21

26. Fruzzetti F, Bitzer J (2010) Review of clinical experience with estradiol in combined oral contraceptives. Contraception 81(1):8–15

27. Palacios S, Wildt L, Parke S, Machlitt A, Romer T, Bitzer J (2010) Efficacy and safety of a novel oral contraceptive based on oestradiol (oestradiol valerate/dienogest): a Phase III trial. Eur J Obstet Gynecol Reprod Biol 149(1):57–62

28. Sitruk-Ware R, Nath A (2010) The use of newer progestins for contraception. Contraception 82(5): 410–417

29. Gerschultz KL, Sucato GS, Hennon TR, Murray PJ, Gold MA (2007) Extended cycling of combined hormonal contraceptives in adolescents: physician views and prescribing practices. J Adolesc Health 40(2):151–157

30. Trussell J, Hatcher RA, Cates W Jr, Stewart FH, Kost K (1990) Contraceptive failure in the United States: an update. Stud Fam Plann 21(1):51–54

31. Brooks TL, Shrier LA (1999) An update on contraception for adolescents. Adolesc Med 10(2): 211–219, v

32. Szarewski A (2002) High acceptability and satisfaction with NuvaRing use. Eur J Contracept Reprod Health Care 7(Suppl 2):31–36; discussion 37–39

33. Audet MC, Moreau M, Koltun WD, Waldbaum AS, Shangold G, Fisher AC, Creasy GW (2001) Evaluation of contraceptive efficacy and cycle control of a transdermal contraceptive patch vs an oral contraceptive: a randomized controlled trial. JAMA 285(18):2347–2354

34. Raine TR, Epstein LB, Harper CC, Brown BA, Boyer CB (2009) Attitudes toward the vaginal ring and transdermal patch among adolescents and young women. J Adolesc Health 45(3):262–267

35. Stewart FH, Brown BA, Raine TR, Weitz TA, Harper CC (2007) Adolescent and young women's experience with the vaginal ring and oral contraceptive pills. J Pediatr Adolesc Gynecol 20(6):345–351

36. Kouides PA, Kadir RA (2007) Menorrhagia associated with laboratory abnormalities of hemostasis: epidemiological, diagnostic and therapeutic aspects. J Thromb Haemost 5(Suppl 1):175–182

37. Coffee AL, Sulak PJ, Kuehl TJ (2007) Long-term assessment of symptomatology and satisfaction of an extended oral contraceptive regimen. Contraception 75(6):444–449

38. Owens K, Honebrink A (1999) Gynecologic care of medically complicated adolescents. Pediatr Clin North Am 46(3):631–642, ix.

39. Gold MA (1999) Prescribing and managing oral contraceptive pills and emergency contraception for adolescents. Pediatr Clin North Am 46(4): 695–718

40. Cole JA, Norman H, Doherty M, Walker AM (2007) Venous thromboembolism, myocardial infarction, and stroke among transdermal contraceptive system users. Obstet Gynecol 109(2 Pt 1):339–346

41. Rice CF, Killick SR, Dieben T, Coelingh Bennink H (1999) A comparison of the inhibition of ovulation achieved by desogestrel 75 micrograms and levonorgestrel 30 micrograms daily. Hum Reprod 14(4):982–985

42. Korver T, Klipping C, Heger-Mahn D, Duijkers I, van Osta G, Dieben T (2005) Maintenance of ovulation inhibition with the 75-microg desogestrel-only contraceptive pill (Cerazette) after scheduled 12-h delays in tablet intake. Contraception 71(1):8–13

43. de Melo NR (2010) Estrogen-free oral hormonal contraception: benefits of the progestin-only pill. Womens Health (Lond Engl) 6(5):721–735

44. Plu-Bureau G, Horellou MH (2008) Therapeutic management of menometrorrhagia in hemostasis disorders. J Gynecol Obstet Biol Reprod (Paris) 37(Suppl 8):S365–367

45. Ottesen S, Narring F, Renteria SC, Michaud PA (2002) Emergency contraception among teenagers in Switzerland: a cross-sectional survey on the sexuality of 16- to 20-year-olds. J Adolesc Health 31(1):101–110

46. Task Force of Postovulatory Methods of Fertility Regulation (1998) Randomised controlled trial of levonorgestrel versus the Yuzpe regimen of combined oral contraceptives for emergency contraception. Task Force on Postovulatory Methods of Fertility Regulation. Lancet 352(9126):428–433

47. Hewitt G, Cromer B (2000) Update on adolescent contraception. Obstet Gynecol Clin North Am 27(1):143–162

48. Glasier AF, Cameron ST, Fine PM, Logan SJ, Casale W, Van Horn J, Sogor L, Blithe DL, Scherrer B, Mathe H et al (2010) Ulipristal acetate versus levonorgestrel for emergency contraception: a randomised non-inferiority trial and meta-analysis. Lancet 375(9714):555–562

49. Haynes KA (2007) An update on emergency contraception use in adolescents. J Pediatr Nurs 22(3):186–195

50. Raine TR, Harper CC, Rocca CH, Fischer R, Padian N, Klausner JD, Darney PD (2005) Direct access to emergency contraception through pharmacies and effect on unintended pregnancy and STIs: a randomized controlled trial. JAMA 293(1):54–62

51. Grimes DA, Lopez LM, Manion C, Schulz KF (2007) Cochrane systematic reviews of IUD trials: lessons learned. Contraception 75(6 Suppl):S55–59

52. Lande RF (1995). New era for injectables. Population Reports, Series K, No. 5. Baltimore, Johns Hopkins School of Public Health, Population Information Program, August

53. Belsey EM (1988) Vaginal bleeding patterns among women using one natural and eight hormonal methods of contraception. Contraception 38(2):181–206

54. Scholes D, Lacroix AZ, Ott SM, Ichikawa LE, Barlow WE (1999) Bone mineral density in women using depot medroxyprogesterone acetate for contraception. Obstet Gynecol 93(2):233–238

55. Cromer BA, Blair JM, Mahan JD, Zibners L, Naumovski Z (1996) A prospective comparison of bone density in adolescent girls receiving depot medroxyprogesterone acetate (Depo-Provera), levonorgestrel (Norplant), or oral contraceptives. J Pediatr 129(5):671–676

56. Harel Z, Cromer B (1999) The use of long-acting contraceptives in adolescents. Pediatr Clin North Am 46(4):719–732

57. Busen NH, Britt RB, Rianon N (2003) Bone mineral density in a cohort of adolescent women using depot medroxyprogesterone acetate for one to two years. J Adolesc Health 32(4):257–259

58. Lara-Torre E, Edwards CP, Perlman S, Hertweck SP (2004) Bone mineral density in adolescent females using depot medroxyprogesterone acetate. J Pediatr Adolesc Gynecol 17(1):17–21

59. Meier C, Brauchli YB, Jick SS, Kraenzlin ME, Meier CR (2010) Use of depot medroxyprogesterone acetate and fracture risk. J Clin Endocrinol Metab 95(11):4909–4916

60. Matkovic V, Jelic T, Wardlaw GM, Ilich JZ, Goel PK, Wright JK, Andon MB, Smith KT, Heaney RP (1994) Timing of peak bone mass in Caucasian females and its implication for the prevention of osteoporosis. Inference from a cross-sectional model. J Clin Invest 93(2):799–808

61. Leiper AD (1998) Osteoporosis in survivors of childhood malignancy. Eur J Cancer 34(6):770–772

62. Arikoski P, Komulainen J, Riikonen P, Parviainen M, Jurvelin JS, Voutilainen R, Kroger H (1999) Impaired development of bone mineral density during chemotherapy: a prospective analysis of 46 children newly diagnosed with cancer. J Bone Miner Res 14(12):2002–2009

63. Meirik O (2002) Implantable contraceptives for women. Contraception 65(1):1–2

64. Glasier A (2002) Implantable contraceptives for women: effectiveness, discontinuation rates, return of fertility, and outcome of pregnancies. Contraception 65(1):29–37

65. Blumenthal PD, Gemzell-Danielsson K, Marintcheva-Petrova M (2008) Tolerability and clinical safety of Implanon. Eur J Contracept Reprod Health Care 13(Suppl 1):29–36

66. Berenson AB, Wiemann CM (1995) Use of levonorgestrel implants versus oral contraceptives in adolescence: a case-control study. Am J Obstet Gynecol 172(4 Pt 1):1128–1135; discussion 1135–1127

67. Weisman CS, Plichta SB, Tirado DE, Dana KH (1993) Comparison of contraceptive implant adopters and pill users in a family planning clinic in Baltimore. Fam Plann Perspect 25(5):224–226

68. Ammerman SD (1995) The use of Norplant and Depo Provera in adolescents. J Adolesc Health 16(5):343–346

69. Cullins VE, Huggins GR (2000). Adolescent contraception and abortion. In: Koehler-Carpenter SE, Rock JA (eds) Pediatric and adolescent oncology. Williams and Wilkins, Philadelphia, Lippincott, pp 364–392

70. Kothari AS, Beechey-Newman N, D'Arrigo C, Hanby AM, Ryder K, Hamed H, Fentiman IS (2002) Breast carcinoma in women age 25 years or less. Cancer 94(3):606–614

71. Perez-Gracia JL, Carrasco EM (2002) Tamoxifen therapy for ovarian cancer in the adjuvant and advanced settings: systematic review of the literature and implications for future research. Gynecol Oncol 84(2):201–209

72. Osterlind A, Tucker MA, Stone BJ, Jensen OM (1988) The Danish case-control study of cutaneous malignant melanoma. III. Hormonal and reproductive factors in women. Int J Cancer 42(6):821–824

73. Hubacher D (2007) Copper intrauterine device use by nulliparous women: review of side effects. Contraception 75(6 Suppl):S8–11

74. Kadir RA, Chi C (2007) Levonorgestrel intrauterine system: bleeding disorders and anticoagulant therapy. Contraception 75(6 Suppl):S123–129

75. Prager S, Darney PD (2007) The levonorgestrel intrauterine system in nulliparous women. Contraception 75(6 Suppl):S12–15

76. Trussell J, Strickler J, Vaughan B (1993) Contraceptive efficacy of the diaphragm, the sponge and the cervical cap. Fam Plann Perspect 25(3):100–105, 135.

77. Mauck CK, Weiner DH, Creinin MD, Archer DF, Schwartz JL, Pymar HC, Ballagh SA, Henry DM, Callahan MM (2006) FemCap with removal strap: ease of removal, safety and acceptability. Contraception 73(1):59–64

78. Rosenberg MJ, Gollub EL (1992) Commentary: methods women can use that may prevent sexually transmitted disease, including HIV. Am J Public Health 82(11):1473–1478

79. Edelman DA, McIntyre SL, Harper J (1984) A comparative trial of the today contraceptive sponge and diaphragm. Am J Obstet Gynecol 150(7):869–876

80. McIntyre SL, Higgins JE (1986) Parity and use-effectiveness with the contraceptive sponge. Am J Obstet Gynecol 155(4):796–801

81. Daly CC, Helling-Giese GE, Mati JK, Hunter DJ (1994) Contraceptive methods and the transmission of HIV: implications for family planning. Genitourin Med 70(2):110–117

82. Bounds W, Guillebaud J, Newman GB (1992) Female condom (Femidom): a clinical study of its use-effectiveness and patient acceptability. Br J Fam Plann 18:36–41

83. Smit J, Beksinska M, Vijayakumar G, Mabude Z (2006) Short-term acceptability of the Reality polyurethane female condom and a synthetic latex prototype: a randomized crossover trial among South African women. Contraception 73(4): 394–398

84. Minnis AM, Padian NS (2005) Effectiveness of female controlled barrier methods in preventing sexually transmitted infections and HIV: current evidence and future research directions. Sex Transm Infect 81(3):193–200

85. Vijayakumar G, Mabude Z, Smit J, Beksinska M, Lurie M (2006) A review of female-condom effectiveness: patterns of use and impact on protected sex acts and STI incidence. Int J STD AIDS 17(10):652–659

86. Pinter B (2002) Continuation and compliance of contraceptive use. Eur J Contracept Reprod Health Care 7(3):178–183

87. Raymond E, Dominik R (1999) Contraceptive effectiveness of two spermicides: a randomized trial. Obstet Gynecol 93(6):896–903

88. Fu H, Darroch JE, Haas T, Ranjit N (1999) Contraceptive failure rates: new estimates from the 1995 National Survey of Family Growth. Fam Plann Perspect 31(2):56–63

89. Schwartz JL, Mauck C, Lai JJ, Creinin MD, Brache V, Ballagh SA, Weiner DH, Hillier SL, Fichorova RN, Callahan M (2006) Fourteen-day safety and acceptability study of 6% cellulose sulfate gel: a randomized double-blind Phase I safety study. Contraception 74(2):133–140

90. Ballagh SA, Brache V, Mauck C, Callahan MM, Cochon L, Wheeless A, Moench TR (2008) A Phase I study of the functional performance, safety and acceptability of the BufferGel Duet. Contraception 77(2):130–137

91. Barnhart KT, Rosenberg MJ, MacKay HT, Blithe DL, Higgins J, Walsh T, Wan L, Thomas M, Creinin MD, Westhoff C et al (2007) Contraceptive efficacy of a novel spermicidal microbicide used with a diaphragm: a randomized controlled trial. Obstet Gynecol 110(3):577–586

92. Centers for Disease Control and Prevention (1988) Condoms for prevention of sexually transmitted diseases. MMWR Morb Mortal Wkly Rep 37(9): 133–137

93. Moreau C, Trussell J, Rodriguez G, Bajos N, Bouyer J (2007) Contraceptive failure rates in France: results from a population-based survey. Hum Reprod 22(9):2422–2427

94. Trussell J (2004) Contraceptive efficacy. In: Hatcher RA et al (eds) Contraceptive technology, 18th revised edn. Ardent Media, New York.

95. Gallo MF, Grimes DA, Lopez LM, Schulz KF (2006) Non-latex versus latex male condoms for contraception. Cochrane Database Syst Rev (1):CD003550

96. Hales BF, Smith S, Robaire B (1986) Cyclophosphamide in the seminal fluid of treated males: transmission to females by mating and effect on pregnancy outcome. Toxicol Appl Pharmacol 84(3):423–430

97. Paladine WJ, Cunningham TJ, Donavan MA, Dumper CW (1975) Letter: Possible sensitivity to vinblastine in prostatic or seminal fluid. N Engl J Med 292(1):52

98. Kahn JA (2001) An update on human papillomavirus infection and Papanicolaou smears in adolescents. Curr Opin Pediatr 13(4):303–309

99. Winer RL, Hughes JP, Feng Q, O'Reilly S, Kiviat NB, Koutsky LA (2009) Comparison of incident cervical and vulvar/vaginal human papillomavirus infections in newly sexually active young women. J Infect Dis 199(6):815–818

100. Castle PE, Schiffman M, Herrero R, Hildesheim A, Rodriguez AC, Bratti MC, Sherman ME, Wacholder S, Tarone R, Burk RD (2005) A prospective study of age trends in cervical human papillomavirus acquisition and persistence in Guanacaste, Costa Rica. J Infect Dis 191(11):1808–1816

101. Moscicki AB (1999) Human papillomavirus infection in adolescents. Pediatr Clin North Am 46(4):783–807

102. Woodman CB, Collins S, Winter H, Bailey A, Ellis J, Prior P, Yates M, Rollason TP, Young LS (2001) Natural history of cervical human papillomavirus infection in young women: a longitudinal cohort study. Lancet 357(9271):1831–1836

103. Malouf MA, Hopkins PM, Singleton L, Chhajed PN, Plit ML, Glanville AR (2004) Sexual health issues after lung transplantation: importance of cervical screening. J Heart Lung Transplant 23(7):894–897

104. Rose B, Wilkins D, Li W, Tran N, Thompson C, Cossart Y, McGeechan K, O'Brien C, Eris J (2006) Human papillomavirus in the oral cavity of patients with and without renal transplantation. Transplantation 82(4):570–573

105. Courtney AE, Leonard N, O'Neill CJ, McNamee PT, Maxwell AP (2009) The uptake of cervical cancer screening by renal transplant recipients. Nephrol Dial Transplant 24(2):647–652

106. Bouwes Bavinck JN, Berkhout RJ (1997) HPV infections and immunosuppression. Clin Dermatol 15(3):427–437

107. Volkow P, Rubi S, Lizano M, Carrillo A, Vilar-Compte D, Garcia-Carranca A, Sotelo R, Garcia B, Sierra-Madero J, Mohar A (2001) High prevalence of oncogenic human papillomavirus in the genital tract of women with human immunodeficiency virus. Gynecol Oncol 82(1):27–31

108. Sun XW, Kuhn L, Ellerbrock TV, Chiasson MA, Bush TJ, Wright TC Jr (1997) Human papillomavirus infection in women infected with the human immunodeficiency virus. N Engl J Med 337(19):1343–1349

109. Bunin N, DiDomenico C, Guzikowski V (2005) Hematopoietic stem cell transplantation. In: Schwartz CL, Hobbie WL, Constine LS, Ruccione

KS (eds) Survivors of childhood and adolescent cancer. Springer, Berlin, Heidelberg, pp 271–282

110. Sasadeusz J, Kelly H, Szer J, Schwarer AP, Mitchell H, Grigg A (2001) Abnormal cervical cytology in bone marrow transplant recipients. Bone Marrow Transplant 28(4):393–397

111. Fujimura M, Ostrow RS, Okagaki T (1991) Implication of human papillomavirus in postirradiation dysplasia. Cancer 68(10):2181–2185

112. Barzon L, Pizzighella S, Corti L, Mengoli C, Palu G (2002) Vaginal dysplastic lesions in women with hysterectomy and receiving radiotherapy are linked to high-risk human papillomavirus. J Med Virol 67(3):401–405

113. Ault KA (2007) Effect of prophylactic human papillomavirus L1 virus-like-particle vaccine on risk of cervical intraepithelial neoplasia grade 2, grade 3, and adenocarcinoma in situ: a combined analysis of four randomised clinical trials. Lancet 369(9576):1861–1868

114. Paavonen J, Jenkins D, Bosch FX, Naud P, Salmeron J, Wheeler CM, Chow SN, Apter DL, Kitchener HC, Castellsague X et al (2007) Efficacy of a prophylactic adjuvanted bivalent L1 virus-like-particle vaccine against infection with human papillomavirus types 16 and 18 in young women: an interim analysis of a phase III double-blind, randomised controlled trial. Lancet 369(9580):2161–2170

115. Centers for Disease and Control Prevention (2009) National, state, and local area vaccination coverage among adolescents aged 13–17 years—United States. MMWR Morb Mortal Wkly Rep 59(32):1018–1023

116. Klosky JL, Gamble HL, Spunt SL, Randolph ME, Green DM, Hudson MM (2009) Human papillomavirus vaccination in survivors of childhood cancer. Cancer 115(24):5627–5636

117. Winer RL, Hughes JP, Feng Q, O'Reilly S, Kiviat NB, Holmes KK, Koutsky LA (2006) Condom use and the risk of genital human papillomavirus infection in young women. N Engl J Med 354(25):2645–2654

118. Killick S (ed) (2000) Contraception in practice. Martin Dunitz Ltd, London, pp 19–28

Sexual Health During Cancer Treatment

5

Linda U. Krebs, PhD, RN, AOCN, FAAN

Heather is a 26 year old single, grade school teacher diagnosed 4 months ago with Stage II breast cancer in her right breast. Initially she was treated with a lumpectomy and sentinel lymph node biopsy with 2 lymph nodes positive for cancer. She began chemotherapy 1 month following her surgery. When she completes this therapy, she will receive radiation therapy to the affected breast and then it is recommended that she take Tamoxifen for 5 years to decrease her risk for recurrence. She was provided with information about the fertility effects related to her treatment, but still hopes to have a family once all treatment is completed. Heather has had several relationships, but is currently not seeing anyone. She is thinking about the prospects of dating again, but is concerned about how she will tell someone that she has had breast cancer or that she may not be able to have children. She has heard that women who have been treated for breast cancer have lots of problems with sexual activity and that she may never be able to find a partner. She is very concerned and wonders what to do.
Heather, Adult Cancer Patient

Introduction

Managing the sexual health of cancer patients has become an increasingly important component of providing comprehensive cancer care. Young adults, those from late adolescence to age 29–39, depending on the author and definition, remain a unique challenge as sexual health is intertwined with the critical developmental tasks of gaining sense of self and one's personal identity, forming healthy intimate relationships, and accomplishing important milestones in the transition from child to mature adult. Unfortunately, much of what is known about this population is gleaned primarily from survivors of childhood cancer [1]. The majority of publications related to the impact of cancer treatment on sexuality and sexual health in young adults generally include adolescents and primarily identify issues and concerns related to fertility and reproduction and providing information on appropriate current management methods. Less is known about strategies to manage the impact of cancer on forming appropriate peer and intimate relationships, managing school and/or early careers, handling a changing body image and associated alterations in changes to self image, becoming independent or maintaining previously gained independence, and developing healthy and safe sexual practices, while dealing with the rigors of cancer treatment. Healthcare providers play an important role in assisting young adults with

L.U. Krebs (✉)
University of Colorado Denver, College of Nursing
Campus, Aurora, CO 80045, USA
e-mail: linda.krebs@ucdenver.edu

G.P. Quinn, S.T. Vadaparampil (eds.), *Reproductive Health and Cancer in Adolescents and Young Adults*, Advances in Experimental Medicine and Biology 732,
DOI 10.1007/978-94-007-2492-1_5, © Springer Science+Business Media B.V. 2012

these concerns through appropriate sexual health assessment, education, counseling, and management [2–6].

Sexual Health and Sexuality

Numerous authors including the World Health Organization have provided definitions of sexuality and sexual health [7–14]. The majority focus on the physical aspects of sexual function/dysfunction and/or fertility and reproduction. These definitions may include a recognition of alterations in body image and sense of sexual self, but few encompass the broader aspects of sexual health that include intimacy, communication, forming and maintaining relationships, and how one views him/herself as a sexual being.

Cleary, Hegarty, and McCarthy suggest a neo-theoretical framework of sexuality that provides a holistic approach to sexual health [15]. Dimensions of the framework include Sexual Self-Concept, Sexual Functioning, and Sexual Relationships, each of which impacts the other dimensions. Sexual Self-Concept includes sexual self-esteem (how one sees him/herself as a sexual partner), body image (how we view ourselves/our bodies and believe others view them) and sexual self-schema (how we see ourselves as sexual beings), while sexual relationships include both intimacy and communication [10]. Sexual Functioning includes the sexual response cycle throughout which numerous alterations in sexual function occur in those diagnosed and treated with cancer. While not tested in young adults, these dimensions have been identified by young cancer survivors as crucial aspects of their survivorship [16].

Tindle, Kelly, and Lilley provide their personal thoughts on the overall impact of cancer on young adults through moving testimonies of being a young adult grappling with a cancer diagnosis and treatment [16]. Through their stories, they share common themes on having and surviving cancer, including: (1) Who am I other than a person with cancer or a number on a chart, (2) Will I ever be attractive to anyone, including

myself, (3) Can anyone ever love me and all of my health issues and cancer baggage, (4) How do I integrate myself back into the world where my peers and life have passed me by and move on with my life? and (5) How do I live with the fact that I may have a recurrence, need further treatment or die? Each provides different experiences including those of having and leaving relationships, separating from parents and going home, and learning to live with altered body images, questions of fertility, and concerns about intimacy, relationships, and sexual function. They note that "an experience of cancer in young adults irrevocably diverts the trajectory of normal identity formation" (p. 281) and as such, affect all aspects of life transitions and maturation including sexual health [16]. This is particularly true as the young adult faces the rigors of cancer treatment, a time filled with uncertainty, discomfort, and grief over a life forever changed.

Impact of Cancer and Cancer Treatment on Sexual Health

Normal Gonadal Function

The pituitary and the hypothalamus regulate gonadal function through secretion of three main hormones: gonadotropin-releasing hormone (GnRH), luteinizing hormone (LH), and follicle-stimulating hormone (FSH); LH and FSH stimulate the testes and ovaries to release the appropriate hormones that allow for sperm and ovum maturation. In the testes, LH stimulates the Leydig cells to produce testosterone while FSH stimulates the Sertoli cells to convert spermatids into sperm. In the ovaries and in conjunction with estrogen and progesterone, FSH is responsible for ovum maturation while LH is necessary for ovulation. When blood levels are sufficient, a negative feedback mechanism is exerted that causes cessation of glandular secretion of these hormones. Any change in hormone production can affect gonadal function which in turn may have a physiological effect on fertility, reproduction, and sexual function [10, 17, 18].

Cancer Treatment Modalities

Mercadante, Vitrano, and Cataia noted that sexual health in those with cancer may be altered by physical, psychological, emotional, and sociocultural issues, including alterations in body image, the ability to give and receive pleasure, changes in roles and relationships, and emotional reactions such as fear, anxiety, and grief [11]. Cancer treatments can affect any or all of these dimensions directly or through short or long-term sequelae of treatment and/or treatment-related side effects [19].

Surgery

The effects of surgery are dependent upon surgical site and structures removed or damaged as a result of surgery. Removal of reproductive organs causes permanent sterility, while damage to nerves, removal of lymph nodes, and postoperative recovery may cause temporary effects, some of which may become permanent over time. Additionally, surgery to body parts associated with sexuality (such as the breast) may alter intimacy, body image, sense of self, and sexual identity while removal of a limb or surgery to the gastrointestinal or genitourinary tract may affect physical function as well as causing associated psychosexual effects [10, 11].

Testicular Cancer

Testicular cancer is relatively common in young men and treatment can have an effect on sexual function and fertility. Current treatment includes orchiectomy and retroperitoneal lymph node dissection (RPLND). If a pelvic mass is present it will be removed. Surgery is generally followed by chemotherapy or radiation therapy. If the orchiectomy is unilateral, previous fertility status should be unchanged and, for the majority, there should be no changes in sexual function, provided the contra-lateral testis is normal. However, infertility before the onset of treatment is well documented and may be a cause of long-term infertility or sterility [20]. With bilateral orchiectomy, decreased libido and sterility will result. Staging or treatment generally includes a RPLND causing temporary or permanent loss of ejaculation or, less frequently, retrograde ejaculation. The ability to have an erection and reach orgasm remains [9, 21]. Nerve-sparing RPLND is associated with preservation of ejaculatory function and fertility and should be undertaken whenever possible [9]. Sexual side effects of RPLND have included decreased libido and arousal and an altered sense of pleasure and intensity of orgasm; if treated solely with unilateral orchiectomy, erectile dysfunction is rare [9, 22, 23]. Discussions about potential alterations in sexual function and fertility are crucial for all patients, but particularly for young adults who may be just beginning sexual relationships and have not yet started or completed their families. Prior to therapy, sperm banking should be discussed and whenever possible, the process completed prior to the onset of therapy [22].

Gynecologic Malignancies

The most common gynecologic cancers seen in young women are cervical and ovarian cancers. Although the surgical treatments are generally invisible to the public, patients experience alterations in sexual identity, self-esteem, femininity, and sexual function. Most surgeries permanently alter fertility and may result in sexual dysfunction. Common alterations in sexual function following gynecologic surgery include: decreased desire, vaginal atrophy and dryness, hot flashes, and other symptoms associated with early menopause and dyspareunia. In some, there is total cessation of all sexual activities. Additionally, emotional responses to loss of fertility and decreased sense of femininity are common. Discussing potential sexual and reproductive alterations prior to surgery is essential and referral to conception specialists may be undertaken to evaluate fertility and childbearing options [9, 24–28].

Cervical Cancer

Multiple surgical and non-surgical procedures are available for treatment of cervical intraepithelial neoplasia and carcinoma in situ. These include laser therapy, cryosurgery, conization, loop electrosurgical excision (LEEP), or simple hysterectomy [29]. While conization may result in cervical incompetence or stenosis, only simple hysterectomy affects future childbearing; none of the surgeries used for non-invasive disease should cause physiological sexual dysfunction although psychoemotional side effects are common [9, 29]. In order to maintain fertility, radical trachelectomy and pelvic lymphadenectomy may be used for early-stage disease [29]. Common side effects of trachelectomy may impact sexual function and include vaginal scarring, dyspareunia, and menstruation difficulties. Sub-fertility is possible, but not common. Neo-cervical stenosis is more common and can be managed by cervical dilation [30].

Invasive disease is usually treated with radical hysterectomy, with or without bilateral salpingo-oophorectomy. Physiologically, sexual side effects are not common if treatment is solely radical hysterectomy. However, following salpingo-oophorectomy, early onset of menopausal symptoms with hot flashes and decreases in vaginal elasticity and lubrication will occur, and may severely affect sexual functioning [31]. Additionally, lack of energy, depression, anxiety, weight gain, and extreme fatigue have been reported in 50% of patients with early-stage cervical cancer, while 10–20% of women complain of dyspareunia and a significant decrease in their sexual relationships and frequency of intercourse [32–34]. Of particular concern to young women are alterations in fertility often before initial child bearing has occurred or families have been completed. When fertility is altered prior to a long term relationship, additional concerns of what information should be disclosed and the optimal timing for disclosure are added to normal grief over loss of fertility and alterations to one's sense of femininity by the inability to bear children.

Ovarian Cancer

Initial management of ovarian cancer is surgery, usually a radical hysterectomy, bilateral salpingo-oophorectomy, and omentectomy. Alterations in body image and sexual self esteem are common, menopausal symptoms occur, and fertility is lost [35, 36]. Fertility in the young woman with a borderline malignant epithelial neoplasia or ovarian teratoma may be maintained if disease is of low grade and confined to one ovary; however, adequate staging and compliance with follow-up are essential [35, 37]. This may be a challenge as these young women attempt to reintegrate themselves into work, school, or home life and previous peer relationships while trying to put "the past behind" them.

Breast Cancer

Breast cancer surgery has undergone a paradigm shift in the last decade with increased use of breast conservation surgery, sentinel lymph node evaluation, and concomitant inclusion of oncoplastic surgery to improve overall cosmetic results through breast remodelling techniques [38]. For young women, the sexual sequelae of a breast cancer diagnosis and treatment can be considerable at a time when relationships are forming and thoughts of initial or further child bearing are paramount in her life. Although surgery to the breast does not alter fertility, loss of a breast or part of a breast can lead to altered sexual self-esteem, feeling less feminine, changes in body image and questions about the safety of childbearing and the possibilities of breastfeeding. Additionally, anxiety about initiating sexual activities and fears of rejection are common and those not in a committed relationship face the concerns of when to disclose the diagnosis and treatment and the potential consequences of this disclosure [39–42]. While treatment choice is not always possible due to stage of disease, size of breasts or other factors, being able to choose the type of surgery (regardless of the surgery chosen) appears to influence body image and psychological adjustment and should be offered, regardless of patient age, whenever possible. Although there is little published information about the use of breast reconstruction surgery in young women with cancer, it should be offered as a component of overall treatment whenever feasible [43, 44].

Radiation Therapy

Radiation therapy (RT) can cause sexual dysfunction through multiple mechanisms. Among these are testicular aplasia and ovarian failure, changes to organ function such as erectile dysfunction and decreased vaginal lubrication and treatment side effects such as diarrhea, skin reactions, or fatigue that may be temporary or permanent. In general, whether an effect is temporary or permanent is related to the total dose received, treatment site and volume, length of treatment, age of patient, and prior fertility status [23, 27, 45].

Fertility in women is related to follicular maturation and ovum release. Radiation to the ovaries damages the intermediate follicles. Temporary or permanent infertility occurs if intermediate follicles are damaged and there are an insufficient number of small follicles remaining [45, 46]. In addition to potential infertility, common side effects include infertility and early menopause as well as vaginal irritation, shortening, or stenosis; decreased lubrication and dyspareunia; and decreases in sexual interest, enjoyment, and the ability to achieve orgasm leading to decreased sexual activity [47–53].

In older women, a radiation dose between 600 and 1,200 cGy can induce menopause; however, younger women may not be permanently infertile until a dose of more than 2,000 cGy is delivered [46]. To maintain fertility and allow for future childbearing, oophoropexy, movement of the ovaries out of the radiation field to either the uterine midline or to the iliac crests, or ovarian transposition to the upper abdomen along with appropriate shielding can be undertaken. Maintenance of menstruation and successful pregnancies have been reported [45, 46].

In men, immature sperm and spermatogonia are radiosensitive while Leydig cells and mature sperm are radio-resistant. As the total dose increases, the potential for permanent infertility increases [46]. Within 6–8 weeks following radiation exposure to the testes, a reduction in the overall sperm count occurs. Temporary infertility occurs at doses less than 500 cGy, while permanent sterility is associated with doses greater than 500 cGy [46, 54]. Return of normal spermatogenesis can take more than 5 years with lower total testicular doses associated with a more rapid recovery [55–57].

Long-term azoospermia is seen in young men receiving below-the-diaphragm irradiation for testicular cancer or Hodgkin's disease. Sperm counts decrease to their lowest point by 6 months. Some men will experience a return of their sperm counts although this may take up to 2 years [57]. When possible, shielding the testicle or repositioning the unaffected testicle to the groin along with appropriate shielding will preserve fertility [58]. Having RT can be a difficult experience for any patient, particularly when a more private body part receives treatment. Ensuring privacy and providing appropriate covering, as allowed by treatment parameters, will decrease the sense of vulnerability that is common in those receiving RT to the breast, testicle, or pelvic region.

Antineoplastic Therapy

The effect of the administration of antineoplastics on sexual and reproductive function may be temporary or permanent. Sexual side effects generally are related to type of drug and dose delivered, length and schedule of treatment, patient age and gender, and concomitant use of more than one chemotherapy drug or other medications that may affect sexuality (such as antiemetics, antihypertensives, or sedatives).

Chemotherapy

Alterations in sexual health including infertility and sterility are common in those receiving chemotherapy. The most common agents to affect fertility include the alkylating agents, with other drugs such as antimetabolites and vinca alkaloids also implicated. Combination therapy and treatments given over a prolonged period of time, as is common in younger patients, are more likely to cause long-term effects. Regardless of age, men are more likely to experience infertility after receiving chemotherapy while women are more likely to experience alterations in fertility and early menopause as they near 40 [59–69]. This is of particular concern to young women who may have delayed childbearing and now are facing a cancer diagnosis and subsequent chemotherapy that may affect fertility.

In men, fertility is altered by chemotherapy-induced depletion of germinal epithelium lining the seminiferous tubules and leading to oligospermia or azoospermia [70–72]. For recovery, the process of spermatogenesis must begin a new; this may take several years [71–74]. In young men treated with chemotherapy for testicular cancer, some authors have reported a decrease in sexual activity, decreased interest in sex and decreased ability to achieve sexual fulfillment while others have reported no adverse effects [60, 62, 64, 75, 76]. In those who attempted to conceive post-treatment, at least 70% were successful, with fertility appearing to improve over time [45, 56, 71, 72, 75]. Despite the fact that infertility is less common in this population, discussions about sperm banking and possible alterations in fertility and sexual health should be part of a routine initial visit prior to the onset of chemotherapy.

In women, sexual dysfunction and infertility most often are related to ovarian fibrosis and destruction of ovarian follicles. Alterations in hormone levels, particularly LH, FSH, and estradiol also play a significant role [56, 60, 70]. Age is a crucial factor as young women, those less than 30, are less likely to experience immediate premature menopause and permanent amenorrhea even when given significantly higher chemotherapy doses, including treatment with an alkylating agent, than those over 30 [73, 77]. However, premature ovarian failure and associated early onset of menopause appear to be merely delayed, occurring in the late 30s or early 40s rather than at the time of chemotherapy

administration [78]. Amenorrhea is common for all ages when treated with combination therapies, especially if an alkylating agent is included [59, 60, 79, 80]. Additionally, amenorrhea has been reported in young women with ovarian germ cell tumors who were treated with fertility-sparing surgery followed by platinum-based chemotherapy [81]. In those under 40, 50% had return of menstruation within 15 months of completing therapy [79]. When amenorrhea becomes permanent, it occurs gradually over time, taking 6–16 months in those under 40 as opposed to 2–4 months in those nearing menopause [45, 56]. Decreased sexual functioning, psychological distress related to infertility, and decreased quality of life are seen in young women with premature menopause. These may be ameliorated though routine discussions about potential sexual health alterations before, during, and following treatment [82].

Of importance, pharmaceuticals used to treat chemotherapy side effects, such as nausea and vomiting, can affect sexual function. Among the potential side effects are decreased sexual desire, sense of fulfillment, and ability to achieve orgasm [60, 62, 64]. The potential for side effects related to other medications should be discussed and modifications made as needed to assure that side effects are managed with the least potential for added sexual difficulties.

Hormonal Therapy

Hormonal therapies, agents such as estrogen receptor antagonists, antiestrogens, aromatase inhibitors, gonadotropin-releasing hormone analogues, and anti-androgens, are used to alter the body's hormonal milieu in order to treat cancer. The choice of hormonal treatment is based on both tumor and patient characteristics. In young adults, the most frequently used hormonal therapy is Tamoxifen which is generally given for 5 years following chemotherapy for breast cancer. Sexual side effects are common and include hot flashes/flushes, menopausal symptoms, decreased interest in sex, altered body image, weight gain, mood disturbances and dyspareunia. In addition, there have been reports of exacerbations of previous HPV warts and genitals herpes lesions with Tamoxifen therapy. Since hormonal therapies impact fertility as well as cause sexual side effects, it is essential that education and counselling occur prior to the onset of therapy and that the young adult be allowed to make an informed choice about taking them [42, 60, 68, 78, 80].

Biological Response Modifiers

Biological response modifiers (BRMs), also referred to as immune system modulators or immunotherapy, include therapeutics such as colony-stimulating factors, monoclonal antibodies, gene therapies, and vaccines. Although biological response modifiers have been available for many years, research remains insufficient related to sexual side effects. Common side effects of these products include fatigue, flu-like symptoms, and body image changes, all of which can have an effect on sexuality and intimacy through decreased interest in sex and sexual function and alterations in sexual self-concept [83, 84].

Targeted Therapies

Use of the novel anticancer therapies that inhibit cancer cell growth is increasing, particularly for those with lymphomas, leukemias, and Ewings sarcoma (and similar bone and connective tissue cancers) [10, 60, 85, 86]. Among these agents are the antiangiogenic agents, epidermal growth factor tyrosine kinase inhibitors, and fusion proteins. While the exact effects of these agents on sexual function remain unclear, their common side effects of fatigue, diarrhea, and rash have the potential to alter body image, sexual self-esteem, and interest in sex and can increase social isolation and separation from peers and normal daily activities [86].

Stem Cell Transplant

Stem cell transplants are fraught with immediate and long-term sexual side effects. In adolescents and adults of all ages, late effects include gonadal dysfunction, infertility, alterations in body image, and chronic fatigue. Premature menopause, difficulty achieving orgasm, vaginal atrophy, decreased vaginal lubrication, and painful intercourse are common among women, while men frequently experience difficulty with erection and ejaculation and may experience gynecomastia [87–91]. Primary gonadal failure is common, with less than 10% of transplant patients recovering gonadal function. Older age and use of concomitant radiation therapy and/or more than one chemotherapeutic agent increase the likelihood that gonadal function will not recover [87, 88, 92, 93]. Immediate effects are particularly noticeable for those experiencing lengthy hospitalizations, as social isolation is common due to limited visitation policies and the rigors of treatment. Intimacy and sexuality can be impacted due to limited privacy and physical contact [87–89, 94]. Additionally, whether at home or hospitalized, concerns about infection and side effects such as fatigue, nausea and vomiting, and pain will further impact sexual function and increase both social isolation and alterations in peer interactions. While difficult for all ages, young adults receiving a stem cell transplant may be particularly impacted by hospitalizations and the side effects of transplant since family and friend visits may be curtailed. Side effects may alter self-esteem, body image, and the willingness or ability to socialize with peers, and others may be altered due to feeling ill or having concerns about not fitting in or looking right in the social situation.

Approach to Managing Sexuality and Sexual Health During Treatment

The majority of publications dealing with sexual health and sexuality in young adults look at an upper age limit ranging from 29 to 39 with some reports of "young women" being any who are less than 50 years of age. In addition, few publications discuss specific issues related to sexual health during treatment, focusing more on long-term effects. This makes understanding the issues of sexual health and sexual and reproductive dysfunction in young adults more difficult and may affect the development of effective, age and maturation-appropriate strategies since developmental tasks and levels of achievement and maturation vary broadly within this age range. Some information and management strategies about sexual health will be appropriate regardless of age, while other common approaches will need to be altered to fit the age, gender maturation, and developmental task attainment levels of the individual young adult.

Communicating About Sexual Health

Talking with any patient about sexual health can be fraught with numerous concerns by patients and healthcare providers alike. This is even truer when discussing sexual issues with young adults. Recent publications have identified that patients of all ages want to know about the impact of cancer treatment on their sexuality, with future fertility of particular concern [10, 19, 94–97]. Unfortunately, providers are often reluctant to raise the topic of sexual concerns due to inadequate education on talking about sexuality, fearing personal or patient embarrassment or overstepping professional boundaries, "opening a can of worms" [98], lack of knowledge about appropriate resources for problems identified, or because other cancer care issues take precedence during brief patient encounters [9, 10, 96, 99–101]. Additionally, with young adults, issues of autonomy and independence are paramount, but may be coupled with the need for parental consent and patient assent for various discussions and disclosures to take place [102].

Many patients are often unwilling to broach sexual topics also fearing embarrassment or that their feelings must be unimportant or taboo since providers did not mention them [10, 19, 103–105]. However, Kotronoulas and colleagues found that patients feel that sexual health is a priority and were willing to discuss sexual issues when given the opportunity, even though many would prefer that healthcare providers take the lead in the initial discussion [96, 97]. Of note, Hordern and Street noted that there is a mismatch between what patients and providers expect in terms of discussions about sexual health with many unmet patient needs experienced [94].

While writing primarily about adult cancer survivors, Wilmoth identified four processes that are key to addressing sexual issues with patients: learning effective communication skills, enhancing one's personal knowledge of sexuality and intimacy issues, increasing one's comfort level with talking about sexuality, and helping patients find and access needed resources related to alterations in sexuality [106]. For young adults, a fifth process should be added: understanding the developmental tasks, strategies, and accomplishments of the individual and providing discussions, education, and information that are age and maturation-level appropriate. Numerous authors have included the need to understand one's own personal sexual attitudes and beliefs to help identify any barriers and to facilitate discussions about sexuality, and particularly sensitive sexual activities or topics, with patients [6, 9, 10, 101]. Because cancer also impacts the family and possibly even the community, a renegotiation of roles and responsibilities and an understanding of the need for care while trying to gain or regain independence is essential [107]. In addition, when discussing sexual health with young adults, knowledge of developmental stages and maturation levels are needed to facilitate timely and open discussions and provide appropriate management strategies and guidance [6, 107].

When discussing sexual issues with patients, a matter-of-fact, yet sensitive approach is essential. Making discussions a routine part of assessment and follow-up allows providers and patients to feel more at ease in the discussion. Approaches that appear to be most successful with all ages include taking cues from the patient as to the timing and nature of the content of discussion; providing non-judgmental, factual information that moves from less to more sensitive issues over time; and avoiding use of both medical jargon and common colloquialisms. Discussion should be neutral to sexual orientation and gender, avoid cultural stereotyping, and move from one topic to another with a normal flow. Clarifying questions or statements should be used and non-verbal as well as verbal communication assessed through all discussions [10, 104, 105]. Additionally, as appropriate and desired by the patient, discussions should include family members and/or significant others and give the patient permission to be sexually active in whatever ways are congruent with the patient's age, lifestyle, and sexual preferences [10, 104, 105]. Goals of care need to be individualized and age-appropriate, focusing on building and/or supporting the young adult's sexual self-esteem and sexual self-schema, facilitating communication about sexuality and sexual health issues, and providing appropriate resources and referrals [10, 103–105].

Young adulthood is a time of developing new relationships, experimenting with personal identification, and exploring one's sexual schema [108]. Katz and others [9, 10, 108, 109] have noted that AYAs with cancer experience alterations in self-esteem and self-image, wide variations in level and characteristics of sexual activity and maturation, changes in relationships with their peers, and delayed or diminished psychosocial development. These changes can affect both the content and direction of discussions of sexuality and sexual health. However, based on current parameters for sexual activity and knowledge of youth, adolescents, and adults, all patients should be assumed to have at least some level of information and experience with sexuality and sexual health. Sexual activity is common in adolescents and sexual knowledge and information about potential risks and safety precautions may or may not be factual. Sexual health discussions with young adults should be held in private settings and include only those individuals desired and welcomed by the patient. Discussions should incorporate assessing sexual attitudes and knowledge, as well as asking about current relationships and sexual practices. While gaining an understanding of the young adult's previous and desired sexual experiences, level of activity, and knowledge, any myths and misinformation should be corrected. Questions and issues that

are likely to be raised during discussions include not only factual information about sexual function/dysfunction and fertility/infertility, but also concerns about body image, peer and parental relationships, when to disclose the diagnosis and treatment to actual or potential romantic partners (and others), and how to deal with the emotions surrounding the diagnosis, treatment, and potential or actual alterations in sexual function and reproduction.

As noted by Zebrack, young adults want information not only about disease, treatment, and side effects but also about ways to be as healthy as possible through exercise and diet, how to access mental health services and complementary/integrative health resources, managing financial issues, finding information via reputable sources from the internet, and information about sexuality, intimacy, fertility, and childbearing [110]. Camps, retreats, and social programs designed specifically for the young adult also were desired, specifically programs that could address the unique needs of this population [110, 111].

Sexual Assessment

Eisner and colleagues [1] state that: "it is not enough to cure the disease at the expense of an individual's physical, social, family, emotional, or cognitive wellbeing [1]." (p. 275). This requires that sexual health issues be valued, assessed, and managed by healthcare providers. Alterations in sexual health are common during cancer treatment. They frequently are due to a combination of factors including the cancer disease process, treatment-related side effects, psychosocial issues and/or management of co-morbidities such as diabetes. While cancer and treatment may alter sexual function as well as body image, sexual self-esteem, and fertility, it cannot alter the fact that each person is a sexual being and that sexuality is a component of all aspects of our lives [10, 53, 103–105]. Potential side effects that will impact sexual health should be discussed prior to the onset of treatment and problems and concerns reassessed throughout treatment and during long-term follow-up visits [10, 103–105, 112]. Assessments and interventions should be individually tailored to the specific age, gender, developmental level, sexual orientation, and disease type, stage, and treatment plan as well as the identified concerns and issues raised by the patient (and parent or partner as appropriate) [10, 103–105]. Whenever possible, a comprehensive assessment model that addresses the full continuum of sexual health should be used and assessment discussions and intervention strategies should address both common sexual concerns such as fertility, reproduction, and the ability to have intercourse as well as issues of body image, intimacy, and relationships. Additionally, direct and open-ended questions may need to be used to assess contraceptive use, risky sexual practices, or the use drugs, alcohol, or other substances or devices. Following the assessment, an intervention plan should be developed and recorded.

Crucial to a comprehensive plan is being aware of community resources, how to access them, and when to refer. Areas of referral for young adults include sperm banking and other fertility-preserving options, and reconstructive surgery and prostheses. Of importance, while not minimizing sexual concerns, providers need to be wary of the possibility of creating concerns when they do not exist, and instead should focus on anticipating, recognizing, advocating, and intervening for those that do have concerns [23, 104, 105]. Geisler et al. used oncology nurse interveners and an interactive computer program to evaluate quality of life in prostate cancer patients [113]. Although not tested with young adults, the use of social media and interactive technology may provide an important avenue for assessing sexual health and other disease and treatment-related side effects in this population and should be investigated further.

Sexual Assessment Models

Multiple models for sexual assessment exist, but few were developed specifically for cancer patients and none were designed or tested

specifically with AYAs. These models can best be divided into three categories: the pure assessment models, the pure intervention models, and those that combine both assessment and intervention. The most frequently recognized model is the PLISSIT model described by Annon in 1974 [114]. It is primarily considered an intervention model although in more recent publications it has been used for both assessment and intervention [103, 104, 106, 115]. In this model, permission (P) is given to the patient to talk about sexual issues and be sexually active, limited information (LI) is provided about potential sexual side effects and alterations in sexual health, specific suggestions (SS) are given to manage identified problems or concerns, and as needed, referral for intensive therapy (IT) by a trained counselor is given when issues are beyond the expertise of the healthcare provider [114]. While this model may be familiar to healthcare providers, it is probably not the best model to use when assessing young adults for alterations in sexual health as it does not take into consideration developmental tasks and maturation levels and thus may not be as comprehensive as is needed for this population.

Mick and colleagues created the BETTER model to meet the sexual assessment needs of those with cancer [116]. Components of the model include bringing (B) up the topic of sexuality and sexual health, explaining (E) your reasons for introducing the topic and offering to help by telling (T) the patient about appropriate strategies and resources to prevent or ameliorate sexual problems, timing (T) discussions to meet the needs of the patient, providing education (E) about potential problems with sexual health, and recording (R) assessment and interventions in the patient's medical record so that others may provide appropriate follow-up. While not evaluated in young adults, it may be more appropriate than PLISSIT for this population.

Hordern notes that most definitions of sexuality and models for assessing sexual health omit important concepts such as intimacy, relationships, body image, and other aspects of sexuality separate from sexual function and fertility [4]. She feels that models should encompass the entire sexual continuum if assessments and interventions are to promote quality sexual health. This is imperative for young adults who may have many myths and misconceptions about sexual health and are struggling not only with understanding their own sexuality, but also attempting to transition to mature, independent selves.

New models need to be developed that address the specific needs of young adults as they transition from childhood to mature adults. Models should focus on identifying completion of developmental tasks and asking questions, holding discussions, and providing strategies that meet the needs of this population. Creating an assessment and intervention model incorporating the dimensions of Cleary and colleagues' neo-theoretical framework may be of benefit in the future for this population, but further research is needed [15].

Barriers and Strategies to Maintaining Sexual Health

Managing sexual health concerns in young adults requires a knowledge of normal gonadal function, potential and actual sexual side effects of the specific cancer diagnosis and treatment, methods to communicate about sexual health, and strategies to assess and prevent, minimize, or treat sexual side effects that occur. Multiple physical and psychological factors can influence sexual health (see Table 5.1), from experiencing infertility and premature menopause to dealing with treatment, side effects, and alterations in sexual function. Psychoemotional effects include dealing with body image changes, grappling with loneliness and social isolation, feeling vulnerable, concerns over rejection/the stigma of having cancer or fears of losing independence, and being a burden on one's family and friends [3, 5, 6, 16, 102, 104, 107, 117–119]. Multiple strategies can support sexual health in young adults. Table 5.2 identifies some possible strategies to enhance sexual health [2, 6, 108, 110, 113, 117, 118, 120–123]. Among them are strategies that directly impact alterations (wigs, prostheses, and evaluations by conception specialists), manage relationship issues (learning communication strategies and coping techniques),

Table 5.1 Common physiologic and psychoemotional factors impact sexual health

Physiologic factors	Psychoemotional factors
Infertility	Body image changes
Premature menopause	Fears of rejection (disclosing diagnosis, treatment)
Dyspareunia	Social isolation/loneliness
Decreased sexual satisfaction	Stigma of having cancer
Difficulty with arousal	Anxiety/depression/distress
Inadequate lubrication	Alterations in what is considered "normal"/loss
Ejaculation difficulties	Mastery/lack of mastery of developmental tasks
Fatigue	Heightened sense of vulnerability/insecurity
Neuropathies	Feeling misunderstood/not supported
Cognitive dysfunction	Gaining/losing autonomy/independence
Alopecia	Inadequate personal coping resources/reserve
Weight loss/gain	Contrasting patient and parental perspectives
Surgical scars/amputations	Feelings of being a burden to family/peers
Medical devices/ports/lines/pumps	Decreased self-esteem, sexual self-concept

Refs: [3, 5, 6, 16, 97, 104, 108, 120–122]

Table 5.2 Strategies to enhance sexual health

Provide accurate information/allow informed choice
Make sexual assessment a component of routine initial and follow-up visits
Intervention/counseling sessions on possible sexual impact, potential means of prevention/treatment of sexual side effects
Identify, evaluate, and provide resources (resource list)
Camps/retreats/special programs specific to needs of young adults
Keep a journal/diary
Teach communication skills (listening, talking, clarifying)
Coping skills investigating flexible coping, alternative ways to view sexuality, sexual reframing
Education for use of alternative positions and devices
Relaxation/visual imagery
Art/music therapy
Discussions/education on methods to foster intimacy

Table 5.2 (continued)

Use interdisciplinary teams with appropriate expertise

Include discussion of safe sex, STDs, contraception (prevent rather than treat)

Encourage use of technology to evaluate symptoms/elicit concerns (interactive computer programs); maintain peer relationships (social media)

Facilitate role play/rehearse to "act out" social situations (i.e., "telling the diagnosis")

Treat in settings that support young adults/plan for transitions

Manage issues such as finances, insurance, childcare, transportation

Refs: [2, 6, 12, 109, 110, 112, 115, 120, 121]

provide information (educating about actual or potential side effects) or those that ease the burden of cancer (financial, spiritual, and social support).

Conclusion

Katz and others [109, 117] have noted that young adults have particular difficulties in sexual health and are faced with challenges that do not occur for older or younger cancer survivors. They may be in the midst of establishing relationships, beginning new lives, thinking about having children or raising young children, facing interruptions to education or work, and are often struggling with issues of independence and leaving home. A cancer diagnosis and treatment may force the newly independent AYA back into a dependent situation, remove him/her from peer groups, and alter hopes and plans for the future. Care may be provided in unfamiliar surroundings far from home and community and in a settings where the young adult is too young or too old, causing or adding to social isolation.

Not only are relationships with peers and family forever changed, but the young adult is also changed, viewing life from a position of vulnerability but also possibly from a position of strength.

In some instances, dealing with cancer may be life-affirming, while at other times the young adult may view the world and those in it as unfriendly and uncaring or see life as hopeless and filled with despair. Side effects of treatment such as alopecia, nausea, diarrhea, and fatigues along with surgical scars, amputations, pumps, lines, and tubes create barriers that may be hard to overcome without significant support, resources, and assistance. Activities previously enjoyed may be no longer possible either because of physical and treatment-related issues or because parents or family are concerned about harm or injury. Anticipatory guidance by providers who understand the life transitions and fears and anxieties of the young adult undergoing cancer treatment are essential. Assisting the young adult in planning for a future that includes intimate relationships, sexual activity, and optimal options for childbearing is essential. Focusing on supporting sexual self-concept, sexual relationships, and quality sexual functioning can allow the provider to meet the sexual health needs of the young adult while also facilitating growth, maturation, and attainment of crucial developmental tasks [117, 118]. Odo and Potter note that "cancer is a crash course in dealing with health crises [3]." Facilitating sexual health in young adults is one strategy for diminishing the impact of that crisis.

Provider Recommendations

1. Cancer treatments can impact sexual functioning both physically and emotionally.
2. The cancer diagnosis itself can impact sexual desire.
3. Oncology healthcare providers may not have received training in sexual health and may be uncomfortable having these discussions with patients.
4. Patients report they do want to talk about sexuality and sexual health issues but are embarrassed or uncertain about how to initiate the conversation.
5. Assessment models, such as BETTER, may assist healthcare providers to assess and attend to their patients' sexual health needs.

References

1. Eiser C, Penn A, Katz E, Barr R (2009) Psychosocial issues and quality of life. Sem Oncol. doi: 10.1053/j.seminoncol.2009.03.005
2. Bolte S, Zebrack B (eds) (2008) Sexual issues in special populations: adolescents and young adults. Sem Oncol Nurs. doi: 10.1016/jsonen.2008.02.004
3. Odo R, Potter C (2009) Understanding the needs of young adult cancer survivors: a clinical perspective. Oncology (Williston Park, NY) 23(11 Suppl Nurse Ed):23(11):23–33
4. Hordern AJ, Street AF (2007) Communicating about patient sexuality and intimacy after cancer: mismatched expectations and unmet needs. Med J Aust 186(5):224–227
5. Evan EE, Kaufman M, Cook AB, Zeltzer LK (2006) Sexual health and self esteem in adolescents and young adults with cancer. Cancer 107(S7): 1672–1679
6. Rosen A, Rodriguez-Wallberg KA, Rosenzweig L (2009) Psychosocial distress in young cancer survivors. Sem Oncol Nurs. doi:10.1016/j.soncn.2009. 08.004
7. Pan American Health Organization WHO. Promotion of sexual health. http://www2.hu-berlin.de/sexology/GESUND/ARCHIV/PSH.HTM
8. Hordern A (2008) Intimacy and sexuality after cancer: a critical review of the literature. Cancer Nurs 31(2):E9–E17
9. Katz A (2005) The sounds of silence: sexuality information for cancer patients. J Clin Oncol 23(1):238
10. Krebs LU (2011) Sexual and reproductive dysfunction. In: Yarbro CH, Wujic D, Goebel BH (eds) Cancer nursing, 7th edn. Jones and Bartlett Publishers, Sudbury, MA, pp 879–911
11. Mercadante S, Vitrano V, Catania V (2010) Sexual issues in early and late stage cancer: a review. Supportive Care Cancer 18(6):659–665
12. Tierney DK (2008) Sexuality: a quality-of-life issue for cancer survivors. Sem Oncol Nurs 24(2):71–79
13. Woods NF (1987) Toward a holistic perspective of human sexuality: alterations in sexual health and nursing diagnoses. Holistic Nurs Pract 1(4):1–11
14. World Health Oraganization (2010) What constitutes sexual health? http://www.who.int/hrp/topics/en/
15. Cleary V, Hegarty J, McCarthy G (2011) Sexuality in Irish women with gynecologic cancer. Oncol Nurs Forum 38(2):E87–E96
16. Tindle D, Denver K, Lilley F (2009) Identity, image, and sexuality in young adults with cancer. Sem Oncol. doi: 10.1053/j.seminoncol.2009.03.008
17. Huether ADS (2008) Structure and function of the reproductive systems. In: Huether SE, McCance KL (eds) Understanding pathophysiology, 4th edn. Mosby, St Louis
18. Marieb EN, Hoehn KN (2009) Human anatomy and physiology, 8th edn. Benjamin/Cummings, Menlo Park, CA
19. Park ER, Norris RL, Bober SL (2009) Sexual health communication during cancer care: barriers and recommendations. Cancer J 15(1):74–77
20. Nonomura N, Nishimura K, Takaha N, Inoue H, Nomoto T, Mizutani Y et al (2002) Nerve sparing retroperitoneal lymph node dissection for advanced testicular cancer after chemotherapy. Int J Urol 9(10):539–544
21. Joly F, Heron J, Kalusinski L, Bottet P, Brune D, Allouache N et al (2002) Quality of life in long-term survivors of testicular cancer: a population-based case-control study. J Clin Oncol 20(1):73
22. Albaugh A, Kellogg-Spadt S, Krebs LU, Lewis JH, Kramer-Levien D (2009) Sexual function and sexual rehabilitation with GU Cancer: what patients want to know. In: Held-Warmkessel J (ed) Site-specific cancer series: urologic cancers. Oncology Nursing Society, Pittsburgh, PA, pp 121–148
23. Bruner DW, Calvano T (2007) The sexual impact of cancer and cancer treatments in men. Nurs Clin North Am 42(4):555–580
24. Gossfield LM, Cullen ML (2000) Sexuality and fertility. In: Moore-Higgs GJ (ed) Women and cancer: a gynecologic oncology nursing perspective, 2nd edn. Jones and Bartlett, Sudbury, MA
25. Stilos K, Doyle C, Daines P (2008) Addressing the sexual health needs of patients with gynecologic cancers. Clin J Oncol Nurs 12(3):457–463
26. Krychman ML, Pereira L, Carter J, Amsterdam A (2007) Sexual oncology: sexual health issues in women with cancer. Oncology 71(1–2):18–25
27. Barton-Burke M, Gustason CJ (2007) Sexuality in women with cancer. Nurs Clin North Am 42(4):531–554
28. Ratner ES, Foran KA, Schwartz PE, Minkin MJ (2010) Sexuality and intimacy after gynecological cancer. Maturitas 66(1):23–26
29. Schlaerth JB, Spirtos NM, Schlaerth AC (2003) Radical trachelectomy and pelvic lymphadenectomy with uterine preservation in the treatment of cervical cancer. Am J Obstet Gynecol 188(1): 29–34
30. Carter J, Sonoda Y, Chi DS, Raviv L, Abu-Rustum NR (2008) Radical trachelectomy for cervical cancer: postoperative physical and emotional adjustment concerns. Gynecol Oncol 111(1): 151–157
31. Andersen BL, Lamb M (1995) Sexuality and cancer. In: Murphy GP, Lawrence W, Lenhard RE (eds) American Cancer Society textbook of clinical oncology, 2nd edn. American Cancer Society, Atlanta, GA, pp 699–713
32. Wilmoth MC, Spinelli A (2000) Sexual implications of gynecologic cancer treatments. J Obstet Gynecol Neonatal Nurs 29(4):413–421
33. Bergmark K, Å Vall Lundqvist E, Dickman PW, Henningsohn L, Steineck G (2002) Patient rating

of distressful symptoms after treatment for early cervical cancer. Acta Obstet Gynecol Scand 81(5): 443–450

34. Jongpipan J, Charoenkwan K (2007) Sexual function after radical hysterectomy for early stage cervical cancer. J Sex Med 4(6):1659–1665
35. DeGaetano C (2001) Ovarian cancer – it whispers... so listen. Nurs Spectrum (South) 2(1):28–32
36. Stead ML, Fallowfield L, Selby P, Brown JM (2007) Psychosexual function and impact of gynaecological cancer. Best Pract Res Clin Obstet Gynaecol 21(2):309–320
37. Fitch MI (2003) Psychosocial management of patients with recurrent ovarian cancer: treating the whole patient to improve quality of life. Semin Oncol Nurs 19(suppl 1):40–53
38. Warren AG, Morris DJ, Houlihan MJ, Slavin SA (2008) Breast reconstruction in a changing breast cancer treatment paradigm. Plast Reconstr Surg 121(4):1116–1126
39. Amichetti M, Caffo O (2001) Quality of life in patients with early stage breast carcinoma treated with conservation surgery and radiotherapy: an Italian monoinstitutional study. Tumori 2:78–84
40. Fialka-Moser V, Crevenna R, Korpan M, Quittan M (2003) Cancer rehabilitation: particularly with aspects on physical impairments. J Rehabil Med 35:153–162
41. Gilbert E, Ussher JM, Perz J (2010) Renegotiating sexuality and intimacy in the context of cancer: the experiences of carers. Arch Sex Behav. doi: 10.1007/s10508-008-9416-z
42. Herbenick D, Reece M, Hollub A, Satinsky S, Dodge B (2008) Young female breast cancer survivors. Cancer Nurs 31(6):417–425
43. Atisha D, Alderman AK, Lowery JC, Kuhn LE, Davis J, Wilkins EG (2008) Prospective analysis of long-term psychosocial outcomes in breast reconstruction. Anna Surg 247(6):1019–1028
44. Temple WJ, Russell ML, Parsons LL, Huber SM (2006) Conservation surgery for breast cancer as the preferred choice: a prospective analysis. J Clin Oncol 24(21):3367–3373
45. Brydøy M, Fosså SD, Dahl O, Bjøro T (2007) Gonadal dysfunction and fertility problems in cancer survivors. Acta Oncol 46(4):480–489
46. Rubin A, Williams JP (2001) Principles of radiation oncology and cancer radiotherapy. In: Rubin A (ed) Clinical oncology: a multidisciplinary approach for physicians and students, 8th edn. Saunders, Philadelphia, PA, pp 99–125
47. Jensen PT, Groenvald M, Klee MC et al (2003) Longitudinal study of sexual function and vaginal changes after radiotherapy for cervical cancer. Int J Radiat Oncol Biol Phys 56:937–949
48. Bakewell RT, Volker DL (2005) Sexual dysfunction related to the treatment of young women with breast cancer. Clin J Oncol Nurs 9(6):697–702

49. Maher EJ, Denton A (2008) Survivorship, late effects and cancer of the cervix. Clin Oncol 20: 479–487
50. White ID (2008) The assessment and management of sexual difficulties after treatment for cervical and endometrial malignancies. Clin Oncol 20:488–496
51. Vistad I, Fossa SD, Kristensen GB, Dahl AA (2007) Chronic fatigue and its correlates in long-term survivors of cervical cancer treated with radiotherapy. BJOG 114:1150–1158
52. Wo JY, Viswanathan AN (2009) The impact of radiotherapy on fertility, pregnancy, and neonatal outcomes of female cancer patients. Int J Radiat Oncol Biol Phys. doi:10.1016/j.ijrobp.2008.12.016
53. Nishimoto PW (2008) Sexuality. In: Gates RA, Fink RM (eds) Oncology nursing secrets, 3rd edn. Mosby, St. Louis, MO, pp 488–501
54. Iwamoto RR, Maher KE (2001) Radiation therapy for prostate cancer. Semin Oncol Nurs 17:90–100
55. Rowley MJ, Leach DR, Warner GA, Heller CG (1974) Effect of graded doses of ionizing radiation on the human testis. Radiat Res 59(3):665–678
56. Tomao F, Miele E, Spinelli G, Tomao S (2006) Anticancer treatment and fertility effects. Lit Rev J Exp Clin Cancer Res 25(4):475
57. Revel A, Revel-Vilk S (2008) Pediatric fertility preservation: is it time to offer testicular tissue cryopreservation? Mol Cell Endocrinol 282(1–2): 143–149
58. Gruschow K, Kyank U, Stuhldreier G, Fietkau R (2007) Surgical repositioning of the contralateral testicle before irradiation of a paratesticular rhabdomyosarcoma for preservation of hormone production. Pediatr Hematol Oncol 24(5):371–377
59. Davis M (2006) Fertility considerations for female adolescent and young adult patients following cancer therapy: a guide for counseling patients and their families. Clin J Oncol Nurs 10(2):213–219
60. Wilkes GM, Barton-Burke M (2010) 2011 Oncology nursing drug handbook. Jones and Bartlett, Sudbury, MA
61. Otto S (2007) Chemotherapy. In: Langhorne ME, Fulton JS, Otto SE (eds) Oncology nursing, 5th edn. Mosby, St. Louis, MO, pp 262–276
62. Prescher-Hughes DS (2008) Nurse's chemotherapy quick pocket reference. Jones and Bartlett, Sudbury, MA
63. Gullatte M (ed) (2001) Clinical guide to antineoplastic therapy: a chemotherapy handbook. Oncology Nursing Society, Pittsburg, PA
64. Chu E (2008) Pocket guide to chemotherapy protocols, 5th edn. Jones and Bartlett, Sudbury, MA
65. Blecher CS (2009) Chemotherapeutic agents. In: Newton S, Hickey M, Marrs J (eds) Mosby's oncology nursing advisor: a comprehensive guide to clinical practice. Mosby, St. Louis, MO, pp 198–223
66. Gobel BH, Mast D (2009) Chemotherapeutic agents. In: Newton S, Hickey M, Marrs J (eds) Mosby's oncology nursing advisor: a

comprehensive guide to clinical practice. Mosby, St. Louis, MO, pp 238–263

67. Krebs LU (2009) Chemotherapeutic agents. In: Newton S, Hickey M, Marrs J (eds) Mosby's oncology nursing advisor: a comprehensive guide to clinical practice. Mosby, St. Louis, MO, pp 263–286

68. Orbaugh K (2009) Hormonal therapy agents. In: Newton S, Hickey M, Marrs J (eds) Mosby's oncology nursing advisor: a comprehensive guide to clinical practice. Mosby, St. Louis, MO, pp 317–325

69. Braun-Inglis C (2009) Chemotherapeutic agents. In: Newton S, Hickey M, Marrs J (eds) Mosby's oncology nursing advisor: a comprehensive guide to clinical practice. Mosby, St. Louis, MO, pp 197, 223–238

70. Schilsky RL, Lewis BJ, Sherins RJ, Young RC (1980) Gonadal dysfunction in patients receiving chemotherapy for cancer. Ann Intern Med 93 (1 Part 1):109–114

71. Schmidt KLT, Carlsen E, Andersen AN (2007) Fertility treatment in male cancer survivors. Int J Androl 30(4):413–419

72. Bashore L (2007) Semen preservation in male adolescents and young adults with cancer: one institution's experience. Clin J Oncol Nurs 11(3):381–386

73. Gospodarowicz M (2008) Testicular cancer patients: considerations in long-term follow-up. Hematol Oncol Clin North Am 22(2):245–255

74. Thaler-DeMers D (2006) Endocrine and fertility effects in male cancer survivors: changes related to androgen-deprivation therapy and other treatments require timely intervention. Cancer Nurs 29(2):66–71

75. Huddart R, Norman A, Moynihan C, Horwich A, Parker C, Nicholls E et al (2005) Fertility, gonadal and sexual function in survivors of testicular cancer. Br J Cancer 93(2):200–207

76. Böhlen D, Burkhard FC et al (2001) Fertility and sexual function following orchiectomy and 2 cycles of chemotherapy for stage I high risk nonseminomatous germ cell cancer. J Urol 165(2):441–444

77. Kurebayashi J (2008) Adjuvant therapy for premenopausal patients with early breast cancer. Curr Opin Obstet Gynecol 20(1):51–54

78. Hickey M, Peate M, Saunders C, Friedlander M (2009) Breast cancer in young women and its impact on reproductive function. Hum Reprod Update 15(3):323–339

79. Minton SE, Munster PN (2002) Chemotherapy-induced amenorrhea and fertility in women undergoing adjuvant treatment for breast cancer. Cancer Control 9(6):466–472

80. Schover LR (2008) Premature ovarian failure and its consequences: vasomotor symptoms, sexuality, and fertility. J Clin Oncol 26(5):753–758

81. Gershenson DM, Miller AM, Champion VL, Monahan PO, Zhao Q, Cella D et al (2007) Reproductive and sexual function after platinum-based chemotherapy in long-term ovarian germ cell tumor survivors: a Gynecologic Oncology Group Study. J Clin Oncol 25(19):2792–2797

82. Knobf M (2006) The influence of endocrine effects of adjuvant therapy on quality of life outcomes in younger breast cancer survivors. Oncologist 11(2):96–110

83. Rieger P (2001) Patient management, 2nd edn. Jones and Bartlett, Sudbury

84. Rothaermel JM, Baum B (2009) Biological response modifiers/Biological response modifier agents. In: Newton S, Hickey M, Marrs J (eds) Mosby's oncology nursing advisor: a comprehensive guide to clinical practice. Mosby, St. Louis, MO, pp 161–182

85. Karosas AO (2010) Ewing's sarcoma. Am J Health Syst Pharm 67(19):1599

86. Remer SE (2009) Targeted therapy/targeted therapy agents. In: Newton S, Hickey M, Marrs J (eds) Mosby's oncology nursing advisor: a comprehensive guide to clinical practice. Mosby, St. Louis, MO, pp 287–313

87. Tierney D (2004) Sexuality following hematopoietic cell transplantation. Clin J Oncol Nurs 8(1): 43–47

88. Lee HG, Park EY, Kim HM, Kim K, Kim WS, Yoon SS et al (2002) Sexuality and quality of life after hematopoietic stem cell transplantation. Korean J Intern Med 17(1):19–23

89. Chatterjee R, Andrews H, McGarrigle H, Kottaridis P, Lees W, Mackinnon S et al (2000) Cavernosal arterial insufficiency is a major component of erectile dysfunction in some recipients of high-dose chemotherapy/chemoradiotherapy for haematological. Bone Marrow Transplant 25(11):1185–1190

90. Chatterjee R, Kottaridis P, McGarrigle H, Linch D (2002) Management of erectile dysfunction by combination therapy with testosterone and sildenafil in recipients of high-dose therapy for haematological malignancies. Bone Marrow Transplant 29(7): 607–610

91. Harris E, Mahendra P, McGarrigle HH et al (2001) Gynaecomastia with hypergonadotrophic hypogonadism of high dose chemotherapy or chemoradiotherapy. Bone Marrow Transplant 28:1141–1114

92. Hammond C, Abrams JR, Syrjala KL (2007) Fertility and risk factors for elevated infertility concern in 10-year hematopoietic cell transplant survivors and case-matched controls. J Clin Oncol 25(23):3511–3517

93. Tauchmanovà L, Alviggi C, Foresta C, Strina I, Garolla A, Colao A et al (2007) Cryptozoospermia with normal testicular function after allogeneic stem cell transplantation: a case report. Hum Reprod 22(2):495–499

94. Syrjala KL, Kurland BF, Abrams JR, Sanders JE, Heiman JR (2008) Sexual function changes during the 5 years after high-dose treatment and

hematopoietic cell transplantation for malignancy, with case-matched controls at 5 years. Blood 111(3):989–996

95. Lally R (2006) Sexuality: everything you might be afraid to ask but patients need to know. ONS New Oncol Nurs Soc 21(9):1, 4, 5

96. Kotronoulas G, Papadopoulou C, Patiraki E (2009) Nurses' knowledge, attitudes, and practices regarding provision of sexual health care in patients with cancer: critical review of the evidence. Support Care Cancer 17(5):479–501

97. Julien JO, Thom B, Kline NE (2010) Identification of barriers to sexual health assessment in oncology nursing practice. Oncol Nurs Forum 37(3):E186–E190

98. Gott M, Galena E, Hinchliff S, Elford H (2004) "Opening a can of worms": GP and practice nurse barriers to talking about sexual health in primary care. Fam Pract 21(5):528–536

99. Magnan MA, Reynolds K (2006) Barriers to addressing patient sexuality concerns across five areas of specialization. Clin Nurse Spec 20(6):285–292

100. Magnan M, Reynolds K, Galvin E (2005) Barriers to addressing patient sexuality in nursing practice. Medsurg Nurs Off J Acad Med Surg Nurses 14(5):282–289

101. Kaplan M, Pacelli R (2011) The sexuality discussion: tools for the oncology nurse. Clin J Oncol Nurs 15(1):15–17

102. Abrams AN, Hazen EP, Penson RT (2007) Psychosocial issues in adolescents with cancer. Cancer Treat Rev 33(7):622–630

103. Krebs LU (2006) What should I say? Talking with patients about sexuality issues. Clin J Oncol Nurs 10(3):313–315

104. Krebs LU (2007) Sexual assessment: research and clinical. Nurs Clin North Am 42(4):515–529

105. Krebs LU (2008) Sexual assessment in cancer care: concepts, methods and strategies for success. Sem Oncol Nurs 24(2):80–90

106. Wilmoth MC (2006) Life after cancer: what does sexuality have to do with it? Oncol Nurs Forum 33(5):905–910

107. Grinyer A (2009) Contrasting parental perspectives with those of teenagers and young adults with cancer: Comparing the findings from two qualitative studies. Eur J Oncol Nurs 13(3):200–206

108. Morgan S, Davies S, Palmer S, Plaster M (2010) Sex, drugs, and rock 'n'roll: caring for adolescents and young adults with cancer. J Clin Oncol 28(32):4825–4830

109. Katz A (2007) The adult with cancer. Breaking the silence on cancer and sexuality: a handbook for healthcare providers. Oncology Nursing Society, Pittsburgh, PA, pp 155–164

110. Zebrack B (2008) Information and service needs for young adult cancer patients. Support Care Cancer 16(12):1353–1360

111. Zebrack B, Oeffinger K, Hou P, Kaplan S (2006) Advocacy skills training for young adult cancer survivors: the Young Adult Survivors Conference at Camp M k-a-Dream. Support Care Cancer 14(7):779–782

112. Thaler-DeMers D (2001) Intimacy issues: sexuality, fertility and relationships. Semin Oncol Nurs 17:255–262

113. Giesler RB, Given B, Given CW, Rawl S, Monahan P, Burns D et al (2005) Improving the quality of life of patients with prostate carcinoma. Cancer 104(4):752–762

114. Annon JS (1974) The behavioral treatment of sexual problems. Mercantile Printing, Honolulu

115. Mick JM (2007) Sexuality assessment: 10 strategies for improvement. Clin J Oncol Nurs 11(5):671–675

116. Mick J, Hughes M, Cohen MZ (2004) Using the BETTER model to assess sexuality. Clin J Oncol Nurs 8(1):84–86

117. Soliman H, Agresta SV (2008) Current issues in adolescent and young adult cancer survivorship. Cancer Control 15(1):55–62

118. Freyer DR, Kibrick Lazear R (2006) In sickness and in health. Cancer: Transition of cancer-related care for older adolescents and young adults 107(S7):1702–1709

119. Carpentier MY, Fortenberry JD (2010) Romantic and sexual relationships, body image, and fertility in adolescent and young adult testicular cancer survivors: a review of the literature. J Adolesc Health 47(2):115–125

120. Brotto LA, Yule M, Breckon E (2010) Psychological interventions for the sexual sequelae of cancer: A review of the literature. J Cancer Survivorship 1–15

121. Canada AL, Schover LR, Li Y (2007) A pilot intervention to enhance psychosexual development in adolescents and young adults with cancer. Pediatr Blood Cancer. doi: 10.1002/pbc.21130

122. Jun EY, Kim S, Chang SB, Oh K, Kang HS, Kang SS (2011) The effect of a sexual life reframing program on marital intimacy, body image, and sexual function among breast cancer survivors. Cancer Nurs 34(2):142–149

123. Reese JB, Keefe FJ, Somers TJ, Abernathy AP (2010) Coping with sexual concerns after cancer: the use of flexible coping. Support Care Cancer. doi: 10.1007/s00520-010-0819-8

The Unique Reproductive Concerns of Young Women with Breast Cancer

6

Kathryn J. Ruddy, MD, MPH and Ann H. Partridge, MD, MPH

I am a 35 year old woman whose boyfriend found a mass in my breast two months ago. A biopsy showed it was breast cancer, and I was ultimately recommended to undergo chemotherapy and tamoxifen in addition to surgery. I told them I would very much like to be able to have children in the future, so my oncologist said I should consider embryo cryopreservation, as my likelihood of being able to conceive naturally after chemotherapy and at age 40, when the tamoxifen was finished, would not be high. However, she acknowledged that no one is sure whether ovarian stimulation prior to treatment, especially when my cancer was hormone sensitive, is safe. I met with a reproductive endocrinologist later that week, and we went over the pros and cons of fertility preservation options. My boyfriend I discussed it and we decided to move forward with embryo cryopreservation. Because my period had recently finished, I started ovarian stimulation quickly and had eggs harvested, fertilized with my boyfriend's sperm, and frozen less than two weeks later. I started chemotherapy the next day. While I realize there is uncertainty about the safety of pregnancy after breast cancer, knowing that I have taken steps to preserve my fertility is very reassuring to me as I begin my treatment.
Diana, Breast Cancer Survivor

Introduction

Approximately 1 in every 250 women is diagnosed with breast cancer before the age of 40 in the United States, and many have not yet completed their desired childbearing at the time of diagnosis. As more women delay childbearing, fertility concerns appear to be increasingly common in young women with breast cancer. Although reproductive health is a crucial issue for all young adults with cancer, young women with breast cancer face unique challenges. While chemotherapies for breast cancer

are not particularly more gonadotoxic than therapies for many other cancers, the theoretic concern that a future pregnancy could increase the risk of breast cancer recurrence is of particular concern in patients with endocrine-responsive malignancies (e.g., breast cancer). Furthermore, the hormonal therapy (e.g., tamoxifen) standardly prescribed for five years to women with hormone-receptor positive breast cancers precludes conception during that time, and allows more natural ovarian aging than would a shorter course of antineoplastic treatment. While menstrual cycling does not imply fertility and amenorrhea does not necessarily indicate that any woman is unable to become pregnant, this is particularly true in women on tamoxifen, a drug that can both cause vaginal bleeding and interrupt menstrual cycling. In addition, recent data suggest that BRCA1 genetic mutations, which predispose to breast

K.J. Ruddy (✉)
Dana-Farber Cancer Institute, Boston, MA 02215, USA
e-mail: kathryn_ruddy@dfci.harvard.edu

G.P. Quinn, S.T. Vadaparampil (eds.), *Reproductive Health and Cancer in Adolescents and Young Adults*, Advances in Experimental Medicine and Biology 732,
DOI 10.1007/978-94-007-2492-1_6, © Springer Science+Business Media B.V. 2012

77

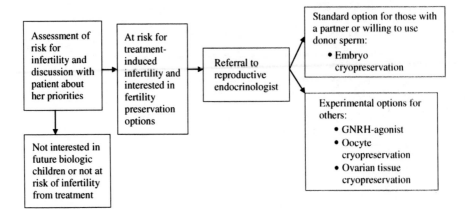

Fig. 6.1 Algorithm for Considering Fertility Issues in Women with Newly Diagnosed Breast Cancer (adapted from Lee et al. [66])

cancer, may also be associated with ovarian dysfunction even apart from breast cancer treatment [1]. Long-term ovarian function is a critical concern for many young breast cancer survivors who are considering the timing and feasibility of childbearing after breast cancer, and for those women who are at risk for infertility, fertility preservation strategies may be considered. Please see Fig. 6.1 for an algorithm for considering fertility issues in women with newly diagnosed breast cancer.

Fertility Concerns

Research suggests that fertility concerns are a major issue for many breast cancer patients both early after diagnosis and later in the survivorship period [2, 3]. In a web-based survey of young breast cancer survivors, the majority, 57%, identified fertility as a major concern at the time of their diagnosis [4]. In a small study comparing breast cancer survivors with regular menses after adjuvant chemotherapy (at least one year after diagnosis) to age-matched, gravidity-matched controls, 80% of survivors but only 25% of controls expressed some concern regarding fertility ($p =$ 0.001) [5]. Ongoing research is investigating how closely fertility concerns at the time of diagnosis are associated with later interest in fertility. A qualitative study of 23 women with early stage

breast cancer who became pregnant after treatment found that pregnancy subsequent to breast cancer is a powerful stimulus for young women to "get well" again [6], but little is known about the psychological impact of surviving cancer and then experiencing infertility. The stress of potential infertility or the experience of infertility may compound the psychological distress of coping with a cancer diagnosis.

Despite the importance of early counseling about fertility issues, according to a survey of 228 women under age 40 when diagnosed with breast cancer, only 71% discussed fertility issues with a health professional as part of oncologic care [7]. This study did not find any relationship between desire for fertility-related information and age, prognosis, or psychological distress. Similarly, a survey of 657 premenopausal women with breast cancer found that only 51% reported that fertility issues had been adequately addressed by their providers [4]. In a slightly older population (less than or equal to 50) of 166 premenopausal breast cancer patients, only 34% recalled a discussion with a physician about fertility, though 68% recalled a discussion about menopause [8]. A recent systematic review of the literature reported that young women with breast cancer prefer to obtain fertility-related information through consultation with a specialist or a decision aid early in the treatment plan [9]. Such decision aids are under development and may inform treatment and fertility preservation choices in young breast cancer patients [10].

Fertility Preservation Techniques for Breast Cancer Patients

Young breast cancer patients who are interested in fertility preservation must make important decisions about whether they wish to actively pursue reproductive technologies before treatment. Embryo cryopreservation, in which oocytes and retrieved, fertilized, and stored as frozen embryos, is the most well-tested method for improving the likelihood of future conception [11]. As in women without cancer, this procedure is most successful when follicular development and oocyte maturation is stimulated hormonally. In vitro maturation has made this technique even more effective than it was previously [12]. However, there are theoretical concerns that the supraphysiologic estradiol levels that occur during conventional ovarian stimulation regimens could stimulate the growth of hormone-receptor positive breast cancers. Therefore, novel stimulation regimens using aromatase inhibitors or tamoxifen have been developed to attempt to minimize the resulting hormonal peak. Oktay and colleagues demonstrated that more embryos were produced using follicle stimulating hormone (FSH) in combination with tamoxifen (3.8 ± 0.8) or letrozole (5.3 ± 0.8) than using tamoxifen alone (1.3 ± 0.2) for ovarian stimulation [13]. Estradiol rates were highest in the group who received tamoxifen in combination with FSH. In this small study, embryo cryopreservation did appear safe, with a breast cancer recurrence rate in the 29 women who underwent embryo cryopreservation that was shown to be similar to that in 31 patients who decided not to undergo the procedure [13]. In a larger sample, Azim et al. [14] found no increase in recurrence or death in 79 breast cancer patients who chose to have embryos stored before treatment using letrozole to stimulate the ovaries compared with 136 patients who were evaluated for but declined the procedure [14]. However, this was a small study with limited follow-up, and meaningful

clinical differences in outcome may not have been detected. Further, the control groups in both of these studies may be biased, as women who are at higher baseline risk may be less likely to want to delay therapy in order to freeze eggs. Thus, the safety of ovarian stimulation and embryo cryopreservation remains controversial in breast cancer patients. Yet, women who strongly value future childbearing sometimes decide that the potential benefits outweigh the risks. Unstimulated egg retrieval is also an option for women who wish to avoid hormonal fluctuations though embryo yield is generally lower than with stimulation. In a recent study of 38 patients who underwent unstimulated egg retrieval, the 18 who stored oocytes had a median of 7 frozen, while the 20 who stored embryos had a median of 4 frozen [15].

Experimental methods such as oocyte cryopreservation and ovarian tissue cryopreservation may be considered for women who do not have a willing male partner and do not wish to use donor sperm to create embryos. Although success rates are lower with oocyte cryopreservation than with embryo cryopreservation (due primarily to intracellular ice formation), techniques have improved recently [16]. Per thawed oocyte, there is currently a 5–6% live birth rate, resulting in more than 500 births to date [17]. Ovarian tissue storage is a promising experimental option for young women with cancer as it does not require ovarian stimulation or a sperm donor at the time of diagnosis. Recently, a case report described healthy twins born to a breast cancer survivor after ovarian cortex extraction, ovarian tissue cryopreservation, ovarian tissue thawing and transplantation, controlled ovarian stimulation (COS), oocyte retrieval, vitrification and in vitro fertilization (IVF), and embryo culture and replacement [18]. This fertility preservation strategy has resulted in few live births to date and there are theoretic concerns that the re-implanted ovarian tissue could harbor cancer cells that might increase the chance of recurrence. Thus, further research to optimize the safety and efficacy of this technique is necessary.

Because stimulation of ovulation is only successful during certain parts of the menstrual cycle, it is essential that cancer patients who are interested in learning about and possibly pursuing embryo or oocyte cryopreservation be referred to a reproductive specialist as soon as possible to minimize treatment delays [19]. Unlike patients with other cancers that require immediate treatment and therefore leave little time for assisted reproduction (e.g., acute leukemias), many women with breast cancer and their physicians are comfortable with a two to six week delay in starting systemic oncologic treatment in order to undergo a cycle of ovarian stimulation and egg harvesting. Furthermore, because most breast cancer patients wait at least several weeks for surgical scheduling and then for healing from surgery before systemic treatment begins, stimulation and egg retrieval can usually be performed within this timeframe and without added delays [20].

Administration of a gonadotropin-releasing hormone agonist (GNRH-a) during chemotherapy (to stop ovarian cycling and hypothetically to reduce susceptibility of ovarian follicles to damage by chemotherapy) is a widely available option for potential fertility preservation, though studies have yielded mixed results to date [21, 22]. Several small non-randomized studies have demonstrated low rates of long-term amenorrhea if GNRH-a is given before and during chemotherapy for breast and other cancers [23–26], but the results of other studies are less promising [21, 27]. Results of larger ongoing studies (such as ZORO and SWOG 0230/POEMS) are awaited to clarify whether this technique actually improves fertility and prevents premature menopause in young survivors after chemotherapy [28, 29].

Predicting Fertility After Breast Cancer Therapy

At this time, it is difficult to predict whether any individual will be able to conceive after her breast cancer therapy is finished. It is also challenging to study subsequent fertility in breast cancer survivors, as only a minority of premenopausal women appear to attempt pregnancy after breast cancer, and menstrual cycling after treatment is an imperfect surrogate for fertility. Some women who experience amenorrhea for months or years after treatment eventually do become pregnant, and others find that they are unable to conceive despite no amenorrhea. Most, but not all, women who are amenorrheic one year after diagnosis remain post-menopausal. However, even women who are menstruating regularly after chemotherapy are likely to enter menopause earlier than they would have otherwise. Modeling data from older adjuvant chemotherapy trials of premenopausal women, Partridge et al. found that even when young women remain premenopausal after treatment, they are still likely to go through menopause prematurely. For example, a woman diagnosed at 25 years old and menstruating 2 years after cyclophosphamide-methotrexate-fluorouracil (CMF) chemotherapy had a 16% risk of menopause 5 years later (at only age 30), and a 75% risk 10 years later (at only age 35) [30]. Despite the imperfect link between menstrual cycling after chemotherapy and potential for future childbearing, amenorrhea is commonly used as a surrogate for fertility in studies of ovarian reserve and fertility.

A number of studies have focused on clarifying what patient or treatment factors predispose to chemotherapy-related amenorrhea. Increasing age is clearly associated with increased likelihood of amenorrhea in survivors of breast cancer, as in survivors of a variety of other cancers. Consistently, studies find that cancer patients who experience amenorrhea are older on average than those who do not [31–34]. Certain chemotherapy regimens are also known to be more likely to cause amenorrhea than others (see section titled The Impact of Specific Chemotherapies on Fertility). However, even amongst women who are all of the same age and receiving the same treatments, there is substantial heterogeneity in whether or not amenorrhea occurs and how long it lasts. This likely reflects individual variability in ovarian reserve or drug metabolism and toxicity.

Research is clearly necessary to improve our understanding of ovarian reserve in breast cancer patients in order to help women who are interested in having future biological children make more informed choices about their treatments and the timing of their childbearing. Those who are trying to decide whether to undergo embryo or oocyte cryopreservation prior to treatment would benefit greatly from a biomarker that could be sent at the time of a breast cancer diagnosis to clarify risk of future infertility or at least, chemotherapy-related amenorrhea [35]. Furthermore, whether or not she receives chemotherapy, a young breast cancer patient may wish to better understand her risk of long-term amenorrhea because this may influence her hormonal therapy choices—some women who desire biologic children may even choose to stop hormonal therapy early in order to attempt pregnancy if they know they are fertile yet have a limited timeframe in which they will remain so [19].

The Impact of Specific Chemotherapies on Fertility

It is well-established that certain chemotherapy drugs are more ovarian toxic than others, but that most regimens used for breast cancer do cause temporary if not permanent amenorrhea in a substantial proportion of premenopausal women. Rates of amenorrhea at one year after treatment have ranged from 16 to 90% in different studies, and vary depending on treatments utilized and age groups of women studied [19]. Alkylating agents such as cyclophosphamide are well-known to impair or destroy ovarian function, with higher cumulative doses associated with greater risk of chemotherapy-related amenorrhea [36–38]. The frequent use of anthracyclines in modern regimens may compound the risk of ovarian toxicity [34]. There are conflicting data regarding whether and how much gonadotoxicity is increased by the addition of a taxane to a given regimen. A retrospective evaluation by Fornier et al. of the addition of a taxane (docetaxel or paclitaxel) to doxorubicin-cyclophosphamide (AC) did not reveal higher amenorrhea rates than historical controls [31]. Abusief et al. similarly reported no difference in amenorrhea rates between AC and AC followed by paclitaxel when confounding variables were controlled [39]. Recently, Sukumvanich et al. reported that patients who received cyclophosphaminde-methotrexate-5-fluorouracil (CMF) were less likely to experience six months of amenorrhea after chemotherapy than were those who received AC or AC-T, but no significant difference was found between AC and AC-T patients [40]. However, another retrospective analysis by Tham et al. did show that three months of a taxane after AC increased the odds of six months of amenorrhea 1.9-fold (95% CI 1.0–3.5, $p = 0.05$) [41], and Han et al. also found that taxane use was a significant predictor for amenorrhea in multivariate analysis of a phase III study of docetaxel-capecitabine (TX) versus AC neoadjuvantly with either AC or fluorouracil with AC (FAC) given adjuvantly. Likewise, Najafi et al. reported that chemotherapy-related amenorrhea was more common in premenopausal women who received taxane in addition to anthracycline than in women who received no taxane (only an anthracycline-based regimen or cyclophosphamide-methotrexate-5-fluorouracil) [42]. Furthermore, a prospective study by Anderson et al. found that regimens that contained taxanes impacted hormonal profiles more than those that did not in a small study of women with early stage breast cancer [43]. A recent evaluation of chemotherapy-induced amenorrhea in China found rates of 45% in 78 patients treated with fluorouracil, epirubicin, and cyclophosphamide (FEC), 30% in 66 patients treated with docetaxel and epirubicin (TE), and 23% in 26 patients treated with Navelbine and epirubicin (NE). Only the difference between the amenorrhea rate on FEC and the rate on NE was statistically significant [44]. The gonadotoxic effects of newer drugs and more modern combinations are less well-studied. Please see Table 6.1 for available data on risk of amenorrhea with adjuvant breast cancer chemotherapy regimens.

Table 6.1 Available data on risk of amenorrhea with adjuvant breast cancer regimens

Regimen	Results from studies including all ages	Age < 40	Age ≥ 40	References
	Percent with CRA (duration varies by study)			
None		<5	20–25	Goldhirsch et al. [37]
Tamoxifen	14	16	74	Goodwin et al. [67], Abusief et al. [39]
AC	53	7–44	28–81	Petrek et al. [38], Bines et al. [36], Burstein and Winer [68], Abusief et al. [39], Sukumvanich et al. [40]
AC-T or AC-D	13–83	10–61	42–85	Petrek et al. [38], Tham et al. [41], Martin et al. [69], Fornier et al. [31], Han et al. [70], Reh et al. [71], Abusief et al. [39], Sukumvanich et al. [40], Swain et al. [72]
AC-TH		14	67	Abusief et al. [39]
CMF	43–82	4–40	36–81	Goldhirsch et al. [37], Bines et al. [36], Levine et al. [73], Petrek et al. [38], Goodwin et al. [67], Parulekar et al. [34], Sukumvanich et al. [40], Najafi et al. [42]
CEF or FEC or ddFEC or FAC	45–93	39–62	75–100	Levine et al. [73], Venturini et al. [74], Goodwin et al. [67], Parulekar et al. [34], Han et al. [70], Zhou et al. [44], Berliere et al. [75], Martin et al. [69]
TX/AC	67–90			Han et al. [70]

AC doxorubicin and cyclophosphamide, *CMF* cyclophosphamide, methotrexate, 5-fluorouracil, *CAF* cyclophosphamide, doxorubicin, 5-fluorouracil, *CEF* cyclophosphamide, epirubicin, 5-fluorouracil, *FAC* 5-fluorouracil, doxorubicin, and cyclophosphamide, *AC-T* AC and paclitaxel, *AC-D* AC and docetaxel, *AC-TH* AC followed by paclitaxel and a year of trastuzumab, *TX/AC* docetaxel and capecitabine (TX) as neoadjuvant therapy and then adjuvant AC or AC as neoadjuvant therapy followed by adjuvant TX, *dd* = dose dense

The Impact of Endocrine Therapy on Fertility

Even women who only receive hormonal therapy may experience infertility related to breast cancer treatment because there is natural waning of ovarian function over time, and because childbearing is contraindicated during hormonal therapy due to risk of teratogenicity. With fertility declining over time, the delay that breast cancer endocrine therapies require is of significant concern to many women. Standard endocrine therapy for premenopausal women entails five years of tamoxifen, during which time natural ovarian

aging can be substantial, though there is no direct damage to the ovaries from tamoxifen or ovarian suppression. A woman who begins tamoxifen at 35 years old is going to be less fertile (and possibly infertile) when she completes her treatment course at age 40. Therefore, some women who are very interested in pursuing pregnancy decide to stop their hormonal therapy early. The timing of this decision is complex, as there is no known accurate indicator of remaining ovarian reserve during tamoxifen therapy. Specifically, menstrual irregularity is not necessarily indicative of waning ovarian function during tamoxifen therapy because the hormonal alterations that are induced by tamoxifen can interfere with regular menses. For example, for a 38-year-old woman who is trying to choose between obtaining optimal tamoxifen benefit by completing 5 years of therapy and stopping tamoxifen at 38 to attempt conception, the data to guide this decision are limited, and the underlying risk of her breast cancer, amount of therapy already received, as well as personal values must be considered.

Measuring Fertility: Ovarian Reserve

Efforts to find biomarkers of ovarian reserve in breast cancer patients have focused on the same hormones that are informative in patients with infertility in the general population. Levels of several hormones that are produced or regulated by the ovaries have shown promise, but those that must be measured at a certain time in the menstrual cycle (e.g., estradiol, FSH, and inhibin B) are less useful in this setting because decisions about fertility preservation for young women with newly diagnosed breast cancer must be made promptly and because of menstrual irregularity that often occurs in survivors on tamoxifen. Anti-mullerian hormone (AMH), expressed by the granulosa cells of the ovaries, can be measured at any point in the menstrual cycle, and therefore may be more practical for this setting [45]. A study by Lutchman Singh et al. showed that AMH levels were comparable between 24 controls and 8 breast cancer patients before chemotherapy, but after chemotherapy, 22 breast cancer patients had lower AMH levels on average [46]. Likewise, Su et al. found that 127 breast cancer survivors had lower AMH levels 2 years post-chemotherapy than age-matched controls [47]. Survivors who were amenorrheic at that time had lower AMH levels than those who were menstruating. Anderson et al. also found that 23 breast cancer patients as old as 52 who became amenorrheic during chemotherapy ($N = 23$) had lower pre-chemotherapy AMH levels than the 19 who continued to menstruate (0.58 vs. 1.9 ng/mL, $p = 0.0007$) [43]. Similarly, Anders et al. found that 16 women under 52 who developed chemotherapy-related

amenorrhea ($N = 16$) had lower AMH levels before chemotherapy (0.16 ng/mL) than 5 women who resumed menses by one year after chemotherapy (0.16 vs. 1.09 ng/mL, $p = 0.02$) [48]. A prospective comparison between 20 breast cancer survivors after chemotherapy and 20 age- and gravidity-matched controls found that antral follicle count, AMH, follicle-stimulating hormone and inhibin B all indicated better ovarian reserve in controls than survivors [49]. However, a recent study of 26 premenopausal women under age 40 suggested that in a younger population, AMH levels before and after chemotherapy were not associated with likelihood of chemotherapy-related amenorrhea at 1 year follow-up (median was 0.98 ng/mL at baseline and 0.06 ng/mL at 1 year in the 11 who had chemotherapy-related amenorrhea at 1 year, comparable to the 0.97 ng/mL and 0.08 ng/mL levels at baseline and 1 year, respectively, in the 15 who had resumed menses) [50]. Thus, more research is needed to clarify whether measuring AMH or other novel biomarkers before chemotherapy can inform our understanding of the likelihood of ovarian function after chemotherapy.

Safety of Pregnancy After Breast Cancer

Studies suggest that 5–15% of young women with breast cancer will later become pregnant [4, 51, 52]. Like most other cancer therapies, breast cancer treatments do not appear to increase the risk of fetal malformations in offspring conceived later [53], though some studies have shown that pregnancies in women who have received cytotoxic chemotherapy for a variety of cancers are more likely to result in low-birth-weight babies and spontaneous abortions [54–56]. A case series found that 22 out of the 23 pregnancies after breast radiation resulted in normal deliveries of healthy infants, and 1 woman delivered a low birth-weight infant [57].

Reassuringly, available data do not support theoretical concerns that recurrence of hormone-receptor positive cancers will be stimulated by elevated estrogen and progesterone levels during pregnancy. Multiple mostly retrospective epidemiologic studies consistently suggest that women who give birth after treatment for breast cancer have equal or better prognoses than those who do not. For example, a study of risk of death in the 2,548 women with a history of breast cancer diagnosed in Finland between 1967–1989 under the age of 40 found that those who had not subsequently delivered a baby were 4.8 times (95% CI 2.2–10.3) as likely to have died in the years following than were those who had given birth to a live child [58]. A similar trend was demonstrated in the Danish Breast Cancer Cooperative Group study, in which 5,725 women diagnosed under 45 with breast cancer were followed for a total of 35,067 patient years of follow-up. The 173 who became pregnant were found to have a statistically non-significant trend toward reduction in risk of death as compared with those who did not become pregnant (RR 0.55, 95% CI 0.28–1.06) [59]. Likewise, in a Swedish study of 2,119 women diagnosed under age 50 with early stage breast cancer between 1971 and 1988, only 8% of the 50 who later became pregnant developed a distant metastasis over the median 7-year follow-up period (median 7 years), compared with 24% of the 2,069 who never became pregnant after breast cancer [60]. The hazard ratio for distant disease recurrence adjusted for node status and age was 0.42 (95% CI 0.16–1.12), with the trend favoring pregnancy, but adjustment for tumor size and ER status was not performed. In a recent study matching 107 members of a Northern California prepaid healthcare plan who became pregnant after a breast cancer diagnosis by age, year and stage at diagnosis, and recurrence status at time when the conception occurred with 344 breast cancer without a subsequent pregnancy, the hazard ratio for death was 1.0 (95% CI 0.6–1.9) [61]. Studying breast cancer survivors who had been age 45 or younger at the time of diagnosis in a single breast center in the United Kingdom, Rippy and colleagues found comparable rates of death between those who did and did not report a pregnancy after breast cancer (6% vs. 10%, respectively),

though sample size was inadequate for statistical testing [62].

Conclusions from these studies are complicated by the potential for a "healthy mother bias" (i.e., women who are less likely to experience recurrence may be more likely to pursue pregnancy). Therefore, it remains unclear whether pregnancy after breast cancer is safe for all women. It is possible that there are subsets of women who may actually benefit from pregnancy after breast cancer and other subsets whose prognoses will be worsened or unchanged by pregnancy-related physiologic alterations. Some physicians recommend that a woman wait at least two years after the cancer diagnosis before attempting to conceive, but this is based primarily on the risk of early recurrence during this time period.

There is, however, evidence that residual ovarian function is associated with an increased risk of recurrence of the cancer. In the International Trial V, women who experienced amenorrhea had a better 4-year disease free survival than those who continued to menstruate regularly (68 vs 61%, $p = 0.05$) [37]. Similarly, Parulekar and colleagues found in a large Canadian clinical trial of CMF versus cyclophosphamide-epirubicin-fluorouracil (CEF) that post-treatment amenorrhea correlated with improved survival in hormone-receptor positive disease [34]. Likewise, Swain et al. found that six months of amenorrhea was associated with improved overall survival in a randomized clinical trial of doxorubicin-cyclophosphamide-docetaxel sequentially versus the same drugs concurrently versus doxorubicin-docetaxel, regardless of treatment group and estrogen-receptor status [63]. Thus, women who are dismayed from a fertility standpoint when they do experience chemotherapy-related amenorrhea can at least be reassured that amenorrhea may improve their prognoses, though definitive data remain outstanding, and it is unclear whether confounders include differential drug metabolism between individuals [64]. The Suppression of Ovarian Function Trial (SOFT), a large international study that randomizes premenopausal breast cancer patients to hormonal therapy with or without ovarian suppressing medication to determine whether five years of no ovarian cycling indeed improves prognosis, should provide more definitive data regarding the potential benefits and risks of allowing ovarian function or not in young breast cancer survivors [65]. This study is unique amongst those of comparable size and scope in that it compares a tamoxifen-alone treatment to tamoxifen with ovarian suppression to an aromatase inhibitor with ovarian suppression. This design will allow investigators to tease out any benefit of the ovarian suppression separately from any benefit of the aromatase inhibitor.

Future Directions for Research

Additional work is needed to clarify the mechanism of chemotherapy-related amenorrhea, and thereby to inform future work to protect against gonadotoxicity from a variety of drugs. Future projects should prospectively evaluate the safety and efficacy of fertility preservation options, develop biomarkers that can be used before and during treatment including hormonal therapy to measure fertility and thus to guide decisions about treatment and reproductive technologies for young breast cancer survivors.

Provider Recommendations

1. Many young women with breast cancer are concerned about fertility.
2. Standard chemotherapy regimens for breast cancer are gonadotoxic, and hormonal regimens allow natural ovarian aging over five years of treatment (during which conception is contraindicated). However, many young women will remain fertile after treatment.
3. Early referral to a reproductive endocrinologist is essential for those who would consider fertility preservation techniques prior to systemic therapy.

References

1. Oktay K et al (2010) Association of BRCA1 mutations with occult primary ovarian insufficiency: a possible explanation for the link between infertility and breast/ovarian cancer risks. J Clin Oncol 28(2):240–244
2. Adams E et al (2011) The experiences, needs and concerns of younger women with breast cancer: a meta-ethnography. Psychooncology 20(8):851–861
3. Hickey M et al (2009) Breast cancer in young women and its impact on reproductive function. Hum Reprod Update 15(3):323–339
4. Partridge AH et al (2004) Web-based survey of fertility issues in young women with breast cancer. J Clin Oncol 22(20):4174–4183
5. Ruddy K et al (2011) Menopausal symptoms and fertility concerns in premenopausal breast cancer survivors. Menopause 18:105–108
6. Dow KH (1994) Having children after breast cancer. Cancer Pract 2(6):407–413
7. Thewes B et al (2005) Fertility- and menopause-related information needs of younger women with a diagnosis of early breast cancer. J Clin Oncol 23(22):5155–5165
8. Duffy CM, Allen SM, Clark MA (2005) Discussions regarding reproductive health for young women with breast cancer undergoing chemotherapy. J Clin Oncol 23(4):766–773
9. Peate M et al (2009) The fertility-related concerns, needs and preferences of younger women with breast cancer: a systematic review. Breast Cancer Res Treat 116(2):215–223
10. Peate M et al (2011) Development and pilot testing of a fertility decision aid for young women diagnosed with early breast cancer. Breast J 17(1):112–114
11. Oktay K, Buyuk E (2004) Fertility preservation in women undergoing cancer treatment. Lancet 363(9423):1830
12. Oktay K et al (2010) In vitro maturation improves oocyte or embryo cryopreservation outcome in breast cancer patients undergoing ovarian stimulation for fertility preservation. Reprod Biomed Online 20(5):634–638
13. Oktay K et al (2005) Fertility preservation in breast cancer patients: a prospective controlled comparison of ovarian stimulation with tamoxifen and letrozole for embryo cryopreservation. J Clin Oncol 23(19):4347–4353
14. Azim AA, Costantini-Ferrando M, Oktay K (2008) Safety of fertility preservation by ovarian stimulation with letrozole and gonadotropins in patients with breast cancer: a prospective controlled study. J Clin Oncol 26(16):2630–2635
15. Huang JY et al (2010) Retrieval of immature oocytes from unstimulated ovaries followed by in vitro maturation and vitrification: A novel strategy of fertility preservation for breast cancer patients. Am J Surg 200(1):177–183

16. Hulvat MC, Jeruss JS (2009) Maintaining fertility in young women with breast cancer. Curr Treat Options Oncol 10(5–6):308–317

17. Porcu E et al (2008) Human oocyte cryopreservation in infertility and oncology. Curr Opin Endocrinol Diab Obes 15(6):529–535

18. Sanchez-Serrano M et al (2010) Twins born after transplantation of ovarian cortical tissue and oocyte vitrification. Fertil Steril 93(1):268 e11–e13

19. Partridge AH, Ruddy KJ (2007) Fertility and adjuvant treatment in young women with breast cancer. Breast 2(16 Suppl):S175–S181

20. Madrigrano A, Westphal L, Wapnir I (2007) Egg retrieval with cryopreservation does not delay breast cancer treatment. Am J Surg 194(4):477–481

21. Giuseppe L et al (2007) Ovarian function after cancer treatment in young women affected by Hodgkin disease (HD). Hematology 12(2):141–147

22. Badawy A et al (2009) Gonadotropin-releasing hormone agonists for prevention of chemotherapy-induced ovarian damage: prospective randomized study. Fertil Steril 91(3):694–697

23. Recchia F et al (2006) Gonadotropin-releasing hormone analogues added to adjuvant chemotherapy protect ovarian function and improve clinical outcomes in young women with early breast carcinoma. Cancer 106(3):514–523

24. Urruticoechea A et al (2008) Ovarian protection with goserelin during adjuvant chemotherapy for premenopausal women with early breast cancer (EBC). Breast Cancer Res Treat 110(3):411–416

25. Blumenfeld Z, Eckman A (2005) Preservation of fertility and ovarian function and minimization of chemotherapy-induced gonadotoxicity in young women by GnRH-a. J Natl Cancer Inst Monogr 34:40–43

26. Sverrisdottir A et al (2009) Adjuvant goserelin and ovarian preservation in chemotherapy treated patients with early breast cancer: results from a randomized trial. Breast Cancer Res Treat 117(3):561–567

27. Ismail-Khan R et al. (2008) Preservation of ovarian function in young women treated with neoadjuvant chemotherapy for breast cancer: a randomized trial using the GnRH agonist (triptorelin) during chemotherapy. In American Society of clinical oncology annual meeting, Chicago, IL

28. Gerber B et al (2009) ZORO: a prospective randomized multicenter study to prevent chemotherapy-induced ovarian failure with the GnRH-agonist goserelin in young hormone-insensitive breast cancer patients receiving anthracycline containing (neo-) adjuvant chemotherapy (GBG 37). In 2009 ASCO annual meeting

29. Southwest Oncology Group: The Group Newsletter (2008) [cited; Volume 22, No. 1: [Available from: http://www.swog.org/Visitors/Download/Newsletters/Newsletter022008.pdf

30. Partridge A et al (2007) Age of menopause among women who remain premenopausal following treatment for early breast cancer: long-term results from International Breast Cancer Study Group Trials V and VI. Eur J Cancer 43(11):1646–1653

31. Fornier MN et al (2005) Incidence of chemotherapy-induced, long-term amenorrhea in patients with breast carcinoma age 40 years and younger after adjuvant anthracycline and taxane. Cancer 104(8):1575–1579

32. Koyama H et al (1977) Cyclophosphamide-induced ovarian failure and its therapeutic significance in patients with breast cancer. Cancer 39(4):1403–1409

33. Minton SE, Munster PN (2002) Chemotherapy-induced amenorrhea and fertility in women undergoing adjuvant treatment for breast cancer. Cancer Control 9(6):466–472

34. Parulekar WR et al (2005) Incidence and prognostic impact of amenorrhea during adjuvant therapy in high-risk premenopausal breast cancer: analysis of a National Cancer Institute of Canada Clinical Trials Group Study–NCIC CTG MA.5.. J Clin Oncol 23(25):6002–6008

35. Ruddy KJ, Partridge AH (2009) Fertility. In: Castiglione M, Piccart MJ (eds) Adjuvant therapy for breast cancer. Springer, The Netherlands, pp 367–385

36. Bines J, Oleske DM, Cobleigh MA (1996) Ovarian function in premenopausal women treated with adjuvant chemotherapy for breast cancer. J Clin Oncol 14(5):1718–1729

37. Goldhirsch A, Gelber RD, Castiglione M (1990) The magnitude of endocrine effects of adjuvant chemotherapy for premenopausal breast cancer patients. The International Breast Cancer Study Group. Ann Oncol 1(3):183–188

38. Petrek JA et al (2006) Incidence, time course, and determinants of menstrual bleeding after breast cancer treatment: a prospective study. J Clin Oncol 24(7):1045–1051

39. Abusief ME et al (2010) The effects of paclitaxel, dose density, and trastuzumab on treatment-related amenorrhea in premenopausal women with breast cancer. Cancer 116(4):791–798

40. Sukumvanich P et al (2010) Incidence and time course of bleeding after long-term amenorrhea after breast cancer treatment: a prospective study. Cancer 116(13):3102–3111

41. Tham YL et al (2007) The rates of chemotherapy-induced amenorrhea in patients treated with adjuvant doxorubicin and cyclophosphamide followed by a taxane. Am J Clin Oncol 30(2):126–132

42. Najafi S et al (2011) Taxane-based regimens as a risk factor for chemotherapy-induced amenorrhea. Menopause 18(2):208–212

43. Anderson RA et al (2006) The effects of chemotherapy and long-term gonadotrophin suppression on the ovarian reserve in premenopausal women with breast cancer. Hum Reprod 21(10):2583–2592

44. Zhou WB et al (2010) Incidence of chemotherapy-induced amenorrhea associated with epirubicin, docetaxel and navelbine in younger breast cancer patients. BMC Cancer 10:281

45. La Marca A et al (2010) Anti-Mullerian hormone (AMH) as a predictive marker in assisted reproductive technology (ART). Hum Reprod Update 16(2):113–130
46. Lutchman Singh K et al (2007) Predictors of ovarian reserve in young women with breast cancer. Br J Cancer 96(12):1808–1816
47. Su HI et al (2010) Antimullerian hormone and inhibin B are hormone measures of ovarian function in late reproductive-aged breast cancer survivors. Cancer 116(3):592–599
48. Anders C et al (2008) A pilot study of predictive markers of chemotherapy-related amenorrhea among premenopausal women with early stage breast cancer. Cancer Invest 26(3):286–295
49. Partridge AH et al (2010) Ovarian reserve in women who remain premenopausal after chemotherapy for early stage breast cancer. Fertil Steril 94(2):634–644
50. Yu B et al (2010) Changes in markers of ovarian reserve and endocrine function in young women with breast cancer undergoing adjuvant chemotherapy. Cancer 116(9):2099–2105
51. Fox KR, Scialla J, Moore H (2003) Preventing chemotherapy-related amenorrhea using leuprolide during adjuvant chemotherapy for early-stage breast cancer [abstract 50]. Proc Am Soc Clin Onc 22:13
52. Ives A et al (2007) Pregnancy after breast cancer: population based study. BMJ 334(7586):194
53. Hawkins MM (1994) Pregnancy outcome and offspring after childhood cancer. BMJ 309(6961):1034
54. Blakely LJ et al (2004) Effects of pregnancy after treatment for breast carcinoma on survival and risk of recurrence. Cancer 100(3):465–469
55. Velentgas P et al (1999) Pregnancy after breast carcinoma: outcomes and influence on mortality. Cancer 85(11):2424–2432
56. Mulvihill JJ et al (1987) Pregnancy outcome in cancer patients. Experience in a large cooperative group. Cancer 60(5):1143–1150
57. Dow KH, Harris JR, Roy C (1994) Pregnancy after breast-conserving surgery and radiation therapy for breast cancer. J Natl Cancer Inst Monogr 16:131–137
58. Sankila R, Heinavaara S, Hakulinen T (1994) Survival of breast cancer patients after subsequent term pregnancy: "healthy mother effect". Am J Obstet Gynecol 170(3):818–823
59. Kroman N et al (1997) Time since childbirth and prognosis in primary breast cancer: population based study. BMJ 315(7112):851–855
60. von Schoultz E et al (1995) Influence of prior and subsequent pregnancy on breast cancer prognosis. J Clin Oncol 13(2):430–434
61. Kranick JA et al (2010) Is pregnancy after breast cancer safe? Breast J 16(4):404–411
62. Rippy EE, Karat IF, Kissin MW (2009) Pregnancy after breast cancer: the importance of active counselling and planning. Breast 18(6):345–350
63. Swain SM et al (2010) Longer therapy, iatrogenic amenorrhea, and survival in early breast cancer. N Engl J Med 362(22):2053–2065
64. Ellis M (2010) Taxane-based chemotherapy for node-positive breast cancer–take-home lessons. N Engl J Med 362(22):2122–2124
65. Puhalla S, Brufsky A, Davidson N (2009) Adjuvant endocrine therapy for premenopausal women with breast cancer. Breast 18(Suppl 3):S122–S1230
66. Lee SJ et al (2006) American Society of Clinical Oncology recommendations on fertility preservation in cancer patients. J Clin Oncol 24(18):2917–2931
67. Goodwin PJ et al (1999) Risk of menopause during the first year after breast cancer diagnosis. J Clin Oncol 17(8):2365–2370
68. Burstein HJ, Winer EP (2000) Primary care for survivors of breast cancer. N Engl J Med 343(15):1086–1094
69. Martin M et al (2005) Adjuvant docetaxel for node-positive breast cancer. N Engl J Med 352(22):2302–2313
70. Han HS et al (2008) Analysis of chemotherapy-induced amenorrhea rates by three different anthracycline and taxane containing regimens for early breast cancer. Breast Cancer Res Treat 115(2):335–342
71. Reh A, Oktem O, Oktay K (2008) Impact of breast cancer chemotherapy on ovarian reserve: a prospective observational analysis by menstrual history and ovarian reserve markers. Fertil Steril 90(5):1635–1639
72. Swain SM et al (2009) Amenorrhea in premenopausal women on the doxorubicin-and-cyclophosphamide-followed-by-docetaxel arm of NSABP B-30 trial. Breast Cancer Res Treat 113(2):315–320
73. Levine MN et al (1998) Randomized trial of intensive cyclophosphamide, epirubicin, and fluorouracil chemotherapy compared with cyclophosphamide, methotrexate, and fluorouracil in premenopausal women with node-positive breast cancer. National Cancer Institute of Canada Clinical Trials Group. J Clin Oncol 16(8):2651–2658
74. Venturini M et al (2005) Dose-dense adjuvant chemotherapy in early breast cancer patients: results from a randomized trial. J Natl Cancer Inst 97(23):1724–1733
75. Berliere M et al (2008) Incidence of reversible amenorrhea in women with breast cancer undergoing adjuvant anthracycline-based chemotherapy with or without docetaxel. BMC Cancer 8:56

Pregnancy and Cancer

7

Celso Silva, MD and Farah S. Chung, MD

My partner and I agreed we wanted a big family so as soon as we agreed we were going to be a couple we wanted to get started on that family. I was thrilled when I got pregnant right away and relieved that the morning sickness wasn't too bad. Except for the odd looking mole I had developed on my growing belly, I felt great and people told me I looked healthy. My OB/GYN said the mole was probably nothing but suggested I see a dermatologist. I made the appointment more out of vanity than real concern and so it didn't occur to me to bring anyone with me to the dermatologist. My partner and my sister had come to every OB/GYN apt with me but I thought I was going to just run in for a quick appointment and the doctor would tell me this mole would go away after pregnancy. But, it didn't happen that way. I was by myself when the dermatologist told me she was concerned and suspected melanoma. My head was spinning as I thought about who to call first – my sister? My partner? My OB-GYN? A priest? So I just sat there in the office not calling anyone and rationalized to myself that everything was fine and there must be a mistake. Hours later I was on the Internet trying to find out what the odds were of getting cancer while pregnant. Whatever those odds were, they had found me. A week later it was confirmed – I had advanced melanoma and I was 5 months pregnant.

I was told I could have surgery right away with no harm to my baby, but the additional treatment I was likely to need could not be administered safely while I was pregnant. My doctor said my chances of long-term survival would be significantly improved if I had chemo right away, but I couldn't do it while I was pregnant. My sister said she just wanted me alive – whatever it took. My partner said he didn't even see what the quandary was because if I didn't survive there would be no baby and no mother to raise the baby.

I wanted this baby as much as I wanted to live, and I didn't want one more or less than the other. I asked my sister if she would promise to raise this baby if anything happened to me and although she said she couldn't bear to think about it, she agreed. That was the tipping point for me. I decided to eschew the medical advice and go on with the pregnancy and delay treatment.

My son was born healthy 3 months later although I eventually agreed to an early inducement so I could begin treatment. My partner thought I was crazy and ended our relationship but I am hopeful he will continue to see his son. I have good days and bad days now. The treatment has been exhausting and my oncologist says he is not seeing the progress he had hoped. I don't regret my decision. Today my son took his first steps and that was such a joy to witness. Will I be here to see him run or go to school or learn to drive? I don't know, and really none of us knows. I may die tomorrow from cancer and you may die in a car accident. What matters is today and for today, my son smiling and laughing and learning how to walk. I just take it one day at a time.
Debbie, Adult Cancer Patient

C. Silva (✉)
Assistant Professor, Director - Center for Fertility
Preservation, USF IVF, Division of Reproductive
Endocrinology and Infertility, Department of Obstetrics
and Gynecology, University of South Florida, Tampa,
FL, USA
e-mail: csilva@health.usf.edu

G.P. Quinn, S.T. Vadaparampil (eds.), *Reproductive Health and Cancer in Adolescents and Young Adults*, Advances in Experimental Medicine and Biology 732,
DOI 10.1007/978-94-007-2492-1_7, © Springer Science+Business Media B.V. 2012

Introduction

Cancer is the second most common cause of death in women of reproductive age, with the incidence of cancer in pregnancy ranging from 0.07 to 0.1% [1]. As cancer therapy is becoming more efficacious and women are waiting later to begin childbearing, cancer in pregnancy as well as pregnancy in cancer survivors are both increasing in prevalence. With the increasing survival of cancer patients, issues regarding the quality of life in cancer survivors are becoming progressively more important. Unfortunately, many of the successful treatment options for cancer lead to infertility. In a time of tragedy, while facing the new diagnosis of cancer, it is very difficult for patients to think about the implications of their therapies. As a healthcare provider, one must weigh a variety of considerations in such circumstances including but not limited to the clinical, biological, ethical, legal and psychosocial issues surrounding cancer and pregnancy.

Through this chapter, it is the intent that the reader will gain a general understanding of the following:

- Basic reproductive physiology,
- Common cancer therapies and their implications on reproductive capacity,
- Methods of fertility preservation,
- Diagnosing cancer in the pregnant patient, and
- Treatment of the most common cancers found in pregnant patients.

A Quick Review

Female reproductive physiology is an integrative, complex chain of events. The female reproductive system must produce gametes while offering a favorable environment for fertilization, implantation and growth of a fetus. During embryogenesis, the first population of primordial germ cells appears in the proximal epiblast of the egg cylinder. During gastrulation, this initial population of germ cells migrate from the anterior to the posterior epiblast, and subsequently migrate through the allantois and hindgut of the embryo, until they arrive in the genital ridge by the sixth week of gestation [2]. Following this migration, rapid mitotic replication occurs and the female embryo reaches the peak number of six to seven million primordial follicles at 16–20 week gestation. At birth the number of primordial follicles decreases to one to two million and at puberty there are only 300,000 oocytes remaining. This process is not completely understood, but it seems to be due to atresia and apoptosis of follicles. Of the follicles present at puberty, only about five hundred will become mature and release oocytes, and the rest will become atretic. At age 51, the average age of menopause in women in developed countries, there are only about 1,000 follicles left [2].

Prior to spontaneous ovulation, there is a degenerative process referred to as oocyte attrition. Every month, a woman develops in general one dominant follicle, and ultimately she ovulates one single mature oocyte. However, during this process there are dozens of follicles that are consumed during the recruitment of this one dominant follicle. As there is a "fixed pool" of primordial follicles endowed at birth that is constantly diminishing, any insult to the ovary that leads to less primordial follicles or an acceleration of the depletion of these follicles may potentially result in early premature ovarian failure and potentially sacrifice fertility. While there are many unknown environmental and genetic causes that may accelerate this process, there are also several iatrogenic factors. Some of these iatrogenic factors include but are not limited to chemotherapy and radiation therapy.

The stark decline in germ cells is mirrored by a decrease in fertility. This is a well-known phenomenon. Women of advanced maternal age have a decline in their fecundity rates as well as a decline in the success rate of assisted reproductive techniques (ART), and this is thought to be secondary to qualitative and quantitative changes in oocytes developmental potential and oocyte numbers. The oocyte can be isolated as the causative agent for the age-related decline in reproductive capacity because, conversely, when older patients use donor oocytes, pregnancy rates after ART are similar to those encountered in young patients. Therefore, often times, reproductive endocrinologists will evaluate a patient's ovarian reserve, by measuring their menstrual cycle day 3 follicle stimulating hormone (FSH) and estradiol levels. Additional techniques to assess ovarian reserve include antral follicle count on transvaginal ultrasound as well as the serum level of anti-mullerian hormone. Prior to embarking on any infertility treatment or fertility preservation strategies, one must evaluate the patient's ovarian reserve to adequately counsel them about their chances of success.

Treating a Woman with Cancer

While making a treatment plan for oncology patients, the patient's future fertility must be considered prior to starting on a path that may negatively affect a patient's reproductive capabilities. In cancer survivors, the issue of fertility is a significant quality of life concern [3]. The American Society of Clinical Oncology and the American Society for Reproductive Medicine champion the importance of healthy survivorship, and they have released recommendations to serve as guidance for oncologists and other providers regarding the importance and availability of fertility preservation techniques [4]. Unfortunately, there are still unknown barriers resulting that only a minority of oncology patients receive adequate counseling and referral before their cancer therapy as far as the potential impact on their reproductive potential and the available options [5–7]. Research has shown that increasing a patient's knowledge and understanding of their disease and treatment confers many long term benefits, including greater satisfaction as well as less anxiety and depression [8]. For women of reproductive age, a large number of whom have not conceived or completed their childbearing, the diagnosis of cancer poses many clinical challenges related to reproductive health.

The majority of chemotherapeutic drugs act by inhibiting the cell replication cycle by interrupting vital cell processes. The ovary itself is extremely chemosensitive [9]. There have been several studies looking at a variety of chemotherapy agents and their effects on reproductive

performance. Frequently, oncologists use a combination of chemotherapeutic agents to attain a synergistic effect. Unfortunately, this can also potentiate their adverse effects. The impact of chemotherapeutic drugs on gonadal function is dependent on the nature and total dosage of medications received by the patient, as well as the length of the treatment and the patient's baseline ovarian reserve which is directly proportional to her age. Therefore, prior to embarking on fertility preservation strategies, one must evaluate the patient's ovarian reserve to adequately counsel them about their potential future fertility. Ovarian reserve testing is also indicated when managing cancer survivors as it will provide a guide for how aggressive one should be in pursuing fertility therapy.

Briefly, we will review a variety of common chemotherapeutic agents and their effects on the gonads. Alkylating agents are associated with the greatest risk among all chemotherapeutic agents for inducing ovarian failure. They are known to have the highest risk of ovarian toxicity and induction of premature ovarian failure. The proposed process by which this occurs is thought to be due to ovarian fibrosis and oocyte depletion [10]. In a study looking at cyclophosphamide, an alkylating agent, when used to treat rheumatological diseases, there was a 26% premature ovarian failure rate. This was highly related to the patient's age at the start of treatment [11]. In a study performed by Warne and colleagues in 1973, ovarian biopsies were performed in patients who were exposed to cyclophosphamide. The biopsies demonstrated a complete absence of oocytes or a small pool of inactive oocytes with fibrosis [12]. Platinum agents, such as cisplatin, have also been demonstrated to promote chromosomal damage in oocytes during early embryogenesis, and it has been associated with embryo mortality and marked aneuploidy [10]. Animal studies have also demonstrated high levels of aneuploidy as a result of vinca alkaloids such as vinblastine [13]. Adriamycin and bleomycin, both anthracycline derivatives, have been demonstrated to be female specific mutagens leading to dominant lethal mutations in maturing and preovulatory oocytes in female mice [10]. Besides its direct effect on the germ cells, systemic chemotherapy can also damage the steroid producing cells of the ovary, particularly the theca and granulosa cells, thereby affecting central hypothalamic-pituitary-ovarian axis by feedback mechanisms [14, 15]. This, in combination with a depleted pool of follicles and abnormal germ cells, may lead to premature ovarian failure and menopause, ultimately rendering survivors infertile [14–16]. It is important to remember that the term "premature ovarian failure" does not equal menopause as there have been case reports of females with premature ovarian failure and sporadic ovulation resulting in pregnancies.

In terms of radiation therapy, ovarian follicles are particularly susceptible to ionizing radiation. The degree and persistence of the damage depends on the dose, irradiation field and the patient's age. Exposure to radiation may induce ovarian atrophy and reduced primordial follicle reserve. Gosden and colleagues demonstrated that there is dose-related depletion of primordial follicles in mouse ovaries after increasing the radiation doses [17, 18]. The total dose of radiation to the pelvis required to increase the risk of premature ovarian failure in a reproductive age female is estimated to be 20 Gy [19]. In a study by Lushbaugh and Casarett, women under the age of 40 years were demonstrated to be less sensitive to radiation induced ovarian damage, and they required 20 Gy to produce permanent ovarian damage as compared to 6 Gy in women >40 years of age [20].

Detrimental radiation effects are not confined to the ovaries. The uterus is also known to be susceptible to radiation effects including but not limited to irreversible changes in the myometrium, endometrium and uterine blood flow, as well as hormone resistant endometrial insufficiency [21]. These changes can be associated with higher rates of obstetrical complications, especially if the pregnancy occurs within 12 months of treatment. It is therefore advisable for women to wait at least 12 months following treatment before trying to conceive [22]. Obstetrical complications that occur as a result of radiation include spontaneous abortions, preterm labor, and low birth weight infants [21, 22]. Teratogenicity is not a problem as long as the patient is not pregnant while receiving radiation.

Non-pelvic radiation can also impact a patient's fertility. One example is cerebral irradiation. Irradiation of the brain may disrupt the patient's central axis leading to hypogonadotropic hypogonadism [23]. Fortunately, these patients are treated relatively simply with replacement of gonadotropins or gonadotropin releasing hormones (GnRH).

Fertility Preservation

The American Society of Clinical Oncology recommends that the impact of cancer therapy on future reproductive function be discussed by the providers with all patients who will need therapy, and those patients who express interest in knowing more about the available options for fertility preservation should be referred to a reproductive endocrinologist for further counseling. It is not possible to predict accurately who will or will not develop reproductive dysfunction after cancer therapy. Furthermore, it is also not possible to predict accurately who, from those who had an initial evidence of reproductive dysfunction, will ultimately resume normal reproductive capacity. A prudent physician cannot provide confident assurance that this will be the case. Numerous studies, both prospective and retrospective, have examined this and demonstrated that many variables such as age, type of chemotherapy and dose (including cumulative doses), and site of radiation therapy influence fertility in the cancer survivor [24–28]. Many patients who experience irregular menses or amenorrhea may regain their pre-treatment menstrual pattern even after a long period of time. Research has also demonstrated that patients with regular menses and a normal reproductive cycle following treatment may still have occult ovarian insufficiency, which may translate into reproductive dysfunction, and these patients are also at a higher risk for premature ovarian failure [13, 29–32]. Researchers have also suggested that patients with normal ovarian function following high dose chemotherapy and/or radiation should not delay childbearing if it is desired. Ovarian function is more likely to return in younger patients, usually within a 2–3 year time frame. Those that strongly desire fertility should be reassessed periodically as the effects can be both acute and cumulative. It is, however, recommended that cancer survivors abstain from pregnancy for the first year following chemotherapy to reduce possible toxic effects of the treatment on maturing oocytes [33]. If fertility is not desired, then appropriate contraceptive options should be undertaken to avoid pregnancy.

As more reproductive-age women survive cancer, the need for viable and successful fertility preservation options has become a priority. Many special interest groups, such as the Lance Armstrong's Livestrong Fertile Hope Foundation and the American Cancer Society, have highlighted and emphasized the importance of patient awareness regarding fertility preservation options. The optimal approach to fertility preservation depends on a variety of variable including: the type of cancer, the type of cancer treatment that is being indicated, the time available before cancer treatment is initiated, and finally the patient's age and partner status.

Fertility preservation and family building strategies can be divided in options to be used before cancer therapy, during cancer therapy and after cancer therapy. Options that can be used before cancer therapy include: embryo cryopreservation, oocyte cryopreservation, ovarian tissue cryopreservation, ovarian transposition and radical trachelectomy. Options used during cancer therapy include: ovarian suppression and ovarian shielding. Options that are used after cancer therapy, in cases where unfortunately premature ovarian failure has already occurred, include donor embryos, donor oocytes, gestational carrier or surrogacy, and adoption.

Embryo cryopreservation is the most widely used method for the past 20 years. Through this technique, women undergo ovulation induction with gonadotropins in order to obtain multifollicular development, allowing that several oocytes are obtained in one single cycle. After the oocytes

are removed, the patient is then allowed to initiate cancer therapy. The oocytes are subsequently fertilized in vitro. The obtained embryos are frozen for future use, at which time they are transferred to the patient's uterus in a relatively simple outpatient procedure. One of the limitations of embryo cryopreservation is the need for sperm for the in vitro fertilization process. Although women have the option of using donor sperm, this may not be an acceptable option for many families or patients.

Fortunately, oocyte cryopreservation has become an acceptable alternative due to procedural advances over the past 15 years, thus eliminating the requirement for donor sperm in patients not currently in a relationship. In this procedure, after the oocytes are obtained, they are frozen before the in vitro fertilization process. Up until recently, the pregnancy rates obtained with oocyte cryopreservation were low, and the procedure was deemed to be experimental. More recently, with the use of new cryopreservation techniques, the success rates have become much higher, approaching the pregnancy rates obtained with embryo cryopreservation.

The results obtained when ovarian downregulation with oral contraceptives or GnRH analogues is used as an option for fertility preservation are controversial. Blumenfield and colleagues were the first to demonstrate that GnRH agonists could make the germinal epithelium less susceptible to the cytotoxic effects of chemotherapy by inhibiting pituitary gonadotropin secretion [34]. However, other studies have failed to achieve the same results [35]. The rationale for this technique is that if the ovarian metabolism is suppressed, potentially any negative effect of the chemotherapy would be minimized, perhaps by inhibition of feedback mechanisms that would stimulate a larger follicular pool. However, the use of oral contraceptives and GnRH agonist do not prevent the physiological atrophy of germ cells via oocyte attrition, and therefore this may explain the overall lack of success.

Ovarian transposition is also a well-known fertility preservation strategy. This technique is indicated in cases where radiation therapy aimed at the pelvic area is to be used. The technique involves the physical relocation of the ovary from its usual pelvic location to a location higher in the abdomen, after the ovarian vessels are mobilized. The procedure requires a surgical intervention, but it can usually be performed laparoscopically. Care must be taken to avoid disruption of the ovarian blood supply which could compromise subsequent ovarian function. Recently, a study by Martin and colleagues suggested a combined approach with the translocation of one ovary and the cryopreservation of the other. It has been suggested that this may lead to less treatment failures as one is employing multiple preservation strategies [36].

Ovarian tissue cryopreservation is one of the most promising methods of preserving fertility. This approach would be extremely valuable for young pre-menarche patients, in whom ovarian superovulation with gonadotropins is not yet possible. The goal of ovarian tissue cryopreservation is to maintain the viability of tissue for an extended storage time. The process involves cooling tissue in a cryoprotectant fluid from the 37°C body temperature to the temperature of liquid nitrogen (−196°C). The tissue is then stored at this temperature in a container of liquid nitrogen.

In general, the technique of cryopreservation is a complex procedure. There are three major mechanisms of damage that occur at different temperature ranges. The first is a chilling injury. This occurs between 15 and −5°C. The next is ice crystal formation between −5 and −80°C. Finally, there is fracture damage. This is the mechanical effect of solidified fluid within the cell that occurs between −50 and −150°C [37].

To prevent cell damage there are numerous ways to avoid the formation of ice crystals. There are permeating and non-permeating agents that allow the cell to freeze without intracellular ice crystal formation. One methodology is to subject the embryos to a slow freeze. In this method, the temperature is lowered at a very slow rate of about 0.33°C/min until reaching −32°C, at which point the tissue is exposed to liquid nitrogen where it is rapidly cooled to −196°C. A second method is vitrification. Vitrification is performed by a rapid freezing. High doses of permeating

cryoprotectants are used and once equilibrated, the sample is placed immediately in liquid nitrogen. These samples must also undergo rapid thawing to prevent the formation of ice crystals [37].

As mentioned, the most widely used and accepted method of fertility preservation is the storage of frozen embryos. Of the methods that involve Assisted Reproductive Techniques, embryo cryopreservation is endorsed by the American Society of Clinical Oncology and the American Society for Reproductive Medicine. Conversely, oocyte cryopreservation and ovarian tissue cryopreservation are considered experimental.

It is important to highlight that in traditional stimulation protocols for ovarian superovulation using gonadotropins, there are exceedingly high levels of estradiol (greater than 10x the normal range). This may be of concern if the patient has a hormonally-sensitive malignancy, such as breast cancer, given the theoretical risk that this supra-physiologic levels of estrogen may stimulate the development of new tumors, decrease the response for therapy, or increase the risk for recurrence. For these patients, there are alternative stimulation protocols that involve drugs which can maintain the estrogen levels at more physiologic levels. These drugs include aromatase inhibitors and selective estrogen receptor modulators.

There are other potential drawbacks with the embryo and oocyte cryopreservation. First, the time requirement for oocyte maturation with ovulation induction is generally about 2 weeks from the onset of menses. Furthermore, follicular and oocyte maturation usually begins within the last few days of the prior menstrual cycle and the first few days of the current cycle. Therefore, depending upon when a patient presents to initiate a cycle of fertility preservation, it may be necessary that she waits for her next menstrual cycle prior to the initiation of the stimulation protocol. Secondly, when embryos are being frozen, an acceptable source of sperm must be available. This can be a predicament if the patient is not currently in a relationship where her partner is willing to donate sperm. Thus, if a patient desires embryo cryopreservation and does not have a partner willing to participate, the difficult decision of using sperm donation must be made. Despite these drawbacks, the pregnancy rates with embryo cryopreservation are good. The survival rates per thawed embryo range from 35 to 90% and implantation rates from 8 to 30% [38]. The cumulative pregnancy rate with this technique has been reported to be up to 60% [16, 39].

An alternative to embryo cryopreservation when a male partner is not available or the patient and/or the family does not want to consider sperm donation is the use of oocyte cryopreservation. With this technology, mature oocytes are obtained by a similar process as described above. Rather than freezing embryos, the oocytes themselves are frozen. Since a mature oocyte is a very large cell that contains a large proportion of cytoplasm, and the cytoplasm is composed mainly of water, there is a concern for damage during cryopreservation secondary to the formation of ice crystal in the cytoplasm. Furthermore, depolymerization of the meiotic spindle has also been demonstrated when the oocyte is exposed to low temperatures, but a number of studies have demonstrated that the spindle can reform in oocytes during the thawing process [40–45]. Another known side effect of oocyte preservation is the hardening of the zona pellucida via premature cortical granule reaction [46]. This can be overcome with the use of intra cytoplasmic sperm injection (ICSI), a procedure by which a single sperm is introduced into each oocyte using a microscopic needle.

Another technique that is gaining force is In Vitro Maturation (IVM). In this technique, immature oocytes can be obtained from the ovaries without any prior gonadotropin stimulation or minimally stimulated ovaries. This is most easily accomplished in patients with polycystic ovarian syndrome as they have a greater number of small follicles in the ovaries. After retrieval, prior to freezing, the oocytes may or may not undergo in vitro maturation. The potential advantage of freezing immature oocytes is that they are smaller in size and less metabolically active than mature oocytes. This technique has several potential advantages over embryo cryopreservation as the time for ovulation induction is diminished (therefore not significantly delaying the initiation of the cancer therapy), and it alleviates the need for gonadotropin stimulation with its resultant supra-physiologic levels of estradiol. Finally, the need for a sperm source is temporarily eliminated.

As mentioned, ovarian tissue cryopreservation is still considered an experimental technique. The ovarian tissue can be obtained through a laparotomy, but in the vast majority of the cases, a laparoscopy is used. Tissue is obtained by either performing several ovarian biopsies, partial oophorectomy, or unilateral versus bilateral oophorectomy. The whole ovary or small sections of the ovary are then cryopreserved. Once the patient is ready to attempt pregnancy, it is then possible to attempt to obtain oocytes from this frozen tissue, which is then in vitro matured, fertilized, and a subsequent uterine embryo transfer is performed. Alternatively, once a patient is in remission, the frozen tissue can be thawed and transplanted back into the patient. There are two methods by which this is performed, orthotopic and heterotopic transplantation [39]. Orthotopic transplantation involves the preserved tissue being transplanted back into the ovarian fossa or ovarian remnant, its initial location. Heterotopic transplantation involves the placement of the preserved tissue in the forearm or anterior abdominal wall. Once transplanted back, it is expected that the harvested tissue will resume endogenous production of hormones and oocytes. There have been two reported cases in the literature of pregnancies following orthotopic transplantation. The controversy surrounding this technique is that it is difficult to ascertain if the oocyte that generated the pregnancy came from the remnant ovary or the transplanted tissue as even quiescent ovaries may ovulate [47]. Furthermore, there is the theoretical risk of reseeding tumor cells at the time of the cryopreserved tissue transplantation. Obviously, the advantage of this technique is that there are no time delays since the tissue can be obtained immediately, there is no need for ovarian stimulation, and no partner is needed at the time of tissue harvesting.

If a patient is not a candidate for any of the above procedures, it is possible that she may use donor oocytes. This technique is employed when the disease is in remission and premature ovarian failure is established. Many patients are not able to undergo the above described fertility preservation options due to a variety of reasons, including but not limited to costs of the procedures, insufficient time before the initiation of the cancer therapy, unwillingness to take the risk of ovulation induction, fear that the fertility preservation procedures will interfere with the cancer therapy or increase the chance for cancer recurrence, lack of a male partner, or fear of reintroducing cancer cells via tissue transplantation. If this is the case, and the patient is rendered with premature ovarian failure after cancer therapy, oocyte donation may be employed. The pregnancy rates with this technique are very high. The Society of Assisted Reproductive Technology quotes that in 2008 the success rate of IVF using fresh donor oocytes was 55% [48]. Nonetheless, using donor eggs provides a plethora of legal, ethical and emotional concerns. These concerns and high cost of treatment may discourage patients from choosing this option.

Cancer in Pregnancy

The most frequently encountered cancers during pregnancy are those that are most common in reproductive age females. These include breast, cervix, melanoma, Hodgkin's disease, and leukemia.

The management of cancer during pregnancy presents an interesting challenge, as any protocol should now take into consideration two patients simultaneously: the mother and the fetus. Often times, the physician's ability to make therapeutic decisions by evidence based medicine is limited as there is a paucity of data about pregnant patients with cancer. There are not double blinded, prospective, randomized control trials involving pregnant women with different diagnostic and treatment modalities. In the paucity of evidence, the physician must still make careful, informed decisions regarding diagnosis and treatment. Although there are no official guidelines, in general, treatments tend to prioritize and benefit the mother's life. Whenever possible, the fetus should be protected against the harmful effects of the treatment. Finally, providers should attempt to preserve the mother's future fertility. With these general guidelines, it is not uncommon that abortions are recommended for patients who were found to be pregnant in early gestation (first to mid second trimester of gestation).

While evaluating a newly diagnosed pregnant patient with cancer, one may need to order additional radiodiagnostic tests. These tests emit ionizing radiation. The effects of radiation on a developing fetus are directly related to dosage as well as the gestational age (see Table 7.1). A dose of <0.1 Gy (10 rads) is considered to have no major effect on the fetus. However, when the doses are higher than 30 Gy (300 rads) it will usually induce an abortion [1]. Likewise, high doses of radiation administered during the preimplantational period or immediately after the

Table 7.1 Effects of radiation in relation to gestation age

Effects of radiation in relation to gestational age

Developmental stage	Time period	Adverse effects
Preimplantation/immediate postimplantation	Conception to day 10	Lethal, failure to implant
Early organogenesis	Weeks 2–6	Increased teratogenecity, growth retardation
Late organogenesis/early fetal period	Weeks 12–16	Mental and growth restriction, microcephaly, malformations
Late fetal stage	Weeks 20–birth	Sterility, malignancies, genetic defects

Modified from Pavlidis et al. [1]

Table 7.2 Imaging procedures and radiation doses

Imaging procedure and associated average uterine/fetal doses

Procedure	Fetal exposure (mGy)
Chest X-ray (2 views)	0.0004
Abdominal film (single view)	0.45–1.0
Mammogram	4
CT Head	<10
CT Chest	<10
CT Abdomen/Pelvis	18–35
Intravenous urography	45
Barium enema	36
ERCP	0.4
Tc99m-MDP bone scan	1st trimester 4.5 2nd trimester 2–4 3rd trimester 1.8–20

10 mGy = 1 rad. Modified from Pentheroudakis et al. [64]

implantation are usually considered lethal for the embryo. The radiation effects also depend on the gestational age, and more detrimental effects are seen in early gestational ages. In pregnancy, the use of staging imaging tests should be limited to those with the least amount of ionizing radiation. As such, abdominal plain films, PET scans, and CT should be avoided; however, chest x-ray and ultrasounds are indicated as their effects on the fetus are limited. In certain cases, magnetic resonance imaging may be recommended as it avoids the use of ionizing radiation (see Table 7.2).

Cervical Cancer

Cervical cancer is the most common malignancy diagnosed during pregnancy. The median age at diagnosis during pregnancy is ages 30–35. Most women are asymptomatic, but sometimes complaints include vaginal bleeding, pelvic pain or discharge. The management of these patients raises several interesting points given the physical proximity to the pregnancy. During routine prenatal screening, a patient receives a pelvic exam and pap smear on her first visit with the obstetrician. At that time, if there is a gross lesion on physical exam, it should be biopsied; however, in the vast majority of the cases, the lesions are not grossly seen. Often abnormalities are found

on the cytology that then prompt a series of tests and diagnostic steps. Colposcopy should be performed during pregnancy as well as biopsies of any lesions suspicious for invasive disease (however, endocervical curettages are usually contraindicated). The risk of hemorrhage from colposcopic biopsies is low. When indicated, a patient should undergo a cold knife conization or Loop Electrosurgical Excision Procedure (LEEP) procedure to rule out microinvasive or invasive disease. These procedures are optimally performed between 14 and 20 weeks gestation.

Squamous cell carcinoma is the most common histological type of cervical cancer, in which 80–90% is found in this population. The remaining 10–20% is largely adenocarcinoma. Once diagnosed with cervical cancer by biopsy, staging should be undertaken. Staging consists of a complete physical examination, chest x-ray, and MRI of the abdomen. The management of cervical cancer during pregnancy largely depends on the gestational age during which the cervical cancer was diagnosed. When diagnosed early, the choice must be made between abortion with immediate therapy or postponing treatment with close monitoring. If a patient elects to continue the pregnancy, laparoscopic staging is recommended to help identify patients that may not benefit from expectant management. This staging should be done during the first and second trimester of gestation. The management and counseling should be tailored to the women's specific case and her stage [49]. Women who have microinvasive cervical cancer, Stage IA, may defer treatment as there is a low likelihood of disease progression [50]. The route of delivery often times depends on the depth of invasion. If the depth of invasion is less than 3 mm, the delivery may be vaginal. If the women has >3 mm depth of invasion and/or lymphovascular space invasion, then she should be delivered by cesarean section. Timing of delivery should include documented fetal lung maturity.

Invasive disease early on demands immediate attention. These women should be counseled regarding the recommendation of termination with immediate initiation of therapy. If invasive disease is diagnosed late in gestation, it is reasonable to opt for delay of therapy until after delivery. However, these patients should receive neoadjuvant chemotherapy. At the time of delivery, the patient should undergo the appropriate therapy. This includes radical hysterectomy with nodal dissection for Stages I-IIA and radiation/chemotherapy for Stages IIB-IVA. In a retrospective study by Van Calsteren and colleagues, pregnancy was not demonstrated to negatively affect patient outcomes when compared to non-pregnant patients [51]. Treatment complications were also noted to be similar in these groups [52]. Fetal outcome was also not significantly different in pregnancies afflicted by cancer versus normal pregnancies [53, 54].

Breast Cancer

Breast cancer is the most commonly diagnosed cancer in reproductive aged females. Although the risk of developing cancer increases with age, about 1 in 3 women are premenopausal at the time of diagnosis [55]. In 2010, the American Cancer Society estimates that there will be 207,090 new cases of breast cancer. The American Cancer Society also quotes 1 in 50 females diagnosed with breast cancer are under age 35 [56]. Breast cancer ranks among the most frequent cancers found during pregnancy. In the majority of cases, its presentation is a painless palpable breast mass. The physiological changes in the breast anatomy during pregnancy, including the increased size and density of the breasts, make the physical diagnosis particularly challenging and lead to delays in diagnosis.

The diagnosis should be made by mammography, ultrasound, or in very difficult cases, breast MRI. Mammographic diagnosis is young pregnant females may have sensitivity as low as 70% [57]. Once a mass is discovered, the next step is to perform a biopsy. Fine needle aspiration is acceptable; however, an open surgical biopsy or core-needle biopsy may be more indicated. The predominant histological type of invasive breast cancer found during pregnancy is ductal adenocarcinoma, followed by lobular adenocarcinoma [49]. The majority of tumors found in pregnancy are high grade malignancies with 60–90% axillary node involvement and 40–70% hormone receptor negative [57–59]. This is not significantly different from the age-matched non-pregnant patients. According to many retrospective studies, pregnancy does not significantly alter the natural course of breast cancer or the clinical outcomes despite the high level of circulating hormones, especially estrogen.

For early stage breast cancers, stages I, II and selected stage III, during the first two trimesters, the treatment of choice is a modified radical mastectomy with axillary node dissection. The use of a radioisotope in sentinel lymph node biopsy is still considered experimental as there are unknown fetal risks. The reported radiation exposure of SLN biopsy is <5–15 mGy [60]. Patients with localized disease in the third trimester of pregnancy, may undergo breast conserving surgery and postpartum radiation. The scatter dose of radiation that the pelvis receives during a typical breast irradiation is considerably less than the dose needed to induce premature ovarian failure or to cause damaging effects on the uterus. Adjuvant chemotherapy is suggested in women with node positive disease, high grade pathology or size greater than 1 cm. It can be administered after the first trimester with relative safety. CMF (cyclophosphamide, methotrexate, 5-fluorouracil) and anthracycline based therapies have been reported with low incidence of fetal malformations when used in the 2nd and 3rd trimester. A study by Berry et al, evaluated a series of 24 patients treated with cyclophosphamide, 5-FU and doxorubicin after 12 weeks of gestation. In that study congenital abnormalities or intra-uterine growth restriction were not reported [61]. The use of methotrexate (MTX), however, in the first trimester has been shown to be harmful. MTX exposure has been associated with mental retardation, poor physical development, spontaneous abortions and even later fetal death in utero [62].

Patients with metastatic disease diagnosed during pregnancy must be appropriately counseled with regards to their disease course, prognosis, and the prognosis of the pregnancy. Women with metastatic breast cancer may be managed with palliative chemotherapy at which time the issue of pregnancy termination should be discussed.

Lymphoma

Lymphoma is also one of the most common diagnosed malignancies during pregnancy. Abortion is often recommended and considered. These cancers can be highly treatable if therapy is initiated early. Curative treatment may require aggressive therapy that has unknown effects on the pregnancy and developing fetus. Often times, the therapies initiated can have severe myelosuppressive effects. This poses a serious risk to the pregnancy, as it increases the probability of maternal infection and vertical transmission. Evidence supporting routine termination is such circumstances is lacking. To the patient, pregnancy termination may have many social, moral and religious implications. Treatment regimens for lymphomas can be extremely gonadotoxic. Therefore, the likelihood of future fertility is low. As previously recommended, avoidance of chemotherapy in the first trimester is preferable. There are higher chances of fetal malformations and spontaneous abortions during this time period.

Hodgkin's lymphoma is the most common lymphoma seen in pregnancy. The median age of diagnosis for Hodgkin's disease is 32 years [63]. Presentation in pregnancy does not differ greatly from non-pregnant patients. The vast majority of patients have painless lymphadenopathy, and 20% develop unspecific symptoms such as night sweats, weight loss, and fever. Diagnosis should be made with excisional lymph node biopsy and subsequent pathological evaluation. Staging should include bone marrow biopsy, chest x-ray, abdominal/pelvic ultrasound, as well as laboratory tests. Patients with Hodgkin's disease can be offered a standardized regimen, including ABVD, starting in the second trimester as there is no evidence of increased adverse fetal events.

Conclusion

As science continues to evolve, great advances are being made in the area of cancer diagnosis and therapy, with more and more patients going on to lead fulfilling lives after a diagnosis of cancer. Concomitantly, we are seeing a social trend of women delaying childbearing in order to first pursue their professional objectives. As a result, we see more and more patients diagnosed with cancer during pregnancy and patients who want to become pregnant after cancer therapy.

With a strong understanding of female physiology, healthcare providers are better able to understand implications of cancer therapies, not only in terms of future reproductive potential but also on the pregnancy itself. While approaching a patient with cancer, it is very important for providers to have an understanding of this patient's future reproductive wishes, and how the cancer itself and its treatment will impact on her wishes. Only when furnished with this information will the provider be able to properly counsel their patients. Each treatment regimen has differing effects on the gonads, and each cancer may also have a different impact on the reproductive potential. During a critical time period where patients are very easily ushered down a path which may negatively affect their fertility, it is important that the patient's health care providers are prudent, and evaluate the patient's future desire for childbearing. It is absolutely the responsibility of the health care provider to identify these patients, educate them on their options, and have the resources to provide fertility preservation options in a timely manner, as not to delay the cancer therapy.

As treatments for cancer are becoming more successful and survival rates are improving, the quality of life of cancer survivors is becoming an area of emphasis. Health care providers are becoming more aware of options available to women newly diagnosed with cancer. As reproductive technologies are becoming more efficient and effective, there is increasing applications for the various technologies. Consultation with a multidisciplinary team seems to be the most reasonable approach under these circumstances. It is important that there is an open line of communication between hematologist/oncologist, reproductive endocrinologist, obstetricians and the patients themselves.

In the situation of cancer during pregnancy, counseling patients during this critical time when they are faced with life threatening disease can be very difficult. However, it is extremely important to empower patients with information. Pregnancy termination may not be a popular option, but in certain circumstances is medically advisable. In patients with moral, social or ethical obligations, it is infinitely more important to educate them on effects of treatment, implications of delays in treatment, as well as a realistic expectation of pregnancy in the setting of a cancer diagnosis.

As the science continues to evolve, so must our understanding of it. The dynamic field of oncofertility is ever expanding. In the interest of the patient, it is important that we, as healthcare providers, continue to educate ourselves.

Provider Recommendations

1. All cancer patients of childbearing age should be informed about potential infertility due to cancer treatments. Interested patients should be referred to reproductive endocrinologist infertility specialist, prior to treatment when possible, to discuss fertility preservation options.
2. Cancer may occur during pregnancy and although uncommon, requires the management of two patients: the woman with cancer and the fetus.
3. Radiation administered for diagnostic tests or treatment can impact the fetus and may cause harm or spontaneous abortion.
4. Chemotherapy can impact the fetus and administration of this treatment must take into account fetal age, type of drug and dose.

5. If termination of pregnancy is warranted, providers should attempt to preserve future fertility.
6. Cancer during pregnancy requires counseling the patient to identify her wishes for the pregnancy and education about the impact of treatment on both her own and fetal morbidity and mortality.

References

1. Pavlidis N (2002) Coexistence of Pregnancy and Malignancy. Oncologist 7(4):279–287
2. Speroff L, Fritz MA (2005) Clinical gynecologic endocrinology and infertility. Lippincott Williams & Wilkins. Available from: http://www.loc.gov/catdir/enhancements/fy0712/2004048582-d.html. Materials specified: Publisher description http://www.loc.gov/catdir/enhancements/fy0712/2004048582-d.html. Philadelphia, Pennsylvania
3. Quinn GP, Vadaparampil ST, Jacobsen PB, Knapp C, Keefe DL, Bell GE (2010) Frozen hope: fertility preservation for women with cancer. J Midwifery Womens Health 55(2):175–180
4. Lee SJ, Schover LR, Partridge AH, Patrizio P, Wallace WH, Hagerty K, Beck LN, Brennan LV, American OK (2006) Society of Clinical Oncology recommendations on fertility preservation in cancer patients. J Clin Oncol 24(18): 2917–2931
5. Quinn GP, Vadaparampil ST, Gwede CK, Miree C, King LM, Clayton HB, Wilson C, Munster P (2007) Discussion of fertility preservation with newly diagnosed patients: oncologists' views. J Cancer Surviv 1(2):146–155
6. Quinn GP, Vadaparampil ST (2009) Fertility preservation and adolescent/young adult cancer patients: physician communication challenges. J Adolesc Health 44(4):394–400
7. Quinn GP, Vadaparampil ST, King L, Miree CA, Wilson C, Raj O, Watson J, Lopez A, Albrecht TL (2009) Impact of physicians' personal discomfort and patient prognosis on discussion of fertility preservation with young cancer patients. Patient Educ Couns 77(3):338–343
8. Thompson SC, Nanni C, Schwankovsky L (1990) Patient-oriented interventions to improve communication in a medical office visit. Health Psychol 9(4):390–404
9. Yap JK, Davies M (2007) Fertility preservation in female cancer survivors. J Obstet Gynaecol 27(4):390–400
10. Maltaris T, Beckmann MW, Dittrich R (2009) Review. Fertility preservation for young female cancer patients. In Vivo 23(1):123–130

11. Mok CC, Lau CS, Wong RW (1998) Risk factors for ovarian failure in patients with systemic lupus erythematosus receiving cyclophosphamide therapy. Arthritis Rheum 41(5):831–837

12. Warne GL, Fairley KF, Hobbs JB, Martin FI (1973) Cyclophosphamide-induced ovarian failure. N Engl J Med 289(22):1159–1162

13. Meirow D, Epstein M, Lewis H, Nugent D, Gosden RG (2001) Administration of cyclophosphamide at different stages of follicular maturation in mice: effects on reproductive performance and fetal malformations. Hum Reprod 16(4):632–637

14. Dowsett M, Richner J (1991) Effects of cytotoxic chemotherapy on ovarian and adrenal steroidogenesis in pre-menopausal breast cancer patients. Oncology 48(3):215–220

15. Mehta RR, Beattie CW, Das Gupta TK (1992) Endocrine profile in breast cancer patients receiving chemotherapy. Breast Cancer Res Treat 20(2):125–132

16. Sonmezer M, Oktay K (2004) Fertility preservation in female patients. Hum Reprod Update 10(3):251–266

17. Gosden RG, Wade JC, Fraser HM, Sandow J, Faddy MJ (1997) Impact of congenital or experimental hypogonadotrophism on the radiation sensitivity of the mouse ovary. Hum Reprod 12(11):2483–2488

18. Meirow D, Nugent D (2001) The effects of radiotherapy and chemotherapy on female reproduction. Hum Reprod Update 7(6):535–543

19. Wallace WH, Thomson AB, Saran F, Kelsey TW (2005) Predicting age of ovarian failure after radiation to a field that includes the ovaries. Int J Radiat Oncol Biol Phys 62(3):738–744

20. Lushbaugh CC, Casarett GW (1976) The effects of gonadal irradiation in clinical radiation therapy: a review. Cancer 37(2 Suppl):1111–1125

21. Critchley HO, Wallace WH (2005) Impact of cancer treatment on uterine function. J Natl Cancer Inst Monogr 34:64–68

22. Fenig E, Mishaeli M, Kalish Y, Lishner M (2001) Pregnancy and radiation. Cancer Treat Rev 27(1):1–7

23. Constine LS, Woolf PD, Cann D, Mick G, McCormick K, Raubertas RF, Rubin P (1993) Hypothalamic-pituitary dysfunction after radiation for brain tumors. N Engl J Med 328(2):87–94

24. Horning SJ, Hoppe RT, Kaplan HS, Rosenberg SA (1981) Female reproductive potential after treatment for Hodgkin's disease. N Engl J Med 304(23):1377–1382

25. Sutton R, Buzdar AU, Hortobagyi GN (1990) Pregnancy and offspring after adjuvant chemotherapy in breast cancer patients. Cancer 65(4):847–850

26. Chatterjee R, Goldstone AH (1996) Gonadal damage and effects on fertility in adult patients with haematological malignancy undergoing stem cell transplantation. Bone Marrow Transplant 17(1):5–11

27. Chatterjee R, Kottaridis PD (2002) Treatment of gonadal damage in recipients of allogeneic or autologous transplantation for haematological malignancies. Bone Marrow Transplant 30(10):629–635

28. Bines J, Oleske DM, Cobleigh MA (1996) Ovarian function in premenopausal women treated with adjuvant chemotherapy for breast cancer. J Clin Oncol 14(5):1718–1729

29. Wallace WH, Shalet SM, Crowne EC, Morris-Jones PH, Gattamaneni HR, Price DA (1989) Gonadal dysfunction due to cis-platinum. Med Pediatr Oncol 17(5):409–413

30. Wallace WH, Shalet SM, Hendry JH, Morris-Jones PH, Gattamaneni HR (1989) Ovarian failure following abdominal irradiation in childhood: the radiosensitivity of the human oocyte. Br J Radiol 62(743):995–998

31. Brewer M, Gershenson DM, Herzog CE, Mitchell MF, Silva EG, Wharton JT (1999) Outcome and reproductive function after chemotherapy for ovarian dysgerminoma. J Clin Oncol 17(9):2670–2675

32. Tangir J, Zelterman D, Ma W, Schwartz PE (2003) Reproductive function after conservative surgery and chemotherapy for malignant germ cell tumors of the ovary. Obstet Gynecol 101(2):251–257

33. Meirow D (1999) Ovarian injury and modern options to preserve fertility in female cancer patients treated with high dose radio-chemotherapy for hemato-oncological neoplasias and other cancers. Leuk Lymphoma 33(1–2):65–76

34. Blumenfeld Z, Haim N (1997) Prevention of gonadal damage during cytotoxic therapy. Ann Med 29(3):199–206

35. Meirow D (2000) Reproduction post-chemotherapy in young cancer patients. Mol Cell Endocrinol 169(1–2):123–131

36. Martin JR, Kodaman P, Oktay K, Taylor HS (2007) Ovarian cryopreservation with transposition of a contralateral ovary: a combined approach for fertility preservation in women receiving pelvic radiation. Fertil Steril 87(1):189 e5–e7

37. Woodruff TK, Snyder KA (2007) Oncofertility: fertility preservation for cancer survivors. Springer, New York, NY

38. Son WY, Yoon SH, Yoon HJ, Lee SM, Lim JH (2003) Pregnancy outcome following transfer of human blastocysts vitrified on electron microscopy grids after induced collapse of the blastocoele. Hum Reprod 18(1):137–139

39. Georgescu ES, Goldberg JM, du Plessis SS, Agarwal A (2008) Present and future fertility preservation strategies for female cancer patients. Obstet Gynecol Surv 63(11):725–732

40. Gao S, Li Y, Gao X, Hu J, Yang H, Chen ZJ (2009) Spindle and chromosome changes of human MII oocytes during incubation after slow freezing/fast thawing procedures. Reprod Sci 16(4):391–396

41. Cobo A, Perez S, De los Santos MJ, Zulategui J, Domingo J, Remohi J (2008) Effect of different cryopreservation protocols on the metaphase II spindle in human oocytes. Reprod Biomed Online 17(3):350–359

42. Ciotti PM, Porcu E, Notarangelo L, Magrini O, Bazzocchi A, Venturoli S (2009) Meiotic spindle recovery is faster in vitrification of human oocytes compared to slow freezing. Fertil Steril 91(6):2399–2407

43. Coticchio G (2006) Sucrose concentration influences the rate of human oocytes with normal spindle and chromosome configurations after slow cooling cryopreservation. Hum Reprod 21:1771–1776

44. Rienzi L, Martinez F, Ubaldi F, Minasi MG, Iacobelli M, Tesarik J, Greco E (2004) Polscope analysis of meiotic spindle changes in living metaphase II human oocytes during the freezing and thawing procedures. Hum Reprod 19(3):655–659

45. Noyes N, Knopman J, Labella P, McCaffrey C, Clark-Williams M, Grifo J (2010) Oocyte cryopreservation outcomes including pre-cryopreservation and post-thaw meiotic spindle evaluation following slow cooling and vitrification of human oocytes. Fertil Steril 94(6):2078–2082

46. Gook DA, Schiewe MC, Osborn SM, Asch RH, Jansen RP, Johnston WI (1995) Intracytoplasmic sperm injection and embryo development of human oocytes cryopreserved using 1,2-propanediol. Hum Reprod 10(10):2637–2641

47. Donnez J, Dolmans MM, Demylle D, Jadoul P, Pirard C, Squifflet J, Martinez-Madrid B, van Langendonckt A (2004) Livebirth after orthotopic transplantation of cryopreserved ovarian tissue. Lancet 364(9443):1405–1410

48. Technologies SfA R (1996–2010) SartCors Online

49. Azim HA Jr., Peccatori FA, Pavlidis N (2010) Treatment of the pregnant mother with cancer: a systematic review on the use of cytotoxic, endocrine, targeted agents and immunotherapy during pregnancy. Part I: solid tumors. Cancer Treat Rev 36(2):101–109

50. Weisz B, Meirow D, Schiff E, Lishner M (2004) Impact and treatment of cancer during pregnancy. Exp Rev Anticancer Ther 4(5):889–902

51. Van Calsteren K, Vergote I, Amant F (2005) Cervical neoplasia during pregnancy: diagnosis, management and prognosis. Best Pract Res Clin Obstet Gynaecol 19(4):611–630

52. Method MW, Brost BC (1999) Management of cervical cancer in pregnancy. Semin Surg Oncol 16(3):251–260

53. Zemlickis D, Lishner M, Degendorfer P, Panzarella T, Sutcliffe SB, Koren G (1991) Maternal and fetal outcome after invasive cervical cancer in pregnancy. J Clin Oncol 9(11):1956–1961

54. Germann N, Haie-Meder C, Morice P, Lhomme C, Duvillard P, Hacene K, Gerbaulet A (2005) Management and clinical outcomes of pregnant patients with invasive cervical cancer. Ann Oncol 16(3):397–402

55. Jemal A, Thomas A, Murray T, Thun M (2002) Cancer statistics, 2002. CA Cancer J Clin 52(1):23–47

56. American Cancer Society (2009–2010) Breast cancer facts & figures 2009–2010. American Cancer Society, Inc, Atlanta, GA

57. Moore HC, Foster RS Jr (2000) Breast cancer and pregnancy. Semin Oncol 27(6):646–653

58. Pavlidis N, Pentheroudakis G (2005) The pregnant mother with breast cancer: diagnostic and therapeutic management. Cancer Treat Rev 31(6):439–447

59. Woo JC, Yu T, Hurd TC (2003) Breast cancer in pregnancy: a literature review. Arch Surg 138(1):91–98; discussion 9

60. Gentilini O, Cremonesi M, Trifiro G, Ferrari M, Baio SM, Caracciolo M, Rossi A, Smeets A, Galimberti V, Luini A, Tosi G, Paganelli G (2004) Safety of sentinel node biopsy in pregnant patients with breast cancer. Ann Oncol 15(9):1348–1351

61. Berry DL, Theriault RL, Holmes FA, Parisi VM, Booser DJ, Singletary SE, Buzdar AU, Hortobagyi GN (1999) Management of breast cancer during pregnancy using a standardized protocol. J Clin Oncol 17(3):855–861

62. Cardonick E, Iacobucci A (2004) Use of chemotherapy during human pregnancy. Lancet Oncol 5(5):283–291

63. Azim HA Jr., Pavlidis N, Peccatori FA (2010) Treatment of the pregnant mother with cancer: a systematic review on the use of cytotoxic, endocrine, targeted agents and immunotherapy during pregnancy. Part II: hematol tumors. Cancer Treat Rev 36(2):110–121

64. Pentheroudakis G, Pavlidis N (2006) Cancer and pregnancy: poena magna, not anymore. Eur J Cancer 42(2):126–140

Preimplantation Genetic Diagnosis for Hereditary Cancers

8

Sioban B. SenGupta, PhD, Susan T. Vadaparampil, PhD, MPH, and Usha Menon, PhD

For some people the thought of 'designing' their offspring is more than science fiction especially if they are carriers of genetic disorders such as cystic fibrosis or Von Hippel-Lindau disease. VHL is a hereditary condition which causes cysts and tumours to grow in different parts of the body. Onset of the disease normally occurs in your mid-twenties and there is no cure, only treatment and management of the symptoms. To some sufferers it's an inconvenience; to others it's a killer. I found out I had VHL when my father got kidney cancer and my sister and I were tested.

There is a 50% chance I'll pass this vicious disease on to my children and the thought of starting a family is a complicated and sensitive issue. I always hoped to have children one day, but I risk passing on VHL and that may be both selfish and irresponsible. Talking about VHL for the first time with a partner is not easy – it's an intensely personal issue and I find I can become incredibly emotional and irrational when discussing it.

My idea of having a baby used to involve vague fantasies of a memorable conception, months of yoga-filled healthy eating and an angelic looking baby somewhere at the end of it. VHL has forced me to take a more pragmatic approach to the whole procreation thing and to plan the best possible future for a child.

Until recently, the only real choices for couples in our position were adoption, donor egg or sperm or prenatal testing followed by a termination decision depending on the outcome of the test, or playing the odds and hoping for the best. However, thanks to the continuing advancement of medical science there is now a treatment available called PGD (pre-implantation genetic diagnosis), which may enable us to have children of our own and all but guarantee that I don't pass my condition on. We would literally be 'designing' our baby using just my good genes, hopefully ensuring that VHL was not passed on to our children.

So should we have our 'designer baby' or not? I'm adamant that I don't want to risk passing my condition on but I also know that I want to at least try to have my own children before I'd consider using a donor or adopting. This leaves PGD as the obvious choice but even if it's successful it still raises several ethical questions. Will we be meddling with nature and is this just the first step towards couples being able to choose things such as eye and hair colour in their children? There's also the issue of what happens to the embryos carrying the genetic fault. Somehow discarding a four cell embryo feels more acceptable than terminating an affected pregnancy, but ultimately every couple's circumstances are different and I believe prospective parents have to make the decision that is right for them.

S.B. SenGupta (✉)
UCL Centre for PGD, Institute for Women's Health,
University College London, WC1E 6HX London, UK
e-mail: s.sengupta@ucl.ac.uk

G.P. Quinn, S.T. Vadaparampil (eds.), *Reproductive Health and Cancer in Adolescents and Young Adults*, Advances in Experimental Medicine and Biology 732,
DOI 10.1007/978-94-007-2492-1_8, © Springer Science+Business Media B.V. 2012

I know my father feels incredibly guilty about passing his illness on, even though it was not in any way his fault. I feel lucky that science and technology have given me the opportunity to at least try to have children without passing on VHL. It's a big decision but I think we'll probably follow the 'designer baby' route. But, I want to be sure our relationship is solid first before I really think about a baby.
Kendra, Adult VHL patient

Introduction

Preimplantation Genetic Diagnosis

Preimplantation Genetic Diagnosis (PGD) is genetic testing of oocytes or embryos. The procedure requires the use of assisted reproductive technologies so that biopsy of polar bodies from oocytes or blastomeres/trophectoderm from preimplantation embryos is possible. Oocytes or embryos are genetically tested to diagnose the presence or absence of specific mutations known to be present in either parental genome. Embryos found not to carry the inherited mutation and not at risk of showing the diseased phenotype are selected for transfer into the mother's uterus to allow implantation and pregnancy [1]. The major benefit of PGD over other forms of prenatal testing (chronic villus sampling or amniocentesis) is that couples do not need to consider the termination of an affected pregnancy. The major drawbacks of PGD are that even fertile couples need to go through in vitro fertilisation and that diagnosis is often based on protocols that are developed for specific couples, adding to the expense and time taken before treatment can be offered.

The first reported cases of PGD were carried out in the UK in 1990 using the polymerase chain reaction (PCR) to sex embryos by the amplification of Y specific sequences from single blastomeres biopsied from cleavage stage embryos [2]. Female embryos were selected for transfer to avoid the development of disorders showing X- lined recessive inheritance. Since that time there has been a rapid increase in the number of indications for PGD, including the detection of chromosomal imbalance using fluorescence in situ hybridisation (FISH) or microarrays [3]. Availability of PGD is largely dependent upon the legislative stance of different nations where some countries restrict testing to oocytes, other countries allow testing on oocytes and embryos but exert control over the particular indications for PGD, while some countries do not enforce any legal boundaries [4]. The application of PGD to hereditary cancers has caused debate as the criteria for the exclusion of embryos is an increased susceptibility to developing cancer rather than the presence of overt disease which is unlike the majority of other indications for PGD [5]. Further controversy rises from the use of PGD for HLA typing for the selection of embryos that could result in child with the potential of being a stem cell donor for a sibling suffering from acquired leukaemia or lymphoma [6, 7].

Genetics of Cancer Predisposition

About 5–10% of all cancers are due to inherited predisposition [8]. Germline mutations usually in tumour suppressor genes result in increased cancer susceptibility. Tumour suppressor genes are associated with the regulation of cell division, differentiation, signalling, DNA repair, and apoptosis. A gemline mutation in any of these genes is present in every cell of the person who inherits it. A second mutation affecting the remaining normal copy of the gene arising in any cell where the gene is expressed can initiate the cancer process. Normal cell regulation breaks down and the cell is prone to acquiring more mutations in other genes. The subsequent mutations in other tumour suppressor genes and proto – oncogenes give a selective growth advantage to the cells resulting in their clonal expansion eventually leading cells with malignant potential. Although both copies of the tumour suppressor gene need to be affected before the cancer process can be initiated these disorders show a dominant pattern of inheritance [9].

Table 8.1 Hereditary Cancer Predisposition Disorders. The causative genes for each disorder are shown and the cancer susceptibilities as listed on OMIM (http://www.ncbi.nlm.nih.gov/omim) are given. Reports of PGD for different cancer predispositions are also listed

Disorder	Gene(s)	Cancers	Reference
Adenomatous polyposis of the colon	APC	Adrenal carcinoma, Thyroid papillary carcinoma, Periampullary carcinoma, Fibrosarcoma, Colon carcinoma, Gastric adenocarcinoma, Medulloblastoma, Hepatoblastoma, Small intestine carcinoid, Desmoid tumor, Astrocytoma	Ao et al. [44], Rechitsky et al. [51], Spits et al. [55], Moutou et al. [50]
Hereditary Breast and Ovarian Cancer	BRCA1, BRCA2	Breast, ovary	Spits et al. [55], Jasper et al. [49], Sagi et al. [52]
Hereditary diffuse gastric cancer	CDH1	Stomach	SenGupta et al. [53]
Multiple endocrine neoplasia type 1	MEN1	Pancreas, adrenal glands, thyroid Carcinoid tumors	SenGupta et al. [53]
Multiple endocrine neoplasia type 2A	RET	Medullary thyroid carcinoma, pheochromocytoma, and parathyroid adenomas.	Harper et al. [48]
Lynch syndrome	PMS1, PMS2	Ovary, small intestine, brain, skin	Harper et al. [48]
Li Fraumeni	TP53	Breast cancer, Soft tissue sarcomas Osteosarcomas, Brain tumors, Acute leukemias. Adrenocortical carcinomas, Lung adenocarcinoma, Colon cancer, Pancreatic cancer, Prostate cancer, Wilms tumor, Phyllodes tumor	Rechitsky et al. [51], Verlinsky et al. [56]
Neurofibromatosis type 1	NF1	Optic glioma, Meningioma Hypothalamic tumor, Neurofibrosarcoma, Rhabdomyosarcoma; Duodenal carcinoid, Somatostatinoma Parathyroid adenoma, Pheochromocytoma, Pilocytic astrocytoma, Malignant peripheral nerve sheath tumors, Tumors at multiple other sites including CNS	Rechitsky et al. [51], Verlinsky et al. [56], Spits et al. [54], Altarescu et al. [42], Vanneste et al. [14]
Neurofibromatosis type 2	NF2	Meningioma, Glioma Vestibular Schwannoma	Abou-Sleiman et al. [41], Rechitsky et al. [51], Spits et al. [55]
Inherited retinoblastoma	RB1	Osteogenic sarcoma, Pinealoma, Leukemia, Lymphoma, Ewing sarcoma	Rechitsky et al. [51], Girardet et al. [47], Fiorentino et al. [46], Xu et al. [57] Dhanjal et al. [45]
Tuberous sclerosis type 2	TSC2	Myocardial rhabdomyoma, Multiple bilateral renal angiomyolipoma, Ependymoma, Renal carcinoma, Giant cell astrocytoma. Benign tumors of the eye, heart, and lungs	Altarescu et al. [43]
von Hippel Lindau syndrome	VHL	Pheochromocytoma, Hemangioblastoma, Hypernephroma, Pancreatic cancer, Paraganglioma Adenocarcinoma of ampulla of Vater	Rechitsky et al. [51], Vanneste et al. [14]

Sporadic cancers tend to arise at an older age as two mutations or epigenetic events in the same tumour suppressor gene in the same cell are required to initiate the cancer process. In inherited cancer, the age of cancer onset is much earlier than sporadic cancer. In addition, multiple primary cancers may develop. Table 8.1 summarises the range of syndromes associated with cancer predisposition. The overall severity of the disorder can be difficult to predict even when the specific germline mutation is known. Some tumour suppressor genes show incomplete penetrance whereby a proportion of individuals with an inherited mutation do not develop cancer in their lifetime. Germline mutations in other tumour suppressor genes such as *NF1* show variable expressivity but high penetrance where almost all individuals express the phenotype but this can range from those who only have few skin lesions to others who develop brain tumours that may be life threatening [10].

Clinical Aspects of PGD

PGD usually involves the collaboration between three specialist laboratories: (1) the clinical genetics laboratory where the inherited gene mutation in the family is identified, (2) the PGD laboratory where the protocol for oocyte/embryo testing is developed and diagnosis on biopsied polar bodies or embryonic cells is carried out, and (3) the IVF laboratory where gametes are collected from the couple, embryos are created, cultured, biopsied and transferred back into the mother.

Inherited predisposition to cancer usually shows a dominant mode of inheritance. This means that the partner carrying the inherited mutation is prone to developing cancer and may be recovering from cancer treatment or prophylactic surgery while preparing for IVF and PGD. The clinical management of the cancer predisposition may have varied affects on PGD outcome ranging from a reduction in fertility or delays in starting PGD cycles. The effect is usually more profound when the germline mutation is present in the female partner as the female partner needs to undergo ovarian stimulation as part of the IVF procedure. In the absence of a surrogate, the female partner should be healthy enough to be able to carry a pregnancy to term if there are embryos suitable for transfer.

The actual risk of a person with a germline mutation in a cancer predisposing gene developing one or more cancers may be difficult to determine and primarily depends upon the gene that is mutated. Therefore appropriate genetic counselling is essential before PGD is considered as a reproductive option. It is important that counselling informs couples that while PGD avoids the high susceptibility to cancers caused by inheritance of a mutated copy of the particular gene being tested, the sporadic environmental risk or low level risk due to polymorphisms in other genes remains [11].

As IVF is intrinsic to PGD, couples need to have the whole process clearly explained to them. Treatment may commence more than six months after initial referral to the IVF unit. Many couples find the prolonged process of PGD difficult, particularly when the affected partner may also have to plan for prophylactic surgery. Only about half of couples who enquire about PGD eventually choose this option [12]. Thus overall PGD for hereditary cancers requires the combined management of the couple between the clinical geneticist, the cancer specialist and the IVF clinician.

Stages of PGD for Inherited Cancers

Identification of the Germline Mutation

The identification of the germline mutation causative of a cancer predisposing syndrome can be difficult. This is because of genetic heterogeneitiy where inherited mutations in different genes can result in the same syndrome. An added problem is that sequence variants that are identified may have unknown functional significance. It is essential that the specific gene and inherited mutation causative of the cancer predisposition in a family is identified before PGD is considered. Referrals for PGD should include a full genetics report about the germline mutation, and a pedigree of the family. Availability of DNA from family members with known mutational status is helpful for the development of a robust PGD protocol for the family.

Protocol Development

Diagnosis in PGD commonly requires analysis of single cells and the results usually need to be reported within 48 h of receiving the biopsied cells so that selected embryos can be transferred at the time when the uterus is optimally prepared for embryo implantation (the implantation window). Therefore PGD protocols need to be designed well in advance of the start of IVF stimulation and optimised to ensure that they are sensitive enough to generate results from single cells [13]. For hereditary cancers (monogenic disorders) direct PCR of lysed biopsied cells is the most common approach. Interphase fluorescence *in situ* hybridisation (FISH) has been reported for the analysis of large deletions [14]. Whole genome amplification (WGA) prior to haplotyping by PCR of short tandem repeat markers (STR) [15] or more recently by arrays for the analysis of single nucleotide polymorphisms (SNP) are being applied [16]. PGD protocols are generally based on linkage analysis. PGD workup involves analysis of genomic DNA from the couple to identify STR markers that are genetically linked (within 1 Mb) to the germline mutation locus and informative whereby each maternal allele can be distinguished from each paternal allele.

Genomic DNA from relatives who have already been tested for the germline mutation are analysed for the STR markers that are informative for the couple. Alleles at linked markers in common between individuals with the germline mutation are on the same chromosome as the mutation. These alleles are known as the phase alleles. Detection of the phase alleles indirectly identifies the presence of the mutation and this can be used diagnostically. The frequency of de novo germline mutations in cancer predisposing genes can be high and for these couples the PGD protocol must include PCR amplification of the mutation site with subsequent analysis of the product with a method such as minisequencing

to distinguish the mutation from the normal gene sequence [17].

Single cell PCR can be prone to error such as amplification failure or allele drop out (ADO) when one allele fails to amplify in a heterozygous sample. Inaccurate PCR can lead to diagnosis failure or misdiagnosis. Inclusion of multiple STR markers flanking the mutation site reduce the chance of misdiagnosis as ADO at one locus may be deduced by the presence of alleles of known phase at other markers in protocol. The smaller the physical distance between the STR marker and the mutation site, the lower is the risk of recombination between the two loci. A recombination event during meiosis will alter the alleles in phase with the mutation in gametes. Using flanking markers allows single recombination events to be identified, meaning that the mutational status of an embryo cannot be determined, but it can prevent a misdiagnosis. The STR markers are also essential in the detection of any DNA contamination. Each embryo should only have one allele from each parent at each locus. The detection of additional alleles indicates contamination.

The final step in protocol development is optimisation of multiplex PCR conditions by testing the protocol on isolated single cells with known genotype. The single cells can be lymphocytes isolated from blood samples from the couple which are lysed using alkaline lysis or proteinase K digestion. A robust protocol should have an efficiency of 90% and ADO less than 10% at each locus when tested on 50 single cells from a sample that is known to be heterozygous at the loci included in the protocol [18].

The PGD workup time can be reduced by doing a whole genome amplification step prior to multiplex PCR. WGA can be PCR based where DNA is fragmented, ligated to synthetic adapter sequences and following which the genomic fragments are amplified by PCR with primers that are directed towards the adaper sequences. A commonly used non-PCR based WGA method is multiple displacement amplification (MDA). This uses Φ29 polymerase in an isothermal reaction. Following WGA multiplex PCR, protocols suitable for genomic DNA can be applied and single cell optimisation is not required. However WGA may introduce some bias in the DNA with some loci excluded and others over represented. ADO rates of multiplex PCR after MDA WGA can be as high as 30% [19]. For this reason several STR markers are used so that sufficient markers flanking the mutation locus give accurate PCR products for diagnosis to be made.

Preimplantation Genetics and Development

Gametogenesis is different between males and females. Male meiosis starts at puberty, while in females, meiosis starts in fetal life. The primary oocyte arrests at the dictyotene of prophase I until puberty. At puberty, primordial follicles are recruited in monthly cycles for growth into pre-antral follicles and maturation of a single antral follicle containing the oocyte surrounded by the zona pellucida (ZP) and cumulus cells. In response to luteinising hormone the primary oocyte completes meiosis I to form a secondary oocyte and extrudes the first polar body into the perivitelline space within the ZP. The oocyte is arrested at metaphase II at the time of ovulation. Fertilisation triggers the completion of female meiosis with the release of the second polar body.

Following fertilization, male and female pronuclei form, the chromosomes condense and with the breakdown of pronuclear membrane syngamy occurs and the first mitotic division of the zygote takes place. This is the cleavage stage of the embryonic cells (blastomeres) without cell growth such that with each division the daughter cells are approximately half the size of the parent blastomeres. Three days post fertilisation between 6 and 8 cells tight, junctions

develop and compaction begins to form a morula by day 4. The embryonic genome is activated at the 4–6 cell stage. However, in these early divisions DNA repair and checkpoint genes are poorly expressed so that errors in mitosis are tolerated [20]. Thus embryos are often mosaic at this stage containing some aneuploid cells [21]. The embryo then begins to differentiate into an inner cell mass (ICM) and the trophecoderm (TE). Cavitation occurs when fluid fills the blastocele and a blastocyst is formed. The ICM will become the fetus and the TE the placenta. By day 5, the blastocyst consists of approximately 120 cells (Fig. 8.1). It actively accumulates fluid and the embryo hatches out of the ZP by day 5/6 ready for implantation into the uterus.

IVF Procedure

Successful PGD requires the production of a large number of embryos to increase the likelihood of identifying an embryo without the germline mutation and that develops sufficiently to allow embryo transfer. Prior to the start of the treatment cycle, fertility checks are carried out to determine ovarian reserve and sperm quality. The most common ovarian stimulation protocol for IVF is the long GnRH agonist protocol which gives effective control over follicular development [22]. The protocol involves administration of gonadotrophin releasing hormone (GnRH) agonist in the cycle preceding stimulation to down regulate the pituitary, followed by daily doses gondanotropins with regular ultrasound and hormone evaluation. When there are two to three mature follicles and estradiol levels are high, human chorionic gonadotrophin (hCG) is given and oocytes are collected 36–37 h later.

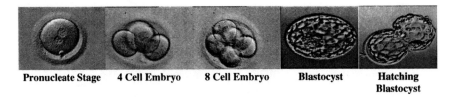

Pronucleate Stage   4 Cell Embryo   8 Cell Embryo   Blastocyst   Hatching Blastocyst

Fig. 8.1 Embryo development from pronucleate stage to hatching blastocyst (Pictures from Alpesh Doshi, Centre for Reproductive and Genetic Health, London, UK)

Progesterone is given from the day of oocyte collection to support the endometrium until a positive hCG pregnancy test.

Oocyte cumulus complexes are isolated from the follicular fluid and incubated for 2–4 h before insemination. A sperm sample is taken from the male partner on the morning of oocyte retrival and prepared usually by density gradient centrifugation and washed and equilibrated in culture media. For single gene disorders, insemination must be carried out by intracytoplasmic sperm injection (ICSI) to avoid contamination by excess sperm that stick to the ZP when IVF is carried out. Cumulus cells surrounding the oocyte must also be removed to prevent contamination and to allow ICSI. Forty hours after hCG the oocytes are denuded by rapid exposure to hyaluronidase. Forty one hours after hCG ICSI is performed by selection of a single sperm, removal of the tail and injection into the oocyte cytoplasm. Fertilisation is checked 16–18 h post ICSI. Two pronuclei and two polar bodies should be detected in the zygote at this stage. Embryo transfer is performed under ultrasound guidance between 2 and 6 days post oocyte retrival.

Biopsy for PGD

Biopsy can take place at three different stages, from the oocyte, the cleavage stage embryo or the blastocyst.

Polar Body Biopsy

Removal of the polar bodies enables analysis of the maternal mutations. The ZP is pierced with a bevelled pipette or drilled with a laser and the polar body is aspirated into a pipette. The first and second polar bodies can be collected sequentially. The first polar can be biopsied straight after ooctye retrival between 36 and 42 h after hCG injection [23] and the second polar body can be removed up to 22 h post insemination [24]. This is important in PGD for monogenic disorders as the chromosomal homologues are separated in the first polar body and the secondary

oocyte. Therefore if the germline mutation and phase alleles of linked markers are identified in the first polar body then the oocyte should be free of the inherited mutation. Sister chromatids are separated in the second polar body and the fertilised ovum. Therefore if mutation and the phase alleles are not present in the second polar body, the ovum should also be free of the mutation. However crossover at the mutation site or errors in meiotic segregation make diagnosis difficult and paternally inherited mutations cannot be detected. Due to these limitations polar body analysis for single gene mutations is restricted to countries where analysis on embryos is not permitted or where couples do not want to discard affected embryos. This requires the use of rapid analysis procedures or freezing of inseminated oocytes prior to syngamy [17]. The advantage of polar body biopsy is that it eliminates the need for micromanipulation of the embryo.

Cleavage Stage Biopsy

Three days post insemination the embryo is at cleavage stage and usually has between 6 and 8 cells (blastomeres). This is the most common stage at which biopsy takes place for PGD. Both maternal and paternal genomes can be analysed and there are up to 48 h available of diagnosis before the embryo transfer needs to take place. A hole is drilled thorough the ZP, usually using a laser and then 1–2 blastomere(s) are aspirated from the embryo. Analysis of two cells improves the diagnosis; however this is may affect the implantation potential of the embryo [25]. The main difficulty in testing at this stage is that the embryo can be mosaic where some cells may be aneuploid due to errors in mitosis [21]. Therefore the results of PCR analysis maybe inconclusive regarding diagnosis of the mutation as one of the parental chromosomes may be missing.

Blastocyst Biopsy

Blastocysts form on 5 to 6 days post insemination. Biopsy at this stage involves removal of

3–0 trophectoderm cells. A small hole is made in the ZP either on Day 3 or on blastocysts 4–10 h before biopsy. The trophectoderm cells close to hole herniate out and these are detached from the blastocyst using a laser. The advantage of blastocyst biopsy is that subsequent analysis is based on more than one cell which means that less optimisation is required for PCR protocols which reduces the time for PGD workup. The major disadvantages are that not all embryos may develop to blastocyst in vitro and that a maximum of 24 h is available for embryos biopsied on day 5 before they need to be transferred. Inspite of this implantation, following blastocyst biopsy is better compared to biopsy at cleavage stage [26]. If diagnosis takes longer than 24 h or the embryos have been biopsied on day 6, then the biopsied blastocysts need to be cryopreserved. The cryopreserved embryos can be thawed and transferred in a medical or natural cycle at a later date.

Tubing of Biopsied Cells and Work Flow

Once biopsied, the cells are individually washed before being transferred into a separate labelled microfuge tubes so that the cell can be linked to embryo from which it was biopsied. The last wash drop from each cell is also put into a tube and processed so that any extraneous DNA contamination can be identified. Contamination is a recognised cause of misdiagnosis in PGD involving molecular analysis [27]. A strict regimen must be maintained both in the IVF laboratory and in the PGD laboratory to minimise the risk of contamination [28]. Maternal contamination of embryos is avoided careful removal of cumulus cells surrounding the oocyte prior to insemination by ICSI to prevent contamination by sperm. In the PGD laboratory, pre and post PCR area are separated to avoid 'carryover' contamination and molecular protocols include STR markers so that contamination can be detected. If contamination is identified then a diagnosis cannot be given for that embryo.

The tubed cells are transferred to the PGD laboratory and the embryos are incubated in the IVF laboratory until the molecular analysis is complete and embryos can be selected for transfer into the uterus. Embryos that are found not to carry the inherited mutation are identified and then the morphologically best embryos are selected for transfer. A maximum of two embryos are transferred, however single embryo transfer is advocated as it avoids the clinical complications of multiple pregnancies. Additional genetically suitable embryos that develop to blastocyst can be cryopreserved. Embryos that carry the inherited mutation can be reanalysed as whole embryos to confirm the result that was diagnosed on single analysis. Such follow up work can be used to assess the risk of misdiagnosis and can be used as a quality indicator for the PGD laboratory [29].

PGD Outcome

Couples undertaking PGD for inherited cancer are generally fertile. However following oocyte retrieval there is loss of sample available for testing at each stage of the PGD process. Thus, not all oocytes collected mature to metaphase II, not all ooctyes inseminated fertilise, and not all embryos develop enough for biopsy. Embryos that are genetically unaffected may arrest and therefore cannot be transferred. Although approximately 81% of cycles that start the PGD process for single gene disorders have an embryo transfer, only 22% of cycles result in a clinical pregnancy [48]. Infertile couples undertaking PGD for inherited cancer with incomplete penetrance and adult onset face difficult choices if the only embryos morphologically suitable for transfer carry the inherited mutation [30].

PGD for Inherited Cancers, Clinical Attitudes and Patient Choice

PGD is a recent addition to the spectrum of familial cancer risk management. Hence it is not widely available and use so far has been limited [48]. However, there has been more recent interest in evaluating patient attitudes and options related to PGD in the context of other hereditary breast and ovarian as well as colorectal cancer syndromes.

In the U.K., a sample of 102 women with a *BRCA* mutation, most were supportive of PGD but only 38% of the women who had completed their families would consider it for themselves and only 14% of women who were contemplating a future pregnancy would consider it [35]. In a study of 77 individuals undergoing *BRCA* testing as part of a multicenter cohort study in Spain, 61% of respondents reported they would consider PGD. Factors associated with PGD acceptance were age >40 and having a cancer diagnosis.

In the U.S., a series of studies have evaluated awareness, acceptance, and attitudes related to PGD among members of Facing Our Risk of Cancer Empowered (FORCE), an advocacy organization focused on persons at increased risk of HBOC [1, 10, 11]. The first study was a web based survey of 283 members [1], the second included 205 attendees of the 2007 annual FORCE conference [10], and the third was a web based survey of 962 members [11, 12]. These studies have documented low levels of awareness, with 20–32% of study respondents reporting having heard of PGD prior to study participation [10, 11]. With respect to acceptance of PGD, Staton et al. [36] found only 13% of women would consider using PGD, whereas, 33% of respondents in the subsequent FORCE studies reported that PGD was an acceptable option [10, 11]. In the third FORCE based study ($n = 962$), multivariable analysis revealed PGD acceptance was associated with the desire to have more children, having previously had a prenatal genetic test, and previous awareness of PGD. With respect to attitudinal factors, respondents who believed that PGD is acceptable for persons at risk for HBOC, PGD information should be given to individuals at risk for HBOC, and endorsed PGD benefits of having children without genetic mutations and eliminating genetic diseases were more likely to accept PGD. Conversely, those who indicated that PGD was "too much like playing God" and reported that they considered PGD in the context of religion were less likely to accept PGD.

With respect to hereditary colorectal cancer, fewer studies have been conducted to assess attitudes toward PGD in the context of Familal Adenomatous Polyposis (FAP). In a study of families from a Dutch FAP registry ($n = 525$), 30% of respondents considered PGD to be an acceptable option. Those that had more favourable attitudes toward PGD were more likely to have higher levels of guilt about the possibility of passing the gene on to their children and a positive attitude toward termination of pregnancy in the context of various situations (in general, if the fetus has Down Syndrome, and if the fetus is a carrier of the FAP associated gene mutation [40]. Conversely, in another study of 20 individuals from a US based clinical sample of individuals affected with FAP, 90% stated they would consider PGD. All participants in this study considered PGD ethical and the 5 participants who reported having "strong religious backgrounds" stated they would consider PGD [34].

In addition to patient factors, the gradual uptake may also be attributed to the knowledge and attitude of referring clinicians to PGD for these disorders [31, 32] especially if penetrance is incomplete and the age of cancer onset is in adulthood [33]. Uptake varies depending upon the specific cancer predisposing syndrome and other treatment options available to patients [34–37].

While a cost benefit analysis of PGD for cystic fibrosis compared to lifelong treatment shows savings, similar studies are yet to be done for cancer predisposition [38, 39]. It is important that individuals with inherited cancers are made aware about PGD so that they are able to make informed reproductive choices [37]. Future developments in array technology and increased understanding of the genetics of cancer may lead to more refined determination of cancer susceptibility that can be applied to embryos.

Conclusion

PGD is an established technology. For couples who are fertile, the chance of a successful pregnancy and subsequently a child unaffected by the inherited germline mutation is good.

Couples with inherited cancer predisposition value the availability of PGD as a reproductive option. Clinical geneticists and cancer specialists therefore need to be knowledgeable about PGD.

Provider Recommendation

1. Patients with hereditary cancer syndromes may benefit from discussions of PGD in the context of family planning.

References

1. Simpson JL (2010) Preimplantation genetic diagnosis at 20 years. Prenat Diagn 30(7):682–695
2. Handyside A et al (1990) Pregnancies from biopsied human preimplantation embryos sexed by Y-specific DNA amplification. Nature 344(6268):768–770. PubMed PMID: 2330030
3. Handyside AH (2010) Preimplantation genetic diagnosis after 20 years. Reprod BioMed Online 21(3):280–282
4. Soini S (2007) Preimplantation genetic diagnosis (PGD) in Europe: diversity of legislation a challenge to the community and its citizens. Med Law 26(2):309–323
5. Clancy T (2010) A clinical perspective on ethical arguments around prenatal diagnosis and preimplantation genetic diagnosis for later onset inherited cancer predispositions. Fam Cancer 9(1):9–14
6. Robertson JA (2003) Extending preimplantation genetic diagnosis: the ethical debate: ethical issues in new uses of preimplantation genetic diagnosis. Hum Reprod 18(3):465–471
7. Van de Velde H et al (2009) The experience of two European preimplantation genetic diagnosis centres on human leukocyte antigen typing. Hum Reprod 24(3):732–740
8. Nagy R, Sweet K, Eng C (2004) Highly penetrant hereditary cancer syndromes. Oncogene 23(38):6445–6470
9. Knudson AG (2002) Cancer genetics. Am J Med Genet 111(1):96–102
10. Lu-Emerson C, Plotkin S (2009) The neurofibromatoses. Part 1: NF1. Rev Neurol Dis 6(2):E47–E53
11. Stadler ZK, Gallagher DJ, Thom P, Offit K (2010) Genome-wide association studies of cancer: principles and potential utility. Oncology Jun;24(7): 629–637
12. Lammens C et al (2009) Attitude towards preimplantation genetic diagnosis for hereditary cancer. Fam Cancer 8(4):457–464
13. Spits C, Sermon K (2009) PGD for monogenic disorders: aspects of molecular biology. Prenat Diagn 29(1):50–56
14. Vanneste E et al (2009) Preimplantation genetic diagnosis using fluorescent in situ hybridization for cancer predisposition syndromes caused by microdeletions. Hum Reprod 24(6):1522–1528
15. Renwick P et al (2010) Preimplantation genetic haplotyping: 127 diagnostic cycles demonstrating a robust, efficient alternative to direct mutation testing on single cells. Reprod Biomed Online 20(4): 470–476
16. Handyside AH, Harton GL, Mariani B, Thornhill AR, Affara N, Shaw MA, Griffin DK (2010) Karyomapping: a universal method for genome wide analysis of genetic disease based on mapping crossovers between parental haplotypes. J Med Genet 2010 Oct;47(10):651–658
17. Fiorentino F et al (2008) Rapid protocol for preconception genetic diagnosis of single gene mutations by first polar body analysis: a possible solution for the Italian patients. Prenat Diagn 28(1):62–4
18. Harton G et al (2011) ESHRE PGD consortium best practice guidelines for amplification-based PGD. Hum Reprod 26(1):33–40
19. Glentis S et al (2009) Molecular comparison of single cell MDA products derived from different cell types. Reprod BioMed Online 19(1):89–98
20. Jaroudi S et al (2009) Expression profiling of DNA repair genes in human oocytes and blastocysts using microarrays. Hum Reprod 24(10):2649–2655
21. Delhanty JDA et al (1997) Multicolour FISH detects frequent chromosomal mosaicism and chaotic division in normal preimplantation embryos from fertile patients. Hum Genet 99(6):755–760
22. Barlow DH (1998) GnRH agonists and in vitro fertilization. J Reprod Med 43(3 Suppl):245–251
23. Verlinsky Y et al (1990) Analysis of the first polar body: preconception genetic diagnosis. Hum Reprod 5(7):826–829
24. Verlinsky Y, Rechitsky S (1997) Preimplantation diagnosis of single gene disorders by two-step oocyte genetic analysis using first and second polar body. Biochem Mol Med 62(2):182–187
25. Goossens V et al (2008) Diagnostic efficiency, embryonic development and clinical outcome after the biopsy of one or two blastomeres for preimplantation genetic diagnosis. Hum Reprod 23(3): 481–492
26. McArthur S et al (2008) Blastocyst trophectoderm biopsy and preimplantation genetic diagnosis for familial monogenic disorders and chromosomal translocations. Prenat Diagn 28(5):434–442
27. Wilton L et al (2009) The causes of misdiagnosis and adverse outcomes in PGD. Hum Reprod 24(5): 1221–1228
28. Harton G et al (2011) ESHRE PGD consortium best practice guidelines for organization of a PGD centre for PGD/preimplantation genetic screening. Hum Reprod 26(1):14–24

29. Harper JC et al (2010) Accreditation of the PGD laboratory. Hum Reprod 25(4):1051–1065
30. Noble R et al (2008) Pandora's box: ethics of PGD for inherited risk of late-onset disorders. Reprod BioMed Online 17:55–60
31. Brandt AC et al (2010) Knowledge, attitudes, and clinical experience of physicians regarding preimplantation genetic diagnosis for hereditary cancer predisposition syndromes. Fam Cancer 9(3):479–487
32. Offit K et al (2006) Cancer genetic testing and assisted reproduction. J Clin Oncol 24(29):4775–4782
33. Julian-Reynier C et al (2009) Professionals assess the acceptability of preimplantation genetic diagnosis and prenatal diagnosis for managing inherited predisposition to cancer. J Clin Oncol 27(27):4475–4480
34. Kastrinos F et al (2007) Attitudes toward prenatal genetic testing in patients with familial adenomatous polyposis. Am J Gastroenterol 102(6):1284–1290
35. Menon U (2007) Views of BRCA gene mutation carriers on preimplantation genetic diagnosis as a reproductive option for hereditary breast and ovarian cancer. Hum Reprod 22(6):1573–1577
36. Staton AD et al (2008) Cancer risk reduction and reproductive concerns in female BRCA1/2 mutation carriers. Fam Cancer 7(2):179–186
37. Quinn GP et al (2009) Physician referral for fertility preservation in oncology patients: a national study of practice behaviors. J Clin Oncol 27(35):5952–5957
38. Davis LB et al (2010) A cost-benefit analysis of preimplantation genetic diagnosis for carrier couples of cystic fibrosis. Fertil Steril 93(6):1793–1804
39. Tur-Kaspa I et al (2010) PGD for all cystic fibrosis carrier couples: novel strategy for preventive medicine and cost analysis. Reprod Biomed Online 21(2):186–195
40. Douma KF et al (2010) Attitudes toward genetic testing in childhood and reproductive decision-making for familial adenomatous polyposis. Eur J Hum Genet 18(2):186–193
41. Abou-Sleiman PM et al (2002) First application of preimplantation genetic diagnosis to neurofibromatosis type 2 (NF2). Prenat Diagn 22(6):519–524
42. Altarescu G et al (2006) Single-sperm analysis for haplotype construction of de-novo paternal mutations: application to PGD for neurofibromatosis type 1. Hum Reprod 21(8):2047–2051
43. Altarescu G et al (2008) PGD on a recombinant allele: crossover between the TSC2 gene and 'linked' markers impairs accurate diagnosis. Prenat Diagn 28(10):929–933
44. Ao A et al (1998) Preimplantation genetic diagnosis of inherited cancer: familial adenomatous polyposis coli. J Assist Reprod Genet 15(3):140–144
45. Dhanjal S et al (2007) Preimplantation genetic diagnosis for retinoblastoma predisposition. Br J Ophthalmol 91(8):1090–1091
46. Fiorentino F et al (2003) The minisequencing method: an alternative strategy for preimplantation genetic diagnosis of single gene disorders. Mol Hum Reprod 9(7):399–410
47. Girardet A et al (2003) First preimplantation genetic diagnosis of hereditary retinoblastoma using informative microsatellite markers. Mol Hum Reprod 9(2):111–116
48. Harper JC et al (2010) ESHRE PGD Consortium data collection X: cycles from January to December 2007 with pregnancy follow-up to October 2008. Hum Reprod 25(11):2685–2707
49. Jasper MJ, Liebelt J, Hussey ND (2008) Preimplantation genetic diagnosis for BRCA1 exon 13 duplication mutation using linked polymorphic markers resulting in a live birth. Prenat Diagn 28(4):292–298
50. Moutou C et al (2007) Strategies and outcomes of PGD of familial adenomatous polyposis. Mol Hum Reprod 13(2):95–101
51. Rechitsky S et al (2002) Preimplantation genetic diagnosis for cancer predisposition. Reprod Biomed Online 5(2):148–155
52. Sagi M et al (2009) Preimplantation genetic diagnosis for BRCA1/2 – a novel clinical experience. Prenat Diagn 29(5):508–513
53. SenGupta S et al (2008) Preimplantation genetic diagnosis for cancer predisposition. Prenat Diagn 28(Supplement S3):2–3
54. Spits C et al (2005) Preimplantation genetic diagnosis for neurofibromatosis type 1. Mol Hum Reprod 11(5):381–387
55. Spits C et al (2007) Preimplantation genetic diagnosis for cancer predisposition syndromes. Prenat Diagn 27(5):447–456
56. Verlinsky Y et al (2002) Preimplantation diagnosis for neurofibromatosis. Reprod Biomed Online 4(3):218–222
57. Xu K et al (2004) Preimplantation genetic diagnosis for retinoblastoma: the first reported liveborn. Am J Ophthalmol 137(1):18–23

Non-traditional Family Building Planning

9

Judith E. Horowitz, PhD

Having cancer has been quite scary and physically exhausting. I felt sick and was worried that I would die. After the treatment put me into remission, I was nervous that I might never have a child. At the same time, I was also concerned I would pass my bad genes to my children and they eventually would get cancer too.

Since finding out that as a result of my cancer treatment I am sterile, many of my friends walk on eggshells when they are around me. I can see by their sideway glances that they are trying to be sensitive and considerate when speaking about their pregnancies and their children. I feel it is my job to reassure them that these are not forbidden topics.

I am quite fortunate. As soon as my oncologist informed me that my cancer treatment would cause infertility, my middle sister told me that when I wanted to become pregnant and have a child, she would like to donate her eggs to me. The reproductive endocrinologist with whom we consulted told us that quite often sisters donate eggs to sisters. Luckily, my middle sister Rita is 23 years old, and is eligible to help me out.

Not to be outdone by Rita, my youngest sister Melody offered to act as our gestational carrier, should I be unable to carry a baby to term. My husband and I will have to wait until Melody first has her own child to see whether she still wishes to be pregnant with our child. However, two of my closest friends who already have children have also volunteered to carry our child.

I am choosing not to disclose to my friends that Rita will act as my egg donor because I believe that the information about my child's conception should belong to my child and that Jake and I have the obligation to be the first ones to explain the facts about his or her conception. Only after I disclose to my child, do I intend to tell others. Of course, everyone will already know that Melody acted as our gestational surrogate because I won't ever be pregnant. My doctor told me that if one of my friends acts as our gestational carrier, I will have to tell her that we used Rita's eggs to conceive.

However, this experience also has been very humbling. I do not think I would have been the type of sister or friend who would have gone through controlled ovarian hyperstimulation or pregnancy for anyone other than me. This has caused me to take a good, hard look at myself and my life. I hope I become a better person as a result of having gone through cancer treatment.
Joanna, Adult Cancer Patient

Introduction

Fertility patients frequently report living in a binary world, one divided between the fertile and the infertile. However, adolescent and young adult (AYA) cancer survivors who later learn they will have difficulty conceiving or bearing children have similar reactions to their diagnosis, but with some marked differences, as the injustices

J.E. Horowitz (✉)
Private Practice, 5551 N University Drive, Suite 204,
Coral Springs, FL 33067, USA
e-mail: jhorowitzphd01@aol.com

G.P. Quinn, S.T. Vadaparampil (eds.), *Reproductive Health and Cancer in Adolescents and Young Adults*, Advances in Experimental Medicine and Biology 732,
DOI 10.1007/978-94-007-2492-1_9, © Springer Science+Business Media B.V. 2012

of their reality are much more complex. They frequently feel betrayed because the very treatments used to save their lives may be the ones that have caused them to be unable to have biogenetic children of their own, unable to fulfill their need for generativity and their longing for a return to normalcy [1].

In 1999, it was predicted that by the time this book is published one in every 250 young adults would be a survivor of cancer [2]. Although the ability to have biogenetically related offspring has been the topic of countless articles and books published in the area of reproductive health and medicine, less than half of adolescent and young adult cancer survivors can recall their oncologist or other members of their medical team discussing fertility related issues, including fertility preservation, prior to commencement of treatment [3–10]. Of those who did remember their physicians providing facts, advice, details, or statistics about fertility, many believed the information they received was inadequate and presented in an untimely manor [8–13]. Age seems to be associated with significant differences in this population: Younger AYA cancer survivors have reported a need for general fertility information and older survivors wanted more age appropriate information, as well as access to psychological counseling [14].

Psychosocial Issues That May Impact Consideration of Fertility Preservation

There are similarities and differences between the general infertile population and AYA cancer survivors whose treatment has caused them to become infertile. Like their infertile counterparts, many AYA male cancer survivors believe if they can ejaculate they are fertile. Similarly, women who continue to menstruate believe their fertility has been unaffected by cancer treatment. However, when they realize their beliefs are wrong they may be quite startled.

In general, fertility patients report feelings of guilt, fear, anxiety, dismay, sadness, helplessness, hopelessness, and, most frequently, extreme anger. They often experience a wide range of somatic symptoms, self-pity, self-blame, and grief. However, AYA cancer survivors worry about their long range prognosis, and, like other infertile individuals, feel a lack of control.

This feeling of being out of control is experienced on two separate and distinct fronts, i.e., not knowing when or if their cancer will recur, as well as whether they will be able to have children. In addition to the stress and various other negative emotions experienced by the infertile population, female AYA cancer survivors report feeling highly anxious that pregnancy with its attendant hormonal changes could cause a recurrence of their cancer. Additionally, both male and female AYA survivors fear their potential children would be at an increased risk for cancer and believe they, themselves, might have a shortened life span, dying before their children are able to live independent of them [15].

Like their counterparts, many AYA infertile cancer patients experience significant depression and anxiety [15]. Additionally, AYA cancer survivors are at an increased risk of depression caused by the pain and changes to the appearance of their sexual organs that often are a direct result of their treatment [16]. Sexual concerns frequently are overlooked by the AYA cancer survivors' medical teams. Cancer treatment often causes sexual dysfunction, including erectile dysfunction, hyposexual desire disorder, inability to climax, vaginal stenosis, and dryness which can cause dyspareunia, numbness, and disfigurement, e.g., surgical removal of breasts, testes, vulva, etc [3].

Additionally, the vomiting, pain, nausea, and obesity that often accompany cancer treatment may leave adolescents and young adults feeling extremely distressed [17]. Visible scars cause AYA cancer survivors to feel considerable self-consciousness (Odo 2009), and they frequently experience fatigue and cognitive changes [18]. Furthermore, along with adjustments to their self-concepts, AYA cancer survivors often feel defective and abnormal, and worry about the likelihood of finding a romantic partner to whom they must disclose not only their history of cancer, but their infertility, as well [18, 19].

Although many AYA cancer survivors have been found to have astonishing resilience, some experience post-traumatic stress disorder, which may cause them to delay fertility treatment, as treatment itself might trigger a recurrence of PTSD symptoms [3, 20, 21]. Due to the late effects of their treatment, AYA cancer survivors may be at increased risk for sexual experimentation and substance abuse, including an addiction to smoking, as well as alcoholism, which are well known contributors to decreased fertility [22–27].

Simultaneously, AYA cancer survivors must negotiate problems with their health insurance and may be saddled with huge debt resulting from their cancer treatment. Moreover, unlike others solely diagnosed with infertility, AYA cancer survivors often find their education and socialization disrupted, and may have difficulty with employment due to frequent absences, not only during treatments but recuperation, as well. Often cancer patients and survivors encounter changes in their relationships with family members, friends, and their peer group. Furthermore, AYA cancer survivors often feel "older" than their peers, causing them to feel disconnected from their contemporaries. Unable to feel the sense of immortality ordinarily experienced by their age group, their developmental tasks may be socially delayed, and subsequently, AYA cancer survivors may put off trying to conceive [6, 26].

Zebrack and Zelter have called upon cancer treatment teams to develop counseling methods to help AYA cancer survivors adopt health promoting behaviors [27]. Practicing healthy behaviors can reduce AYA cancer survivors' fears about the possibility of prematurely dying from cancer, as well as diminish the ill-effects of risky behavior on their potential fertility [28]. As AYA cancer survivors regain some control over their lives, they may be able to more competently cope with infertility.

Informed Decisions

As was previously mentioned, less than half of AYA cancer survivors recall their physicians discussing fertility preservation options. Merz and Fischoff differentiate between mere recall and deeper comprehension, and suggest understanding one's options are very important to good decision-making [29]. Bryan reported that more than 50% of the adult population of the US has low health literacy, and therefore this lack of understanding can lead to questionable informed consent [30].

The debilitating battle with cancer can leave even highly educated and intelligent patients confused and mentally exhausted. Considering the physical repercussions that cancer patients experience, they may feel sense of shame when unable to decipher and make sense of the information their physician is presenting to them, and they may not ask their doctor to provide additional comprehensible explanations.

Peters et al. discuss the concept of numeracy, i.e., the element of health literacy that refers to one's ability to understand numbers, necessary for good decision-making [31]. Less numerate patients give more credibility to immediate benefits than to those that will occur in the future. Therefore, too many AYA survivors may not realize that when certain cancer treatments are employed, infertility is a statistically probable result. Additionally, less numerate patients tend to rely upon nonnumeric sources of information, e.g., their trust of their physician or their emotional state, for their decision-making. Therefore, they may be unable to make good decisions as any conclusions would be derived from *uninformed* sources.

Physicians have a fiduciary duty to obtain informed consent from their patients [32]. Additionally, physicians are trained to identify the best treatments for each patient and then discuss both the benefits and the potential risks involved in each treatment choice. However, it has been estimated that only 12% of adults are considered to possess the ability to understand complex health information [33].

In general, risks for patients can be interpreted as either loss (es) or exposure to the possibility of injury, and fertility risks in the treatment of cancer may mean a temporary or permanent loss of reproductive capabilities [32]. The term *risk communication* refers to the process of communicating information about risks under circumstances involving a combination of low trust, high concern, perceived crisis, or differential interpersonal power. Many of these conditions seem to exist for, among others, AYA cancer patients [34].

AYA cancer patients may find decision-making rather difficult, especially if they never previously considered their fertility at risk. Neither adolescents nor young adults receive training in good decision-making prior to their diagnosis. Provision of sufficient information which permits patients to make knowledgeable choices is necessary for a truly informed consent. However, cancer patients actually may be too ill to consider the benefits of alternative treatments, and therefore the choices they are called upon to make may seem overwhelming.

Many cancer patients may choose to avoid any immediate potential personal risk, i.e., death, and instead may revise their expectations regarding their capacity in the future to have biogenetic children [35]. However, if AYA cancer patients are unable to make good decisions regarding their long-term reproductive health, and should they need to rely upon others for assistance, their decisions could no longer be perceived as having been reached autonomously, presenting an ethical problem. Does this then invalidate their informed consent?

Access to treatment, justice, and fairness are three additional areas of ethical conundrums that bear discussion. AYA cancer survivors' treatments may have depleted their own, as well as their families' monetary resources. ART is very expensive, especially third party collaborative arrangements, and cancer survivors may be unable to afford fertility treatment. Being denied access to fertility treatments seems especially unfair, as AYA cancer survivors have already struggled to survive.

Recently, neuropsychologists have begun to investigate cognitive functioning in adolescents and young adults. Their research helps shed light on the capacity for good decision-making for this population [36, 37]. Sowell and her colleagues found the frontal lobe of the brain, which is responsible for reasoning, as well as

comprehending long-term consequences, undergoes more changes during adolescence than at any other stage of life [38]. In a later study, Sowell and her team of investigators found that the brain continues to mature well into an individual's early 20s [39]. Therefore, a teenager or young adult's inability to plan for the future or think about the consequences of their treatment should be considered when assessing the AYA cancer survivor's decision-making capacity about their future fertility.

Although AYA cancer survivors' immaturity may have an adaptive role when assessing the stress and trauma of their diagnosis, they literally may be unable to wrap their brains around the consequences to their future fertility [20]. It may be that only when AYA cancer survivors attempt to conceive that they will be confronted with the outcome and repercussions of their prior treatment. This is neither *fair* nor *just,* and AYA cancer survivors may require assistance in accepting the reality of infertility, which in all likelihood may cause them to seek non-traditional alternative methods of family building.

Non-traditional Alternatives for Males

Those AYA males with cancer who have a normal sperm count when diagnosed may wish to freeze their sperm for subsequent intrauterine insemination (IUI) cycles with future female partners. However, if they are azoospermic or have a low sperm count at the time of their cancer diagnosis they may choose to freeze sperm obtained through testicular sperm extraction (TESE) for later use with in vitro fertilization (IVF) and intracytoplasmic sperm injection (ICSI), which injects the sperm directly into the egg so fertilization can take place, and offers hope of conceiving biogenetically related offspring [8, 12, 40–50]. Additionally, with respect to those men who have a partner at the time of their diagnosis, ICSI may be used for those who wish to cryopreserve embryos, rather than sperm, alone, prior to the commencement of cancer treatment.

Fearful for their survival, AYA males too often do not think about their lives after cancer treatment ends. A male's fertility may be permanently or transiently affected after treatment ends. As there is no prognostic test available to ascertain who will be left infertile, sperm banking has been urged and cryopreservation should be suggested prior to the beginning of cancer treatment [8, 12, 40, 42, 45, 46, 49–51]. Physicians suggesting sperm banking to those under the age of majority should be particularly sensitive to adolescent embarrassment about masturbation [7]. Additionally, the Ethics Committee of the ASRM recommends that any discussion of sperm banking should take place outside the presence of the adolescent's parents [51]. AYA cancer patients should be told of the potential harmful effects of reproduction on their potential children [51]. Young AYA cancer survivors deciding to cryopreserve their sperm will be forced to make legal decisions about the possibility of posthumous reproduction should they not survive their disease.

According to Shover and her colleagues, most AYA cancer survivors report wanting to have a biogenetically related offspring, and once cancer-free, believe they are healthy enough to be good parents [52, 53]. Additionally, they seem to place a higher value on the family, believing their perspective on life has been radically altered so that they cherish those things that are important and minimize the insignificant. AYA cancer survivors also believe they more easily deal with stress without bearing negative consequences.

Unfortunately, cryopreservation does not guarantee conception. Recently, Dotinga (2010) reported that vitrifying sperm by removing the plasma, suspending them in a sucrose solution, fast-freezing the sperm with liquid nitrogen, and subsequently storing in a deep freeze may improve the survival rate for later use [54]. AYA cancer survivors may be asked to consider sperm recipientcy if they are fearful that their sperm put their future children at greater risk for cancer, if they did not have viable sperm at the time of diagnosis, or if cryopreservation did not occur.

Researchers are developing procedures for male AYA survivors who become infertile as a result of cancer treatment. Recently, Belgian scientists reported that testicular tissue extracted from young, pre-pubescent boys could be successfully converted to sperm precursor cells [55]. Eventually enough cells could grow and repopulate in the adult survivor's testes where they would mature into sperm necessary for conception. This technique is experimental and until it has been found safe, males may decide to use donor sperm.

Sperm Recipientcy

Sperm recipientcy is the most frequently used and successful method of family building available for males. If cryopreservation was not offered or was not possible prior to the beginning of cancer treatment, one might expect the male AYA survivor to feel anger and loss. Researchers have reported that men who need to use donated sperm feel less virile and masculine, and frequently have a diminished sex drive. Often their sexual identities suffer and they feel socially stigmatized [28, 56–61]. Additional psychological and emotional reactions to the need to use donor sperm include; lack of confidence and shame, and low self-esteem [58, 60, 62–69]. Moreover, cancer survivors who need to use donated sperm may feel defective and abnormal and often have an especially difficult time grieving for the loss of their former, healthy selves [19].

When use of their own cryopreserved sperm is not viable, donor sperm in conjunction with IUI offers an alternative fertility treatment. Prior to using donor insemination (DI), the female partner of the male AYA cancer survivor will be medically evaluated. Initially, insemination will be attempted without the use of ovulation stimulating drugs. DI will be synchronized with the woman's menstrual cycle to coincide with ovulation. Should a live birth fail to result from a natural cycle, medications for controlled ovarian hyperstimulation (COH) may be administered in conjunction with DI, which increases the likelihood conception will occur [70].

DI is conducted with the thawed semen of the donor, which is drawn into an insemination catheter with a syringe attached to its end. The syringe is inserted through the woman's cervix and into her uterine cavity where the semen is deposited. If DI is successful, the sperm will travel into his partner's fallopian tubes where fertilization will occur [71].

The donated sperm that is used in IVF procedures with ICSI have to survive the thawing process. The rates of success for this procedure can vary and are influenced by many factors, such as the quality of the sperm, the ova, and the woman's uterine environment [72].

Should the male be a partner in a homosexual relationship, or if he is single, he may elect to use donor sperm, donated oocytes, and a gestational carrier to help him create his family. Because many cancer survivors are fearful they will genetically transmit cancer to their offspring, men in homosexual relationships may prefer to use the sperm of their healthy partner, if available.

Mancini et al. found that AYA cancer survivors who did not preserve their sperm prior to cancer treatment reported a lower physical and mental quality of life [8]. A precautionary tale to physicians emerges from those patients who had not been informed that cryopreservation of sperm was an option, as they universally reported being dissatisfied with their medical treatment [7].

Types of Sperm Donors

Although men unable to conceive with their own sperm rarely disclose their infertility to others, AYA cancer survivors usually do not have the luxury of privacy, as their diagnosis and treatment probably has been the subject of discussion among their families and friends. Consequently, friends and family members might offer to donate their sperm to help the survivor build his family. AYA cancer survivors who are sperm recipients may prefer to use known donors because the donor's medical background and genetics will be familiar. Sperm donated by family members can preserve the genetic link to the recipients. Furthermore, when intrafamilial donation is available, the donors, recipients, and their offspring may enjoy a closer relationship than if the sperm had been provided by an anonymous donor [73].

Known donors, including family members, will be required to submit to the identical medical, genetic, and psychological testing required of anonymous sperm providers. Those tests may reveal problems that were previously unknown to the potential donor, possibly causing him psychologic distress and emotional problems. Additionally, researchers have reported that family members may experience changes in their dynamics, either bringing family members closer or causing a deterioration in their relationship [74, 75]. However, keeping in touch with their sperm donors may be more important to AYA cancer survivors than to the general public because they realize that serious health risks exist and can capriciously strike anyone at anytime.

Researchers have reported the majority of potential sperm donors require anonymity and confidentiality [76–78]. However, mature sperm donors have been found to be more amenable to open donation than younger sperm donors [57, 66]. Many potential sperm donors are willing to provide non-identifying information to their offspring and recipients, and others permit their identities to be released when their offspring reach the age of majority [57, 76–79]. Sperm providers' attitudes toward openness often reflect the attitudes held by the sperm bank personnel [58].

Moreover, Rowland found more than half of the donors surveyed in her study would accept contact from their adult offspring [80]. More recently, sperm donors have reported their willingness to participate in a voluntary sperm donor registry [81]. Momentum and the wishes of the donor conceived children may continue to drive the recent trend toward disclosure and openness.

Alternative Family Building for Females

Although physicians have been strongly urged to discuss fertility preservation with their patients, they infrequently communicate the impact cancer treatment will have on the female's fertility [13, 35, 76, 82]. Many women report that they never received information about the deleterious effects of chemotherapy or radiation on their fertility, nor were they referred to reproductive endocrinologists for fertility treatment prior to undergoing cancer treatment [5, 9–11, 16].

Cancer treatment protocols have improved the long-term survival rates of adolescents and young women, and, following medical intervention, ovarian damage to survivors can be determined by the class of chemotherapeutic agent used, as well as the woman's age, and the dose of pelvic radiation received [83–85]. Anticancer drugs affect a woman's reproductive abilities through both stromal and ovarian follicular damage, but the precise process has yet to be understood [85]. A greater percentage of females than males become infertile as a consequence of their cancer treatment and women usually feel more distressed about their infertility than their male counterparts [4, 13, 86].

The most successful option for women who desire to have children is embryo storage, but cancer treatment would need to be delayed while the woman undergoes controlled ovarian hyperstimulation (COH) and oocyte retrieval, also called egg harvesting. Females with partners at the time of their cancer diagnosis may wish to cryopreserve embryos created with their partner's sperm. Women without partners may chose to use donor sperm with their ova, as embryo cryopreservation currently is the most viable non-traditional alternative of family building. However, if without a partner, she would need to select a sperm donor which may easily overwhelm an adolescent or young adult [87].

Successful family building alternatives for female AYA cancer survivors who have not cryopreserved embryos include oocyte recipientcy, which can be used for those whose ovaries were affected by their cancer treatment, and gestational surrogacy which is appropriate for female AYA cancer survivors whose uteri were affected or removed. Several strategies for fertility preservation are available, but at this time most are experimental. Cryopreservation of ova and other investigational alternatives will be reviewed later in this chapter.

Oocyte Recipientcy

Women are born with a finite number of immature ova. Approximately two million eggs are found in a female infant's ovaries. Although usually as a teenager, 300,000–400,000 ova remain, with about 1,000 dying each month (Silber 2005), Cancer treatment can cause the destruction of an AYA's eggs, and consequently her ovaries will cease to produce estrogen and she will proceed through menopause [88]. The process of ovarian failure is intermittent in women who do not go through cancer therapy [89]. However, in women exposed to radiation, chemotherapy, or a combination of both, ovarian failure is an abrupt event.

Should an AYA cancer survivor wish to have children, she will be asked to consider using donated ova in conjunction with IVF. If she agrees, both the donor's and the AYA cancer survivor recipient's menstrual cycles will be synchronized, and the ovum recipient's endometrial lining will be made ready for implantation of the transferred embryos [90]. Simultaneously, the laboratory staff processes the sperm, which activates them so they can penetrate the eggs. The ova can be fertilized with either her partner's sperm or sperm from a donor. The eggs will be placed in a container with the culture medium, and after several hours the processed sperm will be added to the microenvironments under oil. Once the sperm penetrates the outside of the ovum, consisting of the corona radiata and the zona straita or zona pellucida, fertilization can occur and the embryos are allowed to develop prior to transfer. The petri dishes containing the embryos remain in an incubator at the temperature a woman's body would provide. Once divided, the embryos would be transferred into a catheter and deposited into the recipient's uterus three to five days later [91].

The patient will have a blood test 10–12 days after embryo transfer to determine whether she is pregnant [92]. Any excess embryos that were not transferred to the ovum recipient can be cryopreserved for subsequent IVF cycles. Should the

AYA survivor no longer have a uterus, a gestational surrogate can receive the embryos, and this alternative will be discussed later in this chapter.

Anticipating the need to use donated oocytes, which prevents the intended mother from being biogenetically linked to her child frequently results in feelings of loss, grief, frustration, regret, guilt, ambivalence, and anger at life's injustice. Prior to beginning medical treatment, an oocyte recipient will need to address whether she feels unequal within the parenting unit. Many oocyte recipient patients fearfully fantasize that one day their children will state aloud they are not the "real" mother. These women are distinguishing the difference between being a genetic, rather than gestational mother.

A mental health professional practicing within the realm of reproductive health and medicine can assist the patient to sort through her emotions and help the oocyte recipient come to terms with this differentiation. Psychologists can have the egg recipient AYA cancer survivor acknowledge and accept that for nine months of pregnancy she will nourish, protect, and, in all likelihood, bond with this child. Moreover, the oocyte recipient can learn to see herself as a caring mother even prior to embryo transfer by her efforts to eat well-balanced meals, take prenatal vitamins, and to eliminate caffeine, alcohol, or any drugs that might harm the fetus [70].

Types of Oocyte Donors

There are three possible types of oocyte donors from which AYA cancer survivors can choose. *Known* donors are those known to the recipients at the time of conception. These are usually family members or friends who either approach the recipients or are asked by the recipients to become their potential ovum donors. Recipients are often appreciative of the opportunity to use a known donor because her genetic background and health history are familiar and, in the case of family members, are similar to the recipient herself.

On the other hand, AYA cancer survivors may find *anonymous* donors more suitable because they never wish for their identities to be revealed to the recipient or their offspring. Anonymous donation avoids changes in the relationships among family members or friends. The child or children conceived with gametes from an anonymous donor in this type of collaborative arrangement would not be confused by the biogenetic ties inherent in familial donation, as very definite boundaries would exist. However, there is a growing trend in the field of reproductive health and medicine towards meeting the egg donors.

Identified donors may be particularly attractive to recipients who are cancer survivors, as identified donors are willing to have their identities released to the children conceived from their ova once the offspring have reached the age of legal majority. This would permit the donor conceived children to acquire updated pertinent medical information about their oocyte donors, as well as their biogenetically related families, which, in turn, might allay the recipients' fear of the unknown.

Experimental Procedures

The storage of frozen oocytes for future fertilization has only recently been met with a modicum of success and is still considered an experimental treatment. Other experimental options include freezing ovarian tissue or an entire ovary for future transplantation, the transposition of ovaries prior to radiation, hormonal and pharmacologic protection during cancer treatment, and finally, a complete uterine transplant [87, 93–97]. Patrizio argues that doctors are not ethically obligated to offer experimental services to AYA cancer survivors during a time when they are extremely vulnerable [98]. As more elegant methods for the conveyance of informed consent are established and better educational materials and professional guidelines for fertility preservation are developed, as well as when more successful oocyte cryopreservation methods are devised, women who have had cancer may require donated ova with less frequency [99, 100].

Alternatives for Both Males and Females

The two most popular non-traditional family building methods available to both female and male AYA cancer survivors are traditional and gestational surrogacy. Domestic and international adoptions, which have been employed for decades, also offer AYA cancer survivors the opportunity to have families.

Surrogacy

Surrogacy is a viable option for intended parents who are either unable to carry a baby to term or conceive without assistance. Traditional surrogates use their own eggs and sperm provided by either the intended father or sperm donor, usually using IUI. Traditional surrogacy is less expensive than gestational surrogacy and may not require the surrogate to undergo surgery. However, in the case of single or homosexual AYA male cancer survivors who have previously banked their sperm, IVF with ICSI and embryo transfer with the aid of either a traditional or gestational surrogate offers a good alternative to remaining child-free.

A gestational surrogate, usually called a gestational carrier (GC), does not use her own ova and achieves pregnancy with IVF. After embryo transfer, the GC carries the pregnancy for the intended parent(s). The gametes may be provided by both of the intended parents (IPs), an egg donor and the intended father, donated eggs and donated sperm, donor sperm and the intended mother's oocytes, or donated embryos. Due to the potential for legal and emotional difficulties, traditional surrogacy is being used less frequently than gestational surrogacy. Fewer legal issues arise when using a GC as the surrogate lacks a biogenetic connection to the resulting offspring. AYA female cancer survivors with histories of chemotherapy, radiation, or hysterectomies may find contracting with a GC, an excellent option.

AYA cancer survivors can expect to receive positive reactions from both maternal and paternal parents after they disclose that GCs will be assisting them in the creation of their families

[101]. The majority of IPs perceived their relationship with the surrogates as harmonious [102]. Those surrogates who have a satisfactory relationship with the IP or IPs usually express satisfaction with their experience [101–106].

Adoption

AYA cancer survivors may also elect the adoption alternative. There are many reasons AYA cancer survivors may prefer adoption over participation in the ARTs. AYA survivors may be poor candidates for ART using their own gametes, even those who took advantage of cryopreservation prior to the commencement of cancer therapy, as their reproductive cells would need to survive the thawing process. They may not have sufficient funds to cover both fertility treatment and adoption, especially if the AYA cancer survivor wishes to have more than one child. Therefore, they may choose to adopt as they may feel more confident of building their family with this time honored method. Many kind-hearted individuals and couples prefer to adopt an existing child who might not otherwise have a stable and loving family.

Additionally, after already experiencing the uncertainty of a good prognosis, as well as the toll taken by the lack of personal privacy caused by their cancer treatment, AYA survivors may not wish to be perceived yet again as a patient who is somehow defective. AYA survivors may wish to bypass all additional invasive medical treatments, including those necessary to conceive a child through the ARTs. Moreover, adopting a child who is not biogenetically related to either parent may seem to equitably balance the lack of a biogenetic link between the child and either parent. However, many individuals and couples will decide to adopt after a series of failed attempts to conceive using the options previously discussed. Adoption, which once seemed less desirable, may now be considered their last possible chance to become parents.

Furthermore, current research concludes that children adopted into gay and lesbian families are just as well-adjusted as those raised in heterosexual households [107]. Therefore, AYA gay and lesbian cancer survivors eventually may have an easier time adopting as some countries and states within the US are revising their current laws.

AYA survivors should be cancer free for 5 years (which is the gold standard benchmark) prior to aggressively attempting to adopt. During the time they are cancer free and waiting to build their families, AYA cancer survivors can receive information from their physicians about their chances for long-term survival. Additionally, they can begin to research the various types of adoptions that are available. Survivors could designate who would provide support and be responsible for the child(ren) should they predecease their adopted child.

Individuals do not come with a guarantee that they will live for the 20 plus years necessary to raise children. However, the possibility of living until, and hopefully after, one's child enters college is highly desirable. Furthermore, AYA cancer survivors should prepare a will that provides for the placement of their child upon their death. During this five year wait, AYA cancer survivors can address their fears and psychological concerns about adoption, including the adoption triad comprised of themselves, the birthparent(s), and the adopted child.

Domestic vs. International Adoption

Domestic adoptions involve adoptive parents and children who have the same country of residence and are of the same nationality. International adoptions involve parents who do not reside in the same country as the child who they wish to adopt. There is some disparity in the literature regarding whether it is easier for AYA cancer survivors to adopt domestically or internationally.

Rosen (2005) states that many countries do not consider cancer to be curable and therefore, an AYA cancer survivor's history will exclude him or her from eligibility to participate in an international adoption [109]. However, Moss believes that international adoption is feasible [108]. After providing a well-chosen social worker (one who is well-versed in cancer literature and is sympathetic towards cancer survivors)

with documentation from the cancer survivor's physicians, including their diagnosis and treatment, current medical status, issues of future medical risk, and projected length of survival, the social worker is free to elect not to provide a detailed health history to the birthparents. Often those wishing to become adoptive parents do not know that it is their prerogative to select the social worker with whom they will work. If the social worker chooses to disclose the health status of the AYA cancer survivor to an international agency, it may follow that a domestic rather than international adoption may be easier to achieve. Ineligibility to adopt internationally may cause the survivor to feel further victimized by the unfairness caused by the dual diagnosis of both cancer and infertility.

Birthparents in domestic adoptions, are often permitted to select with whom to place their child. They may chose to discriminate against the AYA cancer survivor once the medical history has been revealed. Therefore, anonymous and closed international adoptions in countries that allow cancer survivors to participate may be preferable. Prospective parents must be prepared to travel at least once, and sometimes more often, to the country from where they wish to adopt. Often lengthy stays are the norm, rather than the exception. This can cause employment disruptions and create additional travel expenses that may be especially onerous for AYA cancer survivors who already may have missed years in the workforce and may face considerable obstacles to their professional development. Moreover, the background and health information about the adoptees that adoptive parents receive from international agencies is often incomplete and unreliable. This may cause anxiety in AYA cancer survivors who already know about the capricious nature of serious, life-threatening diseases.

All domestic adoptions involve home studies which assess the individual or couple's motivations and expectations in their desire to adopt. Family relationships will be examined and unresolved fertility issues will be addressed. Parental education and employment will be scrutinized, and they will be asked to provide financial reports. Applicants' health histories will be taken and sometimes a physical examination by qualified physicians will be required. References must also be supplied to the person conducting the home study. Descriptions of additional types of adoptions follow below.

Agency vs. Independent Adoption

Agency adoptions, e.g., governmental or social service, also help individuals who wish to parent. A governmental agency usually becomes involved when the birthparents' rights have been revoked. Parental rights may be terminated due to abuse, neglect, or inability to provide a home free from exposure to violence, drugs, or other illegal activities. Social service agencies, non-sectarian, as well as those with religious affiliations, e.g., Catholic charities, Jewish Adoption and Foster Care Options (JAFCO), exist in addition to those which are connected to for-profit and non-profit agencies. *Traditional* agency adoptions occur when the birthmother places her child with the agency, and is permitted to select the adoptive parents from that agency's pre-approved list of potential parents.

Independent or private adoptions occur when a potential adoptive individual or couple locates birthparents or a birthmother with the assistance of an attorney or adoption facilitator, who makes arrangements for the placement of a child. Birthmothers can only be reimbursed for the expenses they incur during their pregnancies, the birth of their children, and the care they receive immediately postpartum, as it is illegal to "purchase" a child. Often prospective parents feel some sense of control in independent adoptions because they may be more involved in decision-making.

AYA cancer survivors may prefer independent adoptions, as the restrictions present in other methods of adoption frequently can be bypassed. However, financial risks are greater in independent adoptions and they present the greatest emotional risk because the birthparent(s) can reclaim the child up until the time parental rights have been legally terminated. The time frame for birthmothers (or birthparents) to revoke their rights varies from state to state, and therefore familiarity with adoption laws is essential prior to deciding on an independent adoption.

Closed vs. Open Adoption

Confidential and anonymous adoptions are also called *closed* adoptions. In the past, international adoptions were always closed. However, recently there has been more openness in international adoptions, which slowly are being modified to reflect the changes that have taken place during in the past several decades in domestic adoptions.

Varying degrees of openness exist in open adoptions. The birthparents and the adoptive parents learn identifying information about each other in open adoptions. They are encouraged to meet each other and form a relationship, especially for the benefit of the child. Grotevant (1997) reported open adoptions generally have positive outcomes for the birthparents, adoptees, and the adoptive parents [110].

Birthparents and adoptive parents in *semi-open* adoptions may not permit their identities to be revealed, but they may receive and exchange photographs and information about each other's health background, their educational achievements, type (but not exact location) of employment, etc. A face-to-face meeting (without disclosure of the participants' names, address of residence, or places of employment) may be facilitated in semi-open adoptions by a third party, e.g., social worker, adoption attorney, or representative of an adoption agency.

Furthermore, in both semi-open and open adoptions the birthparents may receive an essay written by the potential adoptive parents explaining why they wish to adopt a child. Frequently, the birthmother is permitted to read potential adoptive parents' portfolios and choose with whom she wishes to place her child, the adoptee. Prospective adoptive parents may be able to choose the degree of openness they want, as well as the extent of future contact, and should memorialize everything in writing. Exchanging emails, photographs, and phone calls, as well as planning to meet in person once or twice a year can help the birthparents move forward in their lives. Open adoptions can help the adoptees have a sense of acceptance rather than abandonment, and may permit the adoptive parents to attach to their children without fearing the unknown.

Adjusting to the Transition to Parenthood

AYA cancer survivors experience significant loss prior to adoption. Survivors' years of medical treatment, psychological upheaval and disappointments, including changes to their self-concept, familial and marital conflicts, narcissistic injury, and stigma will impact their adjustment to parenting after adoption. We can expect AYA cancer survivors to feel a lack of control over their destinies, as well as believing that their world will never again be predictable. However, research supports that adoptive parents usually enjoy an easier transition to parenthood than biogenetic parents, as they have longed for, anticipated, and planned for the arrival of their child [111].

Often infertile individuals and couples fear they will not be able to love an adopted child as much as they could a biogenetically related child. Furthermore, prospective parents frequently are afraid their children will not adequately love them, and will seek out and enjoy a deeper, more loving relationship with their birthparents. AYA survivors may wonder whether their children, knowledgeable about their history of cancer, may wish to find their more robust birthparents with whom they could share a life free from health concerns. However, once informed that most adoptees do want some sort of relationship with their birthparents, parents need not interpret their children's desire as a failure or inadequacy on their part.

Conclusion

In all probability, the ranks of AYA cancer survivors will increase due to advances in treatments, as well as research, especially within the area of genome studies. Individualized cancer treatments will enable medical teams to save more lives, but not necessarily their patients' fertility. However, fertility treatments currently considered experimental hopefully will evolve, significantly improve, and become routine.

Concurrently, psychologists will contribute new research to the existing body of literature regarding how humans learn. Their findings can advise physicians how to better communicate health risks to their AYA patients. Additionally, physicians can present information about fertility in multiple ways, taking into account that people absorb new data through auditory, visual, and kinesthetic means.

Cancer teams can employ an assortment of the above methods and encourage their patients to ask questions in an unhurried and non-judgmental atmosphere, i.e., one that is shame-free. Oncologists and medical team members who heed the advice provided by psychologists can assist AYA cancer survivors and their families, who may not possess adequate health literacy at the time of diagnosis and subsequent treatment. These adaptations in patient education will enable survivors to make truly informed choices. As previously mentioned, ethical decision-making can occur only when patients are able to reach autonomous decisions.

In conclusion, AYA cancer survivors who wish to build families of their own will continue to find assisted reproductive techniques beneficial. Non-traditional methods such as sperm and oocyte recipientcy, as well as traditional and gestational surrogacy will be preferred methods of family building for some, while others will elect the adoption alternative.

Provider Recommendations

1. The medical team should be familiar with the cognitive function of adolescents and young adults so as to enable their patients so they can make good treatment decisions and provide their informed consent.

2. The AYA survivors' oncologists and medical team should provide adequate information regarding fertility related issues, including fertility preservation and the availability of psychological counseling for the emotional difficulties that may arise with the diagnosis of infertility.

3. AYA cancer survivors' medical team should discuss sexual issues with their patients; e.g., disfigurement of sexual organs, various sexual dysfunctions (hyposexual desire disorder, dyspareunia, erectile dysfunction), etc.

4. Physician initiated discussions concerning sexual topics with both male and female AYA cancer patients should take place without the presence of their parents.

5. Prior to treatment, physicians of AYA males should thoroughly explain cryopreservation of sperm, intracytoplasmic sperm injection (ICSI), and testicular sperm extraction (TESE).

6. Male AYA cancer survivors should be informed about sperm recipientcy in conjunction with intrauterine insemination and in vitro fertilization, and, for single and/or homosexual males, the availability of traditional surrogates and gestational carriers.

7. Understanding that more females than males are infertile after cancer treatment and are more upset about being infertile, their medical team should discuss embryo cryopreservation with either their partner's sperm or that obtained from a sperm donor.

8. AYA cancer survivors should be able to distinguish amongst known, anonymous, open, and identified sperm and oocyte donors.

9. Cancer team members should thoroughly explain the experimental medical treatments available to their AYA female patients. These include the storage of frozen oocytes, ovarian tissue and total ovarian transplantation, ovarian transposition, uterine transplants, etc.

10. Both male and female AYA cancer survivors should be aware of the availability of traditional surrogates and gestational carriers. Additionally they should be able to distinguish between the various adoption alternatives, i.e., open vs. closed, agency vs. independent, domestic vs. international.

References

1. Eiser C, Penn A, Katz E, Barr R (eds) (2009) Psychosocial issues and quality of life. Elsevier Seminars in Oncology 36:375–380
2. Ries LAG, Smith MA, Gurney JG, Linet M, Tamra T, Young J et al (1999) Cancer incidence and survival among children and adolescents: United States SEER Program 1975–1995. Bethesda, MD: National Cancer Institute SEER Program NIH Pub no. 994649
3. Algier L, Kav S (2008) Nurses' approach to sexuality-related issues in patients receiving cancer treatments. Turk J Cancer 38(3):135–141
4. Deming S (2007) OncoLog 51. http://www2.mdanderson.org/depts/oncolog/articles/06/1-Jan-06-1.html
5. Forman EJ, Anders CK, Behera MA (2010) A nationwide survey of oncologists regarding treatment-related infertility and fertility preservation in female cancer patients. Fertil Steril 94: 1652–1661
6. Jones BL (2008) Promoting healthy development among survivors of adolescent cancer. Fam Commun Health 31:S61–S70
7. Lee SJ, Schover LR, Partridge AH, Patrizio P, Wallace WH, Hagerty K et al (2006) American Society of Clinical Oncology recommendations on fertility preservation in cancer patients. J Clin Oncol 24(18):2917–2931
8. Mancini J, Rey D, Préau M, Malavolti L, Moatti JP (2008) Infertility induced by cancer treatment: inappropriate or no information provided to majority of French survivors of cancer. Fertil Steril 90(5):1616–1625
9. Nieman CL, Kazer R, Brannigan RE, Zoloth LS, Chase-Lansdale PL, Kinahan K et al (2006) Cancer survivors and infertility: a review of a new problem and novel answers. J Support Oncol 4(4):171–178
10. de Ziegler D, Streuli I, Vasilopoulos I, Decanter C, This P, Chapron C (2010) Cancer and fecundity issues mandate a multidisciplinary approach. Fertil Steril 93(3):691–696
11. Jukkala AM, Azuero A, McNees P, Bates GW, Meneses K (2010) Self-assessed knowledge of treatment and fertility preservation in young women with breast cancer. Fertil Steril 94(6):2396–2398
12. Meseguer M, Molina N, García-Velasco JA, Remohí J, Pellicer A, Garrido N (2006) Sperm cryopreservation in oncological patients: a 14-year follow-up study. Fertil Steril 85(3):640–645
13. Schover LR (1999) Psychosocial aspects of infertility and decisions about reproduction in young cancer survivors: a review. Med Pediatr Oncol 33(1):53–59
14. Zebrack BJ, Mills J, Weitzman TS (2007) Health and supportive care needs of young adult cancer patients and survivors. J Cancer Survivorship 1(2):137–145

15. Schover LR (2005) Motivation for parenthood after cancer: a review. JNCI Monogr 2005(34):2–5

16. Soliman H, Agresta SV (2008) Current issues in adolescent and young adult cancer survivorship. Cancer Control 15(1):55–62

17. Clinton-McHarg T, Carey M, Sanson-Fisher R, Shakeshaft A, Rainbird K (2010) Measuring the psychosocial health of adolescent and young adult (AYA) cancer survivors: a critical review. Cancer 8:25–38

18. Odo R, Potter C (2009) Understanding the needs of young adult cancer survivors: a clinical perspective. Oncology (Williston Park, NY) 23(11 Suppl Nurse Ed) 33:23–27

19. Maier DB, Covington SN, Maier LU (2006) Patients with medically complicating conditions. Cambridge University Press, New York, NY

20. Noll RB, Kupst MJ (2007) Commentary: the psychological impact of pediatric cancer hardiness, the exception or the rule? J Pediatr Psychol 32(9):1089–1098

21. Rourke MT, Hobbie WL, Schwartz L, Kazak AE (2007) Posttrauamatic stress disorder (PTSD) in young adult survivors of childhood cancer. Pediatr Blood Cancer 49(2):177–182

22. Eggert J, Theobald H, Engfeldt P (2004) Effects of alcohol consumption on female fertility during an 18-year period. Fertil Steril 81(2):379–383

23. Gaur DS, Talekar MS, Pathak VP (2010) Alcohol intake and cigarette smoking: Impact of two major lifestyle factors on male fertility. Indian J Pathol Microbiol 53(1):35–40

24. Jensen TK, Hjollund NKI, Henriksen TB, Scheike T, Kolstad H, Giwercman A et al (1998) Does moderate alcohol consumption affect fertility? Follow up study among couples planning first pregnancy. BMJ 317(7157):505–510

25. Silva PD, Cool J, Olson K (1999) Impact of lifestyle choices on female infertility. J Reprod Med 44(3):288

26. Jones L (2008) Surviving childhood cancer – growing up too fast. J Reprod Med 44:288–296

27. Zebrack BJ, Zeltzer LK (2003) Quality of life issues and cancer survivorship. Curr Probl Cancer 27(4):198–211

28. Nielsen AF, Pedersen B, Lauritsen JG (1995) Psychosocial aspects of donor insemination Attitudes and opinions of Danish and Swedish donor insemination patients to psychosocial information being supplied to offspring and relatives. Acta Obstet Gynecol Scand 74(1):45–50

29. Merz JF, Fischhoff B (1990) Informed consent does not mean rational consent. J Legal Med 11:321–350

30. Bryan C (2008) Provider and policy response to reverse the consequences of low health literacy. J Healthcare Manag/Am Coll Healthc Exec 53(4):230–241

31. Peters E, Hibbard J, Slovic P, Dieckmann N (2007) Numeracy skill and the communication,

comprehension, and use of risk-benefit information. Health Aff 26(3):741–748

32. Paterick TJ, Carson GV, Allen MC et al (2008) Medical informed consent: general considerations for physicians. Mayo Clin Proc 83:272–273

33. Education USDo (2003) National assessment of adult literacy. Institute of Education Sciences. http://nces.ed.gov/naal/newsarchives.asp

34. Lundgren RE, McMakin AH (2009) Risk communication: a handbook for communicating environmental, safety, and health risks. Wiley-IEEE Press (4th ed) Hoboken, NJ: John Wiley & Sons

35. Partridge AH (2008) Fertility preservation: a vital survivorship issue for young women with breast cancer. J Clin Oncol 26(16):2612–2613

36. Packard E (2007) That teenage feeling. Monitor Psychol 38:20–21

37. Rosso IM, Young AD, Femia LA, Yurgelun Todd DA (2004) Cognitive and emotional components of frontal lobe functioning in childhood and adolescence. Ann N Y Acad Sci 1021:355–362

38. Sowell ER, Thompson PM, Holmes CJ, Jernigan TL, Toga AW (1999) In vivo evidence for postadolescent brain maturation in frontal and striatal regions. Nat Neurosci 2:859–861

39. Sowell ER, Thompson PM, Tessner KD, Toga AW (2001) Mapping continued brain growth and gray matter density reduction in dorsal frontal cortex: inverse relationships during postadolescent brain maturation. J Neurosci 21(22):8819–8829

40. Agarwal A, Ranganathan P, Kattal N, Pasqualotto F, Hallak J, Khayal S et al (2004) Fertility after cancer: a prospective review of assisted reproductive outcome with banked semen specimens. Fertil Steril 81(2):342–348

41. Crha I, Ventruba P, Zakova J, Huser M, Kubesova B, Hudecek R et al (2009) Survival and infertility treatment in male cancer patients after sperm banking. Fertil Steril 91(6):2344–2348

42. Descombe L, Chauleur C, Gentil-Perret A, Aknin-Seifer I, Tostain J, Lévy R (2008) Testicular sperm extraction in a single cancerous testicle in patients with azoospermia: a case report. Fertil Steril 90(2):443, e1–e4

43. Friedler S, Raziel A, Schachter M, Strassburger D, Bern O, Ron-El R (2002) Outcome of first and repeated testicular sperm extraction and ICSI in patients with non-obstructive azoospermia. Hum Reprod 17(9):2356–2361

44. Gabrielsen A, Fedder J, Agerholm I (2006) Parameters predicting the implantation rate of thawed IVF/ICSI embryos: a retrospective study. Reprod Biomed Online 12(1):70–76

45. Ginsburg ES, Yanushpolsky EH, Jackson KV (2001) In vitro fertilization for cancer patients and survivors. Fertil Steril 75(4):705–710

46. Hallak M (1998) Why cancer patients request disposal of cryopreserved semen specimens post-therapy: a retrospective study. Fertil Steril 69(5):889–893

47. Heidenreich A, Altmann P, Engelmann UH (2000) Microsurgical vasovastomy versus microsurgical epididymal sperm aspiration/testicular extraction of sperm combined with intra-cytoplasmic sperm injection. Eur Urol 37:609–614

48. Kolettis PN (2002) The evaluation and management of the azoospermic patient. J Androl 23(3):293–305

49. Modder TK, Kohler T, Brannigan RE (2007) Fertility preservation: outcomes for Onco-TESE in male cancer patients prior to oncological therapy. Fertil Steril 88:S393–S394

50. Ragni G, Arnoldi M, Somigliana E, Paffoni A, Brambilla ME, Restelli L (2005) Reproductive prognosis in male patients with azoospermia at the time of cancer diagnosis. Fertil Steril 83(6):1674–1679

51. Ethics Committee of the American Society for Reproductive Medicine (2005) Fertility preservation and reproduction in cancer patients. Fertil Steril 83(6):1622–1628

52. Schover LR, Brey K, Lichtin A, Lipshultz LI, Jeha S (2002) Knowledge and experience regarding cancer, infertility, and sperm banking in younger male survivors. J Clin Oncol 20(7):1880–1889

53. Schover LR, Rybicki LA, Martin BA, Bringelsen KA (1999) Having children after cancer. Cancer 86(4):697–709

54. Dotinga R (2010) Fast-freeze may help sperm survive storage, Study finds. http://health.usnews.com/health_news/family-health/womens-health/articles/2010/09/14/fast-freeze

55. Fatimathas L (2010) Hope for post-childhood cancer sperm production. http://wwww.Bio-news.org.uk/page_64914.asp

56. Berger DM (1980) Couples' reactions to male infertility and donor insemination. Am J Psychiatry 137(9):1047–1049

57. Daniels K, Blyth E, Crawshaw M, Curson R (2005) Short communication: previous semen donors and their views regarding the sharing of information with offspring. Hum Reprod 20(6):1670–1675

58. Daniels KR, Thorn P, Westerbrooke R (2007) Confidence in the use of donor insemination: an evaluation of the impact of participating in a group preparation programme. Hum Fertil 10(1):13–20

59. Daniluk JC (1988) Infertility: intrapersonal and interpersonal impact. Fertil Steril 49(6):982–990

60. Petok WD (2006) The psychology of gender specific infertility diagnosis. In: Covington SN, Burns LH (eds) Infertility counseling: a comprehensive handbook for clinicians. 2nd edn. Cambridge University Press, New York, NY, pp 37–60

61. Thorn P (2006) Recipient counseling for donor insemination. In: Covington S, Hammer Burns L (eds) Infertility counselling a comprehensive handbook for clinicians, 2nd edn. Cambridge University Press, Cambridge-New York, NY, pp 305–318

62. Baron A, Pannor R (1993) (2nd ed) Lethal secrets: the psychology of donor insemination, problems, and solutions. Amistad, New York

63. Berger DM, Eisen A, Shuber J, Doody KF (1986) Psychological patterns in donor insemination couples. Can J Psychiatry Revue Canadienne de Psychiatrie 31(9):818–823

64. Carr EK, Friedman T, Lannon B, Sharp P (1990) The study of psychological factors in couples receiving artificial insemination by donor: a discussion of methodological difficulties. J Adv Nurs 15(8):906–910

65. Clarke RN, Klock SC, Geoghegan A, Travassos DE (1999) Relationship between psychological stress and semen quality among in-vitro fertilization patients. Hum Reprod 14(3):753–758

66. Daniels KR (2004) Building a family with the assistance of donor insemination. Dunmore Press, Palmerston N, New Zealand

67. Nachtigall RD, Becker G, Wozny M (1992) The effects of gender-specific diagnosis on men's and women's response to infertility. Fertil Steril 57(1):113–121

68. Van Thiel M, Mantadakis E, Vekemans M, Gillot VF (1990) A psychological study, using interviews and projective tests, of patients seeking anonymous donor artificial insemination. J de gynécologie, obstétrique et biologie de la reproduction 19(7):823–828

69. Hart VA (2002) Infertility and the role of psychotherapy. Issues Mental Health Nurs 23(1):31–41

70. Horowitz JE, Galst JP, Elster N (2010) Ethical dilemmas in fertility counseling. American Psychological Association Books: Washington, DC

71. Goldstein J, Freud A, Solnit A (1973) Beyond the best interests of the child. Wiley Online Library, Free Press, New York

72. Silber SJ, Nagy Z, Devroey P, Camus M, Van Steirteghem AC (1997) The effect of female age and ovarian reserve on pregnancy rate in male infertility: treatment of azoospermia with sperm retrieval and intracytoplasmic sperm injection. Hum Reprod 12(12):2693–2700

73. Ethics Committee of the ASRM (2004) Family members as gamete donors and surrogates. Fertil Steril 82:S217–S223

74. Marshall LA (2002) Ethical and legal issues in the use of related donors for therapeutic insemination. Urol Clin North Am 29(4):855–861

75. Nikolettos N, Asimakopoulos B, Hatzissabas I (2003) Intrafamilial sperm donation: ethical questions and concerns. Hum Reprod 18(5):933–936

76. Lui S, Weaver S, Robinson J, Debono M, Nieland M, Killick S et al (1995) A survey of semen donor attitudes. Hum Reprod 10(1):234–238

77. Mahlstedt PP, Probasco KA (1991) Sperm donors: Their attitudes toward providing medical and psychosocial information for recent couples and donor offspring. Fertil Steril 4(56):747–753

78. Pedersen B, Nielsen AF, Lauritsen JG (1994) Psychosocial aspects of donor insemination: sperm donors-their motivations and attitudes to

artificial insemination. Acta Obstet Gynecol Scand 73(9):701–705

79. Purdie A, Peek J, Irwin R, Ellis J, Graham F, Fisher P (1992) Identifiable semen donors--attitudes of donors and recipient couples. N Z Med J 105(927):27–28

80. Rowland R (1985) The social and psychological consequences of secrecy in artificial insemination by donor (AID) programmes. Soc Sci Med 21(4):391–396

81. Crawshaw MA, Blyth ED, Daniels KR (2007) Past semen donors' view about the use of a voluntary contact register. Reproductive medicine online [serial on the Internet]. http://www.rbmonline.com/4DCG1/Issues/Details. 14:411–417

82. Robertson AD, Missmer SA, Ginsburg ES (2011) Embryo yield after in vitro fertilization in women undergoing embryo banking for fertility preservation before chemotherapy. Fertil Steril 96(1):122–125

83. Abdallah RT, Muasher SJ (2006) Surviving cancer, saving fertility: the promise of cryopreservation. Sex Reprod Menopause 4(1):7–12

84. Lutchman Singh K, Davies M, Chatterjee R (2005) Fertility in female cancer survivors: pathophysiology, preservation and the role of ovarian reserve testing. Hum Reprod Update 11(1):69–89

85. Meirow D (2010) Fertility preservation: New developments. Clin Obstet Gynecol 53(4):727–739

86. Maunsell E, Pogany L, Barrera M, Shaw AK, Speechley KN (2006) Quality of life among long-term adolescent and adult survivors of childhood cancer. J Clin Oncol 24(16):2527–2535

87. Kim SS (2006) Fertility preservation in female cancer patients: current developments and future directions. Fertil Steril 85(1):1–11

88. Silber SJ (2005) How to get pregnant. Hachette Digital, Little Brown, New York

89. Taylor A (2001) Systematic diversities of ovarian failure. J Soc Gynecol Invest 8:S7–S9

90. Sauer MV, Kavic SM (2006) Oocyte and embryo donation 2006: reviewing two decades of innovation and controversy. Reprod Biomed Online 12(2):153–162

91. Balaban B, Urman B, Isiklar A, Alatas C, Aksoy S, Mercan R et al (2001) The effect of pronuclear morphology on embryo quality parameters and blastocyst transfer outcome. Hum Reprod 16(11):2357–2361

92. Sher G, Davis VM, Stoess J (2005) In vitro fertilization: the art of making babies: facts on file, 3rd edn. Checkmark Books, New York

93. Bedaiwy MA, Shahin AY, Falcone T (2008) Reproductive organ transplantation: advances and controversies. Fertil Steril 90(6):2031–2055

94. Clark O (2010) Scientists create 'artificial' ovary. BioNews. http://www.bionews.org.uk/page_70822.as;?dinfo=HM.PYHdDBZDHtfOTuNsZ9gok

95. Sit ASY, Modugno F, Weissfeld JL, Berga SL, Ness RB (2002) Hormone replacement therapy formulations and risk of epithelial ovarian carcinoma. Gynecol Oncol 86(2):118–123

96. Zhang J, Grifo JA, Del Priore G (2005) Gestational carrier pregnancy with oocytes obtained during surgery for stage IIIc ovarian cancer after controlled ovarian stimulation. Fertil Steril 83(5):1547, e15–e17

97. Practice Committee of the ASRM and the Practice Committee of the Society for Assisted Reproductive Medicine (2006) Ovarian tissue and oocyte preservation. Fertil Steril 86(Suppl 3): S241–S246

98. Patrizio P, Caplan AL (2010) Ethical issues surrounding fertility preservation in cancer patients. Clin Obstetrics Gynecol 53(4):717–726

99. Oehninger S (2005) Strategies for fertility preservation in female and male cancer survivors. J Soc Gynecol Invest 12(4):222–231

100. Schover LR (2005) Sexuality and fertility after cancer. Hematology 2005(1):523–527

101. MacCallum F, Lycett E, Murray C, Jadva V, Golombok S (2003) Surrogacy: the experience of commissioning couples. Hum Reprod 18(6):1334–1342

102. Jadva V, Murray C, Lycett E, MacCallum F, Golombok S (2003) Surrogacy: the experiences of surrogate mothers. Hum Reprod 18(10):2196–2204

103. Blyth E (1994) «I wanted to be interesting, I wanted to be able to say «I've done something interesting in my life»: interviews with surrogate mothers in Britain. J Reprod Infant Psychol 12:189–198

104. Ciccarelli JC, Beckman LJ (2005) Navigating rough waters: an overview of psychological aspects of surrogacy. J Soc Issues 61(1):21–43

105. van den Akker OBA (2005) A longitudinal pre-pregnancy to post-delivery comparison of genetic and gestational surrogate and intended mothers: confidence and genealogy. J Psychosom Obstet Gynecol 26(4):277–284

106. van den Akker O (2007) Psychosocial aspects of surrogate motherhood. Hum Reprod Update 13(1):53–62

107. Farr RH, Forssell SL, Patterson CJ (2010) Parenting and child development in adoptive families: does parental sexual orientation matter? Appl Dev Sci 14(3):164–178

108. Moss A (2004) Adoption: challenges and solutions after breast cancer. http://www.lbbc.org/content/newsletter.

109. Rosen A (2005) Third party reproduction and adoption in cancer patients. J Natl Cancer Inst Monogr March 1

110. Grotevant HD (1997) Coming to terms with adoption: the construction of identity from adolescents into adulthood. Adopt Q 1:3–27

111. Brodzinsky D (1990) A stress and coping model of adoption adjustment. In: Brodzinsky D, Schecter M (eds) Psychology of adoption. Oxford University Press, New York, NY, pp 3–24

Parenting with Cancer I: Developmental Perspective, Communication, and Coping

Kristin S. Russell, MD and Paula K. Rauch, MD

Mary is a 45-year-old married mother of three children, 6 year old Sarah, 10 year old Katie, and 15 year old Ethan. She was diagnosed with breast cancer several months ago, and she and her husband have discussed the diagnosis openly with all three children. She comes to the clinic for her first chemotherapy infusion. When the nurse, who knows her well, inquires about how things have been going with her children, Mary starts to cry. She says that Sarah, her youngest daughter, has been asking a lot of questions that are hard to answer; particularly upsetting is the question, "Why did you get cancer mommy and when will I get cancer?" Katie, her middle daughter, has been very anxious about Mary losing her hair and wants her to wear her wig all the time. Mary promised Katie she would, but she wishes she could take the wig off at home. She's not worried about her oldest, Ethan, because he is always out with his friends and never at home. She hasn't been checking in with him, and is hoping he's doing his schoolwork. She appreciates all the calls from neighbors and friends from church, but has been overwhelmed by the constant calls and offers of help.
Mary, Adult Cancer Patient

Introduction

An estimated 2.85 million children in the United States are living with a parent who has been diagnosed with cancer [1]. One-third of patients with breast cancer have dependent children [2]. For these parents, often their biggest worry is what impact their cancer will have on their children. Unfortunately, it is not common for parents to receive support from clinicians about these concerns.

Our aim for this chapter is to familiarize clinicians with the common worries that parents have and empower them with strategies they

can use to help support parents in this difficult time. The content discussed in this chapter is derived from the accumulated clinical experience of the team of clinicians comprising the Parenting at a Challenging Time (PACT) Program at the Massachusetts General Hospital (MGH) [3–21]. This chapter will present information that clinicians can use to take a parenting history, and to use a developmental perspective to guide parents at different stages of illness, including new diagnosis, treatment, survivorship, and end-of-life. Practical strategies for parenting challenges such as communication with children about illness, preserving family time, and harnessing support networks will be addressed so that clinicians are equipped with tools they can use to directly impact parents with cancer.

It goes without saying that families experience considerable distress and pain when a parent has cancer. Despite this stress, children and families

K.S. Russell (✉)
Child and Adolescent Psychiatry, Marjorie E. Korff,
PACT (Parenting At a Challenging Time Program),
Massachusetts General Hospital, Boston, MA, USA
e-mail: ksrussell@partners.org

G.P. Quinn, S.T. Vadaparampil (eds.), *Reproductive Health and Cancer in Adolescents and Young Adults*, Advances in Experimental Medicine and Biology 732,
DOI 10.1007/978-94-007-2492-1_10, © Springer Science+Business Media B.V. 2012

can be profoundly resilient, particularly when supported. For clinicians who are newly working with families facing cancer, the sadness and anxiety can feel overwhelming and prevent clinicians from asking important questions. Our clinical experience has allowed us to see the strength and grace that parents and children so often exhibit when facing such a health crisis. Families return to us, sometimes years later, with insights about this time in their lives. For many families, this experience has been not only one of pain, but also a time of enormous growth, and their children have learned to actively cope with challenges by prioritizing values, appreciating small moments and each other, and working together. With these goals, and the knowledge that these experiences do not have to be traumatic for families, clinicians can begin to feel comfortable and competent to address their patients' parenting concerns.

Parenting with Cancer

While the body of research regarding the impact of parental illness remains small, some important points can be made by reviewing the studies that have been done. For further reading, several recent reviews provide summaries of this work [3–5].

Stress and Family Function

Often, children are significantly stressed when a parent has cancer, and parents often underestimate the psychological distress in their children [22–27]. Maternal depression under these circumstances negatively affects marital relationships, children's coping, and family functioning [28, 29]. Additionally, patients with dependent children were more likely to meet criteria for panic disorder while their spouses were more likely to meet criteria for major depressive disorder and generalized anxiety disorder [30]. Pivotal to successful coping in families is re-establishing normal routines [31]. Interestingly, families in which a parent has

cancer often perceive themselves as functioning in more positive fashion than the norm; these families feel they are more social, expressive, and organized, and less controlling and conflicted than families without parental cancer [32].

Childhood Coping

A child's worry about their parent's cancer fluctuates over time [33]. Developmental stage impacts both style of coping and response to a parent's illness [34]. Children use different strategies to cope with parental cancer, including focusing on normal activities, relying on friends, and seeking to understand medical specifics [35]. Other coping mechanisms include helping others, parentification, distraction, keeping it 'in the head', and wishful thinking. Communication and parental coping were highly correlated with a child coping [36].

Children's lives tend to change with the onset of parental cancer; such changes include increased responsibility, stronger relationships, and learning to value important people and things in life [37]. In a number of studies, approximately one-fourth of children who faced parental cancer experienced clinically significant depression, anxiety, or somatic symptoms compared to approximately 10–15% in normative samples; of note, some studies demonstrated no difference between groups [3]. Some data indicates that adolescent girls of an ill mother may be at highest risk [38, 39].

Communication

Better communication about parental illness improves children's coping, and parents desire guidance to facilitate this communication [40–45]. Studies indicate that children want honest communication about their parent's illness and its treatment, as well as any genetic implications of the disease for them, but they often do not ask directly for this because they worry about upsetting parents [46].

Taking a Parenting History

By taking a basic parenting history as part of an intake interview, clinicians can make great strides in helping patients feel that their concerns about their children are being heard and addressed. Clinicians are often concerned that asking about a patient's children will lead to an emotional conversation that may be overwhelming for both patient and clinician. In fact, patients report that having these discussions helps build an alliance, which may lead to improved adherence. Clinicians often find that parents' concerns are often driving decision-making. Overall, being open to having these conversations leads to improved care that is compassionate and patient-centered.

Clinicians need to lead the way with these conversations. A study of patients receiving palliative chemotherapy demonstrated that while 80% of patients wanted to discuss family-related concerns with their oncologist, many would not bring up the topic themselves, and would only discuss their concerns if the oncologist initiated the conversation [47].

Taking a basic parenting history can start with a question about whether the patient has children, and if so, what their names and ages are. Ask the parent to talk a little bit about the personality of each child. Find out what the children have been told about the cancer and/or treatment, and how they have reacted. Then inquire about how each child is coping with the illness. Find out who are the supports in the parent's life (e.g., a spouse, nearby family, neighbors, school staff) and in particular, who the parent is talking to about their parenting concerns. Table 10.1 summarizes these questions.

Developmental Perspective

Helping parents to look at their children through a developmental lens is a critical step in helping them to support their children. The majority of children pass through predictable developmental stages corresponding to their age, and familiarity with these stages helps parents and clinicians predict the impact of cancer on a particular child. Understanding of the stages can also improve communication and inform decision-making regarding parenting. We will discuss each stage, highlighting the important cognitive, emotional, and social implications of each. Table 10.2 summarizes key elements of each stage.

Infants and Toddlers (0–2)

The primary tasks of this stage are attachment and self-regulation. Children of this age will not have an understanding of the illness itself, but instead will respond to changes in their routines and caregivers. They may be upset by separation from familiar adults, and may be affected by the distress in the home. Signs of this include irritability, difficulty with eating and sleeping, and toddler meltdowns.

Caregivers can support infant and toddlers by helping them feel more secure. This can be achieved by keeping routines to the degree possible, using familiar blankets and stuffed animals, and facilitating communication amongst different caregivers to keep care consistent. Limiting the number of caregivers to a small number is ideal. As much as possible, it is helpful to assist the parent in continuing to feel engaged in the care of their children. Some possibilities include talking

Table 10.1 Brief parenting interview

- Do you have any children? What are their names and ages?
- Can you tell me a bit about each of your children? What are their personalities like?
- What have you told them about your cancer? How have they reacted to these conversations?
- How are they coping?
- Who is a support for you? Who do you talk to about your worries about your children?

Table 10.2 Key points and parenting tips by developmental stage

Developmental stage	Key issues	Parenting tips
Infancy (birth to $2\frac{1}{2}$ years)	Attachment Self regulation	Maintain familiar routines Keep number of caretakers to a minimum
Pre-school years (3–6 years)	Immature thinking + egocentricity = magical thinking (e.g., "I am to blame")	Focus on consistency and loving limits Repeatedly remind the child that the illness is not their fault
Latency (7–12 years)	Mastery of skills Focus on rules and fairness	Attend to the details of their daily life and accomplishments Protect family time
Adolescence (13–18 years)	Separation	Foster safe independent behavior Support relationships with trustworthy adults
Older adolescents (19–23 years)	Living away from home	Provide information so they can make decisions regarding when and how to be with family

to or hearing messages from caregivers with daily updates, and viewing videos.

Pre-schoolers (3–6)

As with infants and toddlers, pre-schoolers are more impacted by changes in routines than by information about the cancer. Children at this stage may be most distressed by the parent not being present for parts of the day like bedtime, if a routine involving that parent had been important. Other changes in family rhythms, like changes at dinnertime, new caregivers in the home, or mom or dad's absence at other key parts of the day are likely to be upsetting.

Pre-schoolers use magical thinking to intermingle fantasy and reality without a cogent understanding of cause and effect. They are appropriately egocentric at this stage, and the combination of this with immature thinking can lead them to conclude that something they did, said, or thought caused the illness. For instance, a four-year-old girl, after learning her mother has breast cancer, might conclude that she caused this by coming into her mother's bed and sleeping on her chest. Children feel anxiety at the ideas that they have this power. They may become aggressive and push limits in response. To help dispel these misconceptions, it is helpful to discuss with

children what they think caused the parent's illness, and then to discuss the etiology of the illness in an age-appropriate way. For instance, children of this age can be given the metaphor of a garden; weeds in the garden represent the cancer, and the medication helps get rid of the weeds. Reminding children with some regularity that nothing they did (or anyone else did) caused the cancer is important.

In response to changes at home, it is common for pre-schoolers to regress; behaviors such as wetting themselves may re-emerge. Children may express their distress about changes by complaining of headaches or stomachaches. In general, these behaviors are transient and do not persist. Maintaining routines and familiar people and objects is very helpful for pre-schoolers. Additionally, consistency with age-appropriate limits is critical, and caregivers should overcome their temptation to relax discipline because the child is already going through so much. Loving limits help children understand the world to be a predictable, safe place. Parents may be concerned when they see medical themes in their children's pretend play; however, this is generally an appropriate and constructive way for children to grapple with their feelings about the illness.

As children progress through these stages, their understanding of death and dying becomes more mature. At this stage, if conversations involve any discussion of death, it is important to be aware that pre-schoolers see death as a temporary state that is reversible and may require many reminders that this is not the case.

Latency/School-Aged Children (7–12)

At this stage, the mastery of new skills is central. School-aged children tend to feel strongly that everything, including cancer, should be "fair" and they may become angry at the unexpected and unfair sequalae of the illness. It can be useful to address this directly with them, for instance with the phrase "cancer doesn't fight fair." Although children can now make connections between cause and effect, they may well regress with the stress of the situation and feel responsible for a parent's illness. Reminding them, as with younger children, that this is not the case is very important. Even when cognitively able to use their cause-and-effect logic, their reasoning tends to be concrete and inflexible such that they may insist, for instance, that cancer is contagious or that cancer is always caused by smoking.

School-aged children commonly care deeply about appearances, as they are developmentally programmed to figure out where they themselves fit into their social milieu. This may lead to particular embarrassment around physical changes caused by the cancer (e.g., hair loss from chemotherapy) and they may beg parents to hide these issues (e.g., wear a wig). Parents may understandably have their own opinions about this, and they should take these into account. Honoring and validating the child's strong feelings about fitting in is more important than the ultimate outcome.

Regarding death, children at this stage are now able to understand that death is both permanent and universal. It can be disarming for parents to see children being surprisingly matter-of-fact and intellectualized about death rather than affectively connected. In fact, children of this age are often quite curious about the details of death and dying. Preparing parents for these

possibilities may help them feel more comfortable engaging with their child when a question arises.

Adolescents

Adolescents now have the capacity to reason in a more mature and abstract way. They can appreciate the effect of the situation and can think about, for instance, feared potential consequences of death such as changes in finances and loneliness of the surviving spouse. Given these changes in their cognitive and emotional capacities, parents may overestimate the behaviors that adolescents will have in response to the situation. For instance, adolescents may react by spending more time away from home with peers or engaged in outside activities. Parents may feel the teen is self-absorbed or uncaring, when in fact they are desperately trying to regulate their distress over the impact of the cancer and potential losses that may ensue.

A central developmental task of this stage is to negotiate a balance between separation and connectedness to their parents. It is particularly poignant for teens to navigate this while a parent is seriously ill as the developmental pull to separate may feel disloyal and dangerous given their fear of losing a parent. The adolescent will likely need help to translate these opposing pressures into a reasonable balance between safe, independent behavior and time with the family. Teens may often be caught up in the shifting roles and routines at home, and may be expected to help more than is appropriate with younger siblings. Shifting parental responsibilities to adolescents is especially common with girls, and although teens should be expected to help with chores and pitch in during a crisis, parents should be cautious about overburdening teens with developmentally inappropriate responsibilities. Teens should be encouraged to foster relationships with trustworthy non-parental adults who may be easier to confide in about intense feelings and existential thoughts. It is can relieve guilt for the teen to feel the parent supports these outside relationships.

Young Adults

Young adults may be living away from home and may be unsure about whether to return home when they receive news about the parent's diagnosis or a change in their illness. It is common for young adults to feel conflict about having a life outside the family, and they may well feel a mixture of relief, guilt, and isolation. Younger siblings may feel resentment towards the young adult who is avoiding the turmoil and tension at home. If the young adult is a new parent themselves, they may feel anger, fear, and loss at not having the help and attention they had hoped for from the ill parent.

Communication

It is important for parents to begin a dialogue with children about the illness sooner rather than later. If parents have just received a diagnosis, it may be sensible to take a few days to allow their emotions to settle enough that they can help their child process his or her own emotions. Children cope better when parents initiate communication about the illness in a timely way, before children have the opportunity to overhear conversations or pick up on changes in the emotional tone at home. If children find out indirectly about the illness, they may think that they are not being told because the information is too terrible to discuss, or that they are not valued or trusted enough to be involved in the discussion. Children will not trust future information if they think their parents are not being honest and straightforward, and going forward, they will tend to search for clues that their parents are lying to them. Also, children who overhear information are often confused by what they have heard and may be reluctant to tell the parent that they were listening, so an opportunity to clarify the situation may not come until after a long, anxious period for the child.

Parents can begin by finding out whether their children have noticed anything. Oftentimes, children may have picked up on changes in the parent or in the home, and it is useful to be aware of this. Parents should call the illness by its real name (e.g., "breast cancer" as opposed to "a lump"). They can follow with an age-appropriate explanation of the illness. For instance, for a school-aged child this could involve discussion about the parent having "sick cells" in the body that are "like weeds in a garden that get in the way of the healthy cells." During the discussion, it is important to not make promises that cannot be kept. Instead, parents can say they are just not sure. As difficult as it is for everyone, showing children that the parent can tolerate uncertainty is helpful. Parents may put off these conversations, feeling that they need to be prepared for every possible question before diving in. However, parents should be reassured that it is all right to answer a question by saying "that's a great question, I need to think about that and get back to you" or "I'm not sure, but I will ask my doctor about that."

While some children tend be comfortable talking about varied topics, others are not, and the illness is unlikely to change these tendencies. Parents should give children ample opportunities to discuss the illness, but particularly for children who tend to process things internally, resistance to talking should be respected. For these children, parents can help by wondering aloud about some of the questions that the child might have, and noticing whether the child becomes engaged. If so, parents can continue talking, even if the conversation is mostly one-sided. Children are generally quick to communicate whether they want the conversation to stop; parents should respect these signals, which may be non-verbal. It can be helpful to try these conversations at moments when the child is more likely to be receptive. This may be when driving in the car, cooking together, or at bedtime with the lights out. All of these are times when eye contact and intensity is lower, and this can help children titrate their emotions and responses. All children tend to do better with more specific and focused questions rather than questions that pull for emotional responses. For instance, asking them how it is going having a friend's mother drive them to soccer practice will likely be more fruitful than asking them how they are feeling about the illness. When children ask questions, it can be helpful to find out what the child really wants to know before

Table 10.3 Tips for communicating with children about parental illness

Be honest

Share information promptly as the worst way to hear difficult news is to overhear it

Welcome all questions warmly

Find out what the child is really wondering before answering difficult questions

Feel free to say "that's a great question, let me think about it and get back to you"

Encourage children to share things they hear from others

Remind children not to worry alone

embarking on a long answer that may provide more or different information than the child was hoping for.

Parents should encourage children to share what they hear from others about the illness. Neighbors, teachers, and other children may have good intentions when they share their own experiences with cancer, but it can be easy for these comments to be frightening. It is helpful to remind children that there are many different types of cancer and that "only Mom, Dad, and Mom's doctors know about Mom's cancer." If children are expecting these moments and know to bring them up with their parents, it can help make them easier when they happen.

One of the worries children commonly have is about death. Parents are often very apprehensive about their children asking a question such as "are you going to die," and it can help decrease parental anxiety about this conversation to have some responses ready. Parents need to appreciate their stage of illness and prognosis, as well as their own degree of hopefulness to be best equipped for these conversations. Under most circumstances, parents can let their children know that nobody knows for sure when they might die, but that the parent plans to get the best possible treatment and take very good care of themselves, and that they and their doctors are not worried about them dying now. Table 10.3 summarizes some of these communication strategies.

Coping

The following sections outline practical suggestions for parents regarding daily routines and family life. General principles include keeping routines as consistent as possible, preserving family time, and using support wisely.

Routines

To the highest degree possible, follow regular family routines. Children are reassured that their lives are stable and secure when daily life is predictable and consistent. For younger children, keeping routines for mealtimes, bath time, and bedtime the same from day to day is important. For older children, help structure caretaking so that they are able to continue their usual activities such as soccer or dance. Let children and caretakers know what each day holds by posting schedules or using calendars. Children of all ages are highly attuned to changes at home such as a change in parental roles, dinnertime routines, and even who is answering the phone. Children who are asked often identify these types of changes as the most upsetting part about the cancer. Remembering how important this consistency is to children can help parents honor details that may seem trivial. For instance, keeping chores the same or dinnertime at 6 p.m. every night may be important priorities.

Family Time

Keeping family time firmly off-limits from visits, phone calls, and other interruptions is crucial to keeping the focus on togetherness. This may also protect children from overhearing unnecessary detail about the illness. It is important to have plenty of time when the cancer is not the focus, and staying up-to-date about the child's school projects, friends, and daily activities helps the child feel loved and understood, and gives them permission to pursue these things even though the parent is ill.

Creating new family rituals can be a silver lining in the midst of the turmoil. It is often surprisingly meaningful for children to have these new routines to count on and look forward to. Innovations might include such things as having a certain meal each day of the week or Friday as movie-and-popcorn night.

Limit-Setting

Children are reassured when parents enforce consistent limits. During such difficult times, parents, relatives, and other caregivers are often compelled to make "errors of kindness" by relaxing discipline and indulging children when they otherwise would not. Despite their good intentions, children often perceive this as reminders that all is not normal and that the world is less consistent and therefore less secure than it used to be. Parents will likely need to speak about this to caregivers to ensure that everyone is on the same page.

Harnessing Support

Particularly in the time following a new diagnosis, families may be overwhelmed by well wishers in their communities. Appointing a "captain of kindness" to organize this support so that volunteers are not contacting the family directly about ways to help can be important. When families are contacted directly, parents may be distracted and drained by the time-consuming job of coordinating help. While a parent might be reluctant to speak up, the designated captain can effectively direct volunteers to provide help that is attuned to the needs of the family, such as driving help or vegetarian meals.

Along the same lines, a friend or relative can act as the "minister of information" to organize communication, providing updates to concerned friends while allowing the immediate family to

focus their energy on their children. It may be helpful to have volunteers in several domains such as extended family, school, church, and work to keep others updated while buffering the family. Websites may provide a way to communicate efficiently, and families find sites such as carepages.com helpful.

Caring for Self

Although their attention and focus may be on their children, parents with cancer and their spouses and loved ones need to ensure that they are also taking care of their own physical and emotional needs. It may be useful to remind parents of the familiar warning on airplanes to "be sure to fasten your own oxygen mask before attending to the masks of others" as parents who are out of commission are of little use to their children. Children will benefit from the model their parents are providing to care for themselves. Furthermore, children feel more secure when they see their parents caring for themselves. The ill parent must make time to get necessary medical care and to follow treatment recommendations. If either parent or a loved one is feeling overwhelmed or hopeless, seeking additional support is important. The cancer center may have support groups, social workers, and/or counselors, or may be able to recommend resources in the community.

School Support

Parents should let their child's school know about the illness and should provide guidance about how they would like the school and teacher to proceed. Children usually do best when school is a protected haven, and well-meaning teachers and administrators who ask the child how they or their parent is doing, can disrupt the child's ease and sense of normalcy at school. Parents should tell the child's teachers to let the child lead the way with such conversations (children are in fact quite unlikely to bring the topic up at school), and they should make clear that they want to hear about how the child is doing at school, both emotionally and academically. Sometimes teachers avoid "bothering" parents with information, thinking they are coping with enough already. It can help to be explicit that parents would like to hear all information, as this is a time that parents need to be on top of any emerging problems or warning signs.

Provider Recommendations

1. For many parents, their biggest worry is what impact their cancer will have on their children.
2. Taking a basic parenting history is essential to quality care.
3. Children pass through predictable developmental stages and understanding of how children cope at these various stages can help guide parents.
4. Open, honest, and age-appropriate communication helps children cope.
5. Children do best when daily life is consistent, family time is protected, and parents take care of themselves.
6. Parents will benefit from strategies to maximize family and community supports.
7. All clinicians should be knowledgeable about practical parenting strategies as well able to guide parents to additional resources as needed.

References

1. Weaver K, Rowland J, Alfano C, McNeel T (2010) Parental cancer and the family: a population-based estimate of the number of US cancer survivors residing with their minor children. Cancer 116:4395–4401
2. Bloom J, Kessler L (1994) Risk and timing of counseling and support interventions for younger women with breast cancer. J Natl Cancer Inst Monogr (16):199–206
3. Moore C, Rauch P (2006) Addressing parenting concerns of bone marrow transplant patients: opening (and closing) Pandora's box. Bone Marrow Transplant 38(12):775–782
4. Moore CW, Pirl WF et al (2005) Adult cancer patients as parents: what do oncologists and primary care providers know? Psychooncology 14(1):S58
5. Moore CW, Beiser ME et al (2006) Parenting concerns among adult cancer patients: a pilot study. Psychooncology 15(S1):S47
6. Moore CWRP (2006) Current pediatric therapy. W.B. Saunders Company, Philadelphia, PA
7. Muriel AC (2004) Learning to bear witness. J Palliat Med 7(5):720–722
8. Muriel AC, Rauch PK (2003) Suggestions for patients on how to talk with children about a parent's cancer. J Support Oncol 1(2):143Y5
9. Muriel ACRP (2006) Quick reference for oncology clinicians: the psychiatric and psychological dimensions of cancer symptom management. IPOS Press Charlottesville, VA
10. Pirl WF, Beiser M et al (2005) Comparison survey of oncology and primary care providers on psychosocial distress. Psychosomatics 46:164
11. Pirl WF, Beiser M et al (2005) Differences between primary care and oncology providers in managing depression. Psychooncology 14(Suppl 1):57
12. Muriel AC, Rauch PK (2003) A pilot parent guidance program for parents with cancer. Psychooncology 12(Suppl 4):S151
13. Rauch P (1998) Saunders manual of pediatric practice. W.B. Saunders Company, Philiphelphia
14. Rauch P (2000) Comment: supporting the child within the family. J Clin Ethics 11(2):169
15. Rauch P, Arnold R (2002) Fast facts and concepts# 47. What do I tell the children? J Palliat Med 5(5):740
16. Rauch PK (2007) You are only as happy as your most unhappy child. Psycho Oncol 16(2):99–100
17. Rauch PK, Muriel AC (2004) The importance of parenting concerns among patients with cancer. Crit Rev Oncol Hematol 49(1):37–42
18. Rauch PK, Muriel AC, Cassem NH (2002) Parents with cancer: who's looking after the children? J Clin Oncol 20(21):4399
19. Rauch PKDS (2004) Facing cancer: a complete guide for people with cancer, their families, and caregivers. McGraw-Hill, New York, NY
20. Rauch P (1999) Helping the children cope when a parent has cancer. Prim Care and Cancer 6–9
21. Swick SD, Rauch PK (2006) Children facing the death of a parent: the experiences of a parent guidance program at the massachusetts general hospital cancer center. Child Adolesc Psychiatr Clin North Am 15(3):779
22. Siegel K, Mesagno FP, Karus D, Christ G, Banks K, Moynihan R (1992) Psychosocial adjustment of children with a terminally ill parent. J Am Acad Child Adolesc Psychiatry 31(2):327–333
23. Christ GH, Siegel K, Freund B, Langosch D, Hendersen S, Sperber D et al (1993) Impact of parental terminal cancer on latency age children. Am J Orthopsychiatry 63(3):417–425
24. Christ GH, Siegel K, Sperber D (1994) Impact of parental terminal cancer on adolescents. Am J Orthopsychiatry 64(4):604–613

25. Compas B, Worsham N, Ey S, Howell D (1996) When mom or dad has cancer: II. Coping, cognitive appraisals, and psychological distress in children of cancer patients. Health psychology: official journal of the Division of Health Psychology. Am Psychol Assoc 15(3):167

26. Compas BE, Worsham NL, Epping-Jordan JAE, Grant KE, Mireault G, Howell DC et al (1994) When mom or dad has cancer: markers of psychological distress in cancer patients, spouses, and children. Health Psychol 13(6):507

27. Wellisch D, Gritz E, Schain W, Wang H, Siau J (1992) Psychological functioning of daughters of breast cancer patients. Part II: characterizing the distressed daughter of the breast cancer patient. Psychosomatics 33(2):171

28. Watson M, James-Roberts IS, Ashley S, Tilney C, Brougham B, Edwards L et al (2005) Factors associated with emotional and behavioural problems among school age children of breast cancer patients. Br J Cancer 94(1):43–50

29. Lewis FM, Hammond MA, Woods NF (1993) The family's functioning with newly diagnosed breast cancer in the mother: the development of an explanatory model. J Behav Med 16(4):351–370

30. Nilsson ME, Maciejewski PK, Zhang B, Wright AA, Trice ED, Muriel AC et al (2009) Mental health, treatment preferences, advance care planning, location, and quality of death in advanced cancer patients with dependent children. Cancer 115(2): 399–409

31. Hilton B, Elfert H (1996) Children's experiences with mothers' early breast cancer. Cancer Pract 4(2):96

32. Gazendam-Donofrio S, Hoekstra H, Van der Graaf W, van de Wiel H, Visser A, Huizinga G et al (2007) Family functioning and adolescents' emotional and behavioral problems: when a parent has cancer. Ann Oncol 18(12):1951–1956

33. Helseth S, Ulfsæt N (2003) Having a parent with cancer: coping and quality of life of children during serious illness in the family. Cancer Nurs 26(5):355

34. Christ GH, Christ AE (2006) Current approaches to helping children cope with a parent's terminal illness. CA Cancer J Clin 56(4):197

35. Issel L, Ersek M, Lewis F (1990) How children cope with mother's breast cancer. Oncol Nurs Forum 17(Suppl 3):5–12

36. Thastum M, Johansen MB, Gubba L, Olesen LB, Romer G (2008) Coping, social relations, and communication: a qualitative exploratory study of children of parents with cancer. Clin Child Psychol Psychiatry 13(1):123

37. Kennedy VL, Lloyd Williams M (2009) How children cope when a parent has advanced cancer. Psycho Oncol 18(8):886–892

38. Huizinga GA, Visser A, van der Graaf WTA, Hoekstra HJ, Klip EC, Pras E et al (2005) Stress response symptoms in adolescent and young adult children of parents diagnosed with cancer. Eur J Cancer 41(2):288–295

39. Welch AS, Wadsworth ME, Compas BE (1996) Adjustment of children and adolescents to parental cancer: Parents' and children's perspectives. Cancer 77(7):1409–1418

40. Nelson E, Sloper P, Charlton A, While D (1994) Children who have a parent with cancer: a pilot study. J Cancer Educ 9(1):30–36

41. Rosenheim E, Reicher R (1985) Informing children about a parent's terminal illness. J Child Psychol Psychiatry 26(6):995–998

42. Kroll L, Barnes J, Jones AL, Stein A (1998) Cancer in parents: telling children. BMJ 316(7135):880

43. Barnes J, Kroll L, Burke O, Lee J, Jones A, Stein A (2000) Qualitative interview study of communication between parents and children about maternal breast cancer. BMJ 321(7259):479

44. Keeley D (2000) Telling children about a parent's cancer. Br Med J 321(7259):462

45. Shands M, Lewis F, Zahlis E (2000) Mother and child interactions about the mother's breast cancer: an interview study. Oncol Nurs Forum 27(1):77–85

46. Kennedy VL, Lloyd-Williams M (2009) Information and communication when a parent has advanced cancer. J Affect Disord 114(1–3):149–155

47. Detmar S, Aaronson N, Wever L, Muller M, Schornagel J (2000) How are you feeling? Who wants to know? Patients' and oncologists' preferences for discussing health-related quality-of-life issues. J Clin Oncol 18(18):3295

Parenting with Cancer II: Parenting at Different Stages of Illness

Kristin S. Russell, MD and Paula K. Rauch, MD

Brian is a 54-year-old father of two boys (6 and 8) with pancreatic cancer. Alexandra, his oncology social worker, has met with Brian and his wife, Nancy, several times over the past year to discuss parenting issues. In their first meeting, Brian had just been diagnosed and the couple had not yet talked to their children. In the next meeting, Brian was about to have surgery and they discussed how to best prepare the children to visit him in the hospital. In preparation for her next meeting with the couple, Alexandra approaches Brian's medical team for information regarding the status of Brian's treatment and whether there will be a shift to end-of-life care this month. Alexandra needs input from the team in order to provide information about legacy leaving, end-of-life care, and funeral planning at an appropriate time.
Brian, Adult Cancer Patient

New Diagnosis

In the period immediately following a new diagnosis, parents often describe being in a state of shock, similar to the aftermath of a traumatic event. This overwhelming distress may cause parents to feel that they cannot think straight, their world has turned upside down, or that their sense of time and space has been altered [1]. During this time, caring for themselves and gathering medical information are priorities. As much as possible, steadying themselves with reminders to take one day at a time, or even one hour at a time, can be crucial. It may be important to wait until this acute period has passed and parents once again have their feet underneath them

before attempting to discuss the diagnosis with their children. It can be challenging to find an appropriate balance between allowing time for some emotional stabilization, while not letting too much time go by that parents risk children picking up on cues or overhearing conversations about the illness.

As soon as is feasible, parents should begin to have conversations with their children about the diagnosis. There are important elements to these conversations, including naming the illness and letting children know that they have found the very best doctors that have a lot of experience treating this type of cancer. More details regarding communication during this difficult time can be found in the "Communication" section of chapter 10 [2–11].

Another important step to take during this time is organizing and bolstering support systems. This is a critical time to mobilize support—family members and close friends can provide loving emotional support, while other friends, acquaintances, or neighbors can provide

K.S. Russell (✉)
Child and Adolescent Psychiatry, Marjorie E. Korff,
PACT (Parenting At a Challenging Time Program),
Massachusetts General Hospital, Boston, MA, USA
e-mail: ksrussell@partners.org

G.P. Quinn, S.T. Vadaparampil (eds.), *Reproductive Health and Cancer in Adolescents and Young Adults*, Advances in Experimental Medicine and Biology 732,
DOI 10.1007/978-94-007-2492-1_11, © Springer Science+Business Media B.V. 2012

logistical support. Further discussion of strategies to facilitate coping during this difficult time is available in the "Coping" section of chapter 10 [1, 12–21].

Treatment

Parents with cancer may be facing surgery, chemotherapy, or radiation. It is important for parents and their medical team to communicate so that the parent is equipped with information about what to expect during treatment. For instance, asking about recovery time from surgery, impacts of treatment on driving, or expectations about hair loss can help parents plan and prepare their family. When talking to children about upcoming treatment, it is helpful to provide a brief explanation about what the treatment is doing. For instance, describing chemotherapy as "very, very, very, very strong medicine that gets rid of the cancer cells" can help children distinguish chemotherapy from other types of medications they may need to take. Because chemotherapy has significant side effects such as nausea, fatigue, and hair loss, it is important to help children understand that the medication they may need to take for ear infections, for instance, will not cause these same side effects.

It is useful to anticipate with children the side effects that may develop from chemotherapy and radiation and explain to them that these are side effects from the treatment and not symptoms of the cancer. Seeing a parent in distress from these effects is more alarming when children think this is the disease process than it is when they can be reassured that the effects are from the treatment, which is in fact making the parent better in the long run. An explanation such as "because the medicine needs to be very, very strong to get rid of the cancer cells, sometimes it also hurts healthy cells" can be helpful. Finding out what side effects are the most distressing to children and why can help parents and children strategize about how to minimize the impact of these effects. For instance, middle-school children may be particularly self-conscious about a parent's bald head and discussing this and planning for the

parent to wear a wig at certain events may relieve anxieties [13, 14].

It may be useful to help children anticipate that schedules may not be certain during this time. While it is very helpful to keep routines as consistent as possible, this is not always feasible during a busy treatment schedule that may have unexpected changes, side effects, or other factors requiring the family's schedule to change. If children can anticipate that changes may be required, they may be less disrupted when this occurs [22–25].

Hospital Visits

In general, children who want to visit a parent in the hospital should be helped to do so. Parents often worry about their child seeing them looking ill or attached to tubes, and wonder if it is better for them to stay home. In reality, however, children seem to do much better with real images rather than imagined ones. It is important to prepare children for the visit by describing what the child will see; for instance, how the parent looks (e.g., if they are wearing a hospital gown, if they have any tubes attached) and how the hospital room looks. Parents can even take advantage of cell phone cameras to send a quick photo to help prepare their child for what to expect. It is often helpful to bring a familiar adult who is available to step outside with the child if they need a walk or break, particularly if there are multiple children or if the other parent wants time to visit with the ill parent. This way, the child can help determine the length of the visit. Bring quiet activities and snacks to occupy children during the visit, as children may become bored after the initial curiosity subsides. Children may want to bring something to play with or show the parent, such as a new game or a school project. After leaving, is important for children to have the opportunity to discuss their impressions of the visit and to ask any questions they may have.

There are a limited number of situations in which a visit may not be a good idea. For instance, when parents are delirious, children may be frightened or confused by the parent's

Table 11.1 Tips for hospital visits

Describe what the child will see before entering the room and discuss the visit after leaving
Bring a familiar adult who is available when the child is ready to go and let the child determine the length of the visit
Bring play materials

agitation and/or disorientation. If a parent is weak and feeling lousy from a recent intervention, but is expected to be feeling and looking much better quickly, it may be prudent to defer the visit. Phone calls and even videophone calls can replace visits when logistics or circumstances dictate. Table 11.1 summarizes key tips for hospital visits.

Bone Marrow Transplant

Parents often have significant anxiety about the impact of bone marrow transplant (BMT) on their children [26]. Factors including long hospitalizations and recovery times, risk of the procedure and potential for serious complications, and need to avoid infection contribute to this worry. There are large hurdles to be overcome during the transplant process, and parents can take specific steps to help their children cope during this time. As with all phases of cancer treatment, open and honest communication about the upcoming intervention is crucial. The oncologist can play an important role by empowering parents with information about what to expect in terms of length of hospital stay and estimated recovery times, as well as potential side effects and need for post-transplantation precautions regarding infection.

During transplantation, hospital stays can be extensive and span many months. Parents and families may even have to temporarily relocate so they are close to the hospital where the transplant is being received. Children can be helped with these transitions by helping keep their daily schedule as consistent as possible, and by helping them to anticipate the changes that may be required. During the hospitalization, visits, phone calls, and Skype may be used to help maintain contact. Children can be helped to keep track of the things they want to share with their parent by storing drawings and projects in a shoe

box, and the contents can be shared during visits. During and after transplantation, infection control measures may have to be strict. Children should be reminded that these steps are designed to help keep the parent healthy, and not because they may catch something from the ill parent. Many parents worry that children may struggle with obsessive compulsive symptoms because of these measures; however, our experience suggests that children quickly return to their usual comfort with germs when the measures are no longer needed.

Survivorship

Family members may differ greatly in how they feel about discussing and revisiting the fact of the cancer, and anticipating this can help family members respect these differences. Individuals may have processed the events differently during active treatment, leaving them in very different places in terms of how they feel about moving forward versus continuing to actively process the experience. It can be especially difficult for the patient themselves to make a transition from the crisis modes of diagnosis and active treatment to the very different phase of survivorship. Patients may not feel ready to put this behind them and may feel that the cancer is still looming, consuming their thoughts.

Both parents and children may be surprised by the degree of emotional stress caused by ongoing, cancer-related appointments and scans. Families are trying hard to put the cancer experience behind them, and these visits are stark reminders that this is not entirely possible. For parents, it may help to anticipate that this may be a very stressful time so they can allow themselves space to be worried and sad. Being aware of their own fears during this time will help parents be empathic to their children, who may also be undergoing significant stress. As with other phases of treatment, communication and preparation for the visit and news that will come are important elements in helping children cope.

Family members may have many residual feelings left from the prioritization that has had to happen during the course of treatment. Immediate crises where physical and emotional resources have had to be focused on the parent likely left other family members drained and maybe resentful. These crises may have been followed by "make up" times where parents or other relatives have been hyper-focused (i.e., with time, gifts, relaxing of limits and expectations) on the children to compensate. Parents may have residual guilt about not having "been there" as much as they would have liked, while children may have stored up anger about sacrifices they have had to make or may now feel guilty about fusses they have made. It may take time for families to re-quilibrate from these shifts and find a more consistent pace and focus.

Just because treatment is done does not mean everything will go back to the way it was, and this is a harsh reality for families to come to terms with. Both small and large things may be permanently altered, and adjusting to the "new normal" can be a bumpy process for parents and children alike. At the same time, there may have been positive changes that occurred during treatment, such as children taking on new roles and responsibilities (e.g., childcare, cooking) that they are truly ready for. Allowing them to continue to make these contributions may help them feel valued and needed.

Children may appear to be coping well during the crisis, only to become unglued around seemingly minor challenges after the acute crisis of diagnosis/treatment has passed. Anticipating this pattern may help families understand and manage better. Another thing that is helpful to anticipate with families is that children's understanding of cancer changes as they develop, and it will be necessary to continue to have conversations over time to continue to process and update their understanding about the diagnosis and its implications.

End-of-Life

When a parent's medical care shifts from life-extending treatment to end-of-life care, several parenting considerations come to the forefront. These may include choosing the location for end-of-life care, giving children the opportunity to say goodbye, and leaving a legacy, and planning for funerals and memorial services.

Location of Care

Parents may have a choice about where to receive their care; options generally include care at a hospital, hospice, or at home. There are pros and cons to each. In an institutional setting, there is less burden of caretaking on family, but it is more difficult for family members to visit with the parent. Caring for the parent allows for easier and more frequent visits. Families are often concerned about the nursing needs, pain management, and equipment required. It's best to have a room with a door to allow privacy for the parent. Parents may also be concerned about death occurring in the home; for instance, where the children will be at the time and whether the family will have discomfort about the room after the parent has died there. Making this choice is emotional and difficult. Although it may be daunting, it is important to include children in the decision-making process so they can offer their own perspective and concerns [10, 27].

Saying Goodbye

It is important for children to be given the opportunity to visit with a parent at the end of life. Children who are uncomfortable about seeing a parent at this time can be offered the option of being nearby, for instance in a waiting room. If a parent is not responsive at the time, it can be enormously helpful to let children know that although we do not know what someone may hear while in that state, we believe that patients can sense that loved ones are nearby. Children can be encouraged to say something to the parent, to hold their hand, or to think something they want the parent to know. Children who are not comfortable being in the room can think thoughts for their parent while nearby, or can write a message for someone to read to the parent. Telling the child that the parent loved the child—and knew the child loved them—is important. In the event that the relationship was conflicted, it can be helpful to acknowledge this and then reassure the child that despite this, the parent loved them and knew they were loved by the child. Literally saying "goodbye" is not the important part at this time, but rather the expressions of love and opportunity to be close to the parent that can be so helpful in this final stage.

Receiving input in advance from the child about how they would like to be told about a parent's death can be useful. For instance, if the death happens in the middle of the night, would they prefer to be awakened or told in the morning? This can help make these decisions at the time of death easier on family members and help the child feel some semblance of control during this period.

Leaving a Legacy

Parents often feel that they would like to leave something for their child to treasure after their death. There is a great deal of variation in how parents feel about this, and what they feel would be significant to leave. It may be helpful to think about leaving a legacy as a way to communicate to the child that they were loved. Parents who are not interested—or not able—to do so should be reassured that there are many ways to communicate these feelings to their children and that leaving something is not necessary for children to feel well loved.

Parents may be inspired to write a letter to their child describing their feelings, sharing favorite memories of the child, or detailing the ways they see their child as special. Letters can also encourage children to attach to new loved ones without feeling disloyal. While some parents think about writing a letter for the child to open at various special occasions (e.g., graduation, wedding, birth of a child), children who have received such letters sometimes relate that these letters feel out-of-tune with the person the child has become and can feel disappointing. Instead, a single letter for the child to open when they are older that describes feelings and memories may serve a useful purpose without risking misattunement.

Other parents may leave treasured belongings, such as a piece of jewelry, or may leave scrapbooks, CDs, recipes, or funds for the child to use for something specific. Something that can be very meaningful is for a parent to leave a list of friends for the child to contact who knew the parent well at different phases of their life.

Financial and Legal Planning

Taking time to address financial and legal issues is an important aspect of caring for children. Leaving these spheres as well-prepared and considered as possible can help children feel that the parent worked hard to create as much safety and security as they were able to, even if difficult consequences nevertheless ensue. Financial issues to address can involve assessing current income and expenses, as well as looking carefully at insurance policies and how best to ensure the children's financial welfare after the parent's death. This may feel insurmountable to parents tackling it alone, and family, friends, and professionals can all be of assistance.

In terms of legal issues, the advance preparation of relevant documents is vital (e.g., a will, health-care proxy, power of attorney, and living will). Particularly when there are issues involving custody of the child, consultation with a family law attorney may be essential. A full consideration of the custody issues at play is beyond the scope of this chapter and varies from state to state. However, there are several outcomes that are common. When parents are married and one dies, custody will go to the surviving parent. If the parents are not married, custody will typically go to the surviving parent unless there is clear reason it should not. In situations where the custodial parent is approaching death and feels strongly that the non-custodial parent is inappropriate, several options are available. These include contacting the other parent and asking them to voluntarily give up their parental rights (and financial responsibility), or requesting the court to appoint a guardian *ad litem* to evaluate the best interests of the child.

Funerals and Memorial Services

Families are often left with questions about how to plan for a service and how best to include the children. Ideally, planning should begin before the parent's death, allowing the parent to share their wishes and helping to minimize family conflict after the fact. Some general child-centered guidelines for the service itself include having a familiar person preside, having the service in a familiar location, and providing children with the opportunity to participate however they are comfortable. Some may want to speak, to play an instrument, or just listen. If a child does not want to participate actively, this should be respected and the child should be reassured that the parent would want them to do what is most comfortable, and that they are not failing the parent or the expectation of family and friends by choosing to stay on the sidelines.

It is important for a familiar adult to help prepare the child with as many specifics as possible before the service. Questions should be answered or answers tracked down so the child can feel as comfortable as possible. Younger children should have someone specifically designated to support them and to take them outside, if needed, and all children should have a familiar adult check in with them after the event to share feelings and reactions. Although children differ in their wishes and developmental readiness, a usual recommendation would be that by the age of 4, most children can benefit from attending all or some of a funeral or memorial service. In contrast, children of this age are often not ready be taken to the cemetery itself, as they may have trouble understanding the idea that death is irreversible and they may be especially distressed at the image of the parent being buried.

Supporting Parents and Children

Seeking Outside Help for Children

In most situations, children prove resilient; they are often able to adjust fairly well given supportive caregivers. In cases where children are not able to adjust, further evaluation and perhaps support by child mental health providers may be helpful. How do you gauge when to recommend this? These are some guidelines [15–18, 21, 28].

In situations where a child specifically requests to speak to someone outside the family, this should be facilitated. Children with previous psychiatric challenges are at higher risk for new or recurring difficulties when a parent is ill and so it is a good idea to connect these children with their previous providers when possible. Children with ADHD and/or executive functioning deficits may have particular difficulty concentrating during an illness in the family or while grieving. Children with symptoms of depression and/or anxiety that interfere with their daily activities (e.g., school, friendships, and family life) for more than a few weeks should have a consultation. These symptoms may include depressed, anxious, or irritable mood for more than a few weeks, and may manifest with change in sleep, appetite, energy, and/or concentration. Children who are having thoughts of suicide should have an urgent evaluation. Finally, children who are engaging in risky behaviors such as substance abuse, unsafe relationships, or fighting should be referred for consultation.

Access to mental health supports for children varies by location. Contacting a child's pediatrician and/or school guidance counselor can be a useful place to start.

PACT Team: A Parent Guidance Model

There are many possibilities for individual or groups of clinicians to support parents with cancer. At Massachusetts General Hospital, the Parenting at a Challenging Time (PACT) program is one such example [29]. The PACT program is composed of child psychiatrists and psychologists who provide expert consultation to families who are referred. Referrals are made through any member of the medical team, or by the patient themselves. The most common times for consultation include the time of initial diagnosis, if recurrence occurs, and at end of life.

Consultations typical consist of one to several initial visits; families often initiate further contact at a later phase of illness, when new parenting concerns emerge, or after the patient dies. Discussion commonly focuses on one of three areas: communication with the children, behavior issues of a child, and general family coping. Clinicians meet with the patient, and if the situation warrants, with children, spouses, and other family members. Consultations occur on inpatient units, in outpatient offices, during chemotherapy infusion or dialysis, or by telephone. Patients and families who need more extensive intervention or psychiatric treatment are referred for treatment.

Table 11.2   Resources for cancer patients

People Living with Cancer, from the American Society for Clinical Oncology (ASCO)
   Offers educational information for patients and families. (www.plwc.org)

American Psychosocial Oncology Society (APOS)
   Provides a free Helpline to connect patients and families with local counseling services, as well as webcasts for professionals on topics such as "Cancer 101 for Mental Health Professionals," and "Psychosocial Aspects of Cancer Survivorship" (co-sponsored by the Lance Armstrong Foundation). (www.apos-society.org)

American Cancer Society (ACS)
   Provides information on talking to children about cancer, as well as numerous other cancer-related topics. (www.cancer.org)

The Wellness Community
   A national, nonprofit organization that provides free online and in-person support and information to people living with cancer and their families. (www.thewellnesscommunity.org)

Living Beyond Breast Cancer
   A national education and support organization with the goal of improving quality of life and helping patients take an active role in ongoing recovery or management of the disease. (www.lbbc.org)

Young Survival Coalition
   Through action, advocacy and awareness, this nonprofit seeks to educate the medical, research, breast cancer, and legislative communities and to persuade them to address breast cancer in women 40 and under—and serves as a point of contact for young women living with breast cancer. (www.youngsurvival.org)

Breast Cancer.org
   This organization offers medical information about current treatments and research in breast cancer care and survivorship. (www.breastcancer.org)

Hurricane Voices Breast Cancer Foundation
   Among other breast-cancer related resources, this organization offers a family reading list of books and stories for children of all ages dealing with cancer, in particular with breast cancer. (www.hurricanevoices.org)

CancerCare
   The mission of this national nonprofit is to provide free professional help to people with all cancers through counseling, education, information, and referral and direct financial assistance. They offer online, telephone, and face-to-face support groups to those affected by cancer. (www.cancercare.org)

Lance Armstrong Foundation (LAF)
   LAF offers information and services to cancer survivors and the professionals who care for them. (www.livestrong.org)

The Life Institute
   This organization's online publication "Conversations from the Heart" provides an annotated list of resources for parents and professionals who want to learn more about how to have developmentally appropriate conversations with children about serious illness and death. (www.thelifeinstitute.org)

The PACT team meets in weekly rounds to discuss challenging cases. Oncology team members attend these rounds to collaborate around complicated families. Consultations are provided free of charge and funding is secured through the MGH Cancer Center and through philanthropic donations (see www.mghpact.org).

Resources

Direct and online resources for parents with cancer can provide additional support and information.

Table 11.2 summarizes useful resources for parents with cancer.

Provider Recommendations

1. In order to feel ready to have conversations with their children, parents need specific guidance at each stage of illness, including new diagnosis, recurrence, and end-of-life care.
2. At each stage of illness, parents will be adjusting to a "new normal" and can be supported in learning how their child's past reactions can guide current parenting approaches.
3. Guidance regarding when and how parents might communicate with their child's school staff can be important in helping children cope.
4. Children will benefit from being prepared for hospital visits; describing any changes in a parent's appearance and/or capacities and the arrangement of the hospital room can help them anticipate what to expect at their visit.
5. When a parent transitions to end-of-life care, families may need guidance about how to choose the location for care, how to help children say goodbye, and whether to leave a legacy gift or letter.
6. In most situations children are resilient and adjust fairly well given supportive caregivers. In some cases, children may benefit from extra help, and mental health support can be accessed through schools, pediatricians, and other resources.

References

1. Visser A et al (2004) The impact of parental cancer on children and the family: a review of the literature. Cancer Treat Rev 30(8):683–694
2. Thastum M et al (2008) Coping, social relations, and communication: a qualitative exploratory study of children of parents with cancer. Clin Child Psychol Psychiatry 13(1):p. 123
3. Welch AS, Wadsworth ME, Compas BE (1996) Adjustment of children and adolescents to parental cancer: parents' and children's perspectives. Cancer 77(7):1409–1418
4. Nelson E et al (1994) Children who have a parent with cancer: a pilot study. J Cancer Educ 9(1):30–36
5. Rosenheim E, Reicher R (1985) Informing children about a parent's terminal illness. J Child Psychol Psychiatry 26(6):995–998
6. Kroll L et al (1998) Cancer in parents: telling children. BMJ 316(7135):880
7. Barnes J et al (2000) Qualitative interview study of communication between parents and children about maternal breast cancer. BMJ 321(7259):479
8. Keeley D (2000) Telling children about a parent's cancer. Br Med J 321(7259):462
9. Shands M, Lewis F, Zahlis E (2000) Mother and child interactions about the mother's breast cancer: an interview study. Oncol Nurs Forum 27(1):77–85
10. Kennedy VL, Lloyd-Williams M (2009) Information and communication when a parent has advanced cancer. J Affect Disord 114(1–3):149–155
11. Detmar S et al (2000) How are you feeling? Who wants to know? Patients' and oncologists' preferences for discussing health-related quality-of-life issues. J Clin Oncol 18(18):3295
12. Siegel K et al (1992) Psychosocial adjustment of children with a terminally ill parent. J Am Acad Child Adolesc Psychiatry 31(2):327–333
13. Christ GH et al (1993) Impact of parental terminal cancer on latency age children. Am J Orthopsychiatry 63(3):417–425
14. Christ GH, Siegel K, Sperber D (1994) Impact of parental terminal cancer on adolescents. Am J Orthopsychiatry 64(4):604–613
15. Compas B et al (1996) When mom or dad has cancer: II. Coping, cognitive appraisals, and psychological distress in children of cancer patients. Health psychology: official journal of the Division of Health Psychology. Am Psychol Assoc 15(3):167
16. Compas BE et al (1994) When mom or dad has cancer: markers of psychological distress in cancer patients, spouses, and children. Health Psychol 13(6):507
17. Wellisch D et al (1992) Psychological functioning of daughters of breast cancer patients. Part II: Characterizing the distressed daughter of the breast cancer patient. Psychosomatics 33(2):171

18. Watson M et al (2005) Factors associated with emotional and behavioural problems among school age children of breast cancer patients. Br J Cancer 94(1):43–50
19. Lewis FM, Hammond MA, Woods NF (1993) The family's functioning with newly diagnosed breast cancer in the mother: the development of an explanatory model. J Behav Med 16(4):351–370
20. Issel L, Ersek M, Lewis F (1990) How children cope with mother's breast cancer. Oncol Nurs Forum 17(Suppl 3):5–12
21. Kennedy VL, Lloyd Williams M (2009) How children cope when a parent has advanced cancer. Psycho Oncol 18(8):886–892
22. Hilton B, Elfert H (1996) Children's experiences with mothers' early breast cancer. Cancer Pract 4(2):96
23. Gazendam-Donofrio S et al (2007) Family functioning and adolescents' emotional and behavioral problems: when a parent has cancer. Ann Oncol 18(12):1951–1956
24. Helseth S, Ulfsæt N (2003) Having a parent with cancer: coping and quality of life of children during serious illness in the family. Cancer Nurs 26(5):355
25. Christ GH, Christ AE (2006) Current approaches to helping children cope with a parent's terminal illness. CA Cancer J Clin 56(4):197
26. Moore C, Rauch P (2006) Addressing parenting concerns of bone marrow transplant patients: opening (and closing) Pandora's box. Bone Marrow Transplant 38(12):775–782
27. Nilsson ME et al (2009) Mental health, treatment preferences, advance care planning, location, and quality of death in advanced cancer patients with dependent children. Cancer 115(2):399–409
28. Huizinga GA et al (2005) Stress response symptoms in adolescent and young adult children of parents diagnosed with cancer. Eur J Cancer 41(2):288–295
29. Rauch PK, Muriel AC (2004) The importance of parenting concerns among patients with cancer. Crit Rev Oncol Hematol 49(1):37–42

Pediatric Oncology and Reproductive Health

12

James L. Klosky, PhD, Rebecca H. Foster, PhD, and Alexandra M. Nobel, BA

I am now sterile because of the chemo, radiation, and the bone marrow transplant. I found out several months ago definitively that I am sterile. There was some question because often all of the cancer drugs will put a woman into temporary menopause that reverses once she is off of the meds. Since I was 18 when I was diagnosed, I never had a chance to have a child, and now I never will. That is very upsetting to me. And, yes, I realize that there are other options like adoption or in vitro, but cancer has robbed me of the chance to have a child of my own. That is probably the hardest thing I have had to deal with as a result of my cancer. I get sick more often than other people, and I stay sick longer, and I have less energy all around, but being sterile is the hardest thing to accept. I still often feel broken and stolen from because of the cancer. It took three years of my life, my fertility, and the opportunity to live a normal life. I think I do pretty well at life, but I think it's harder for me than it is for normal people. I have had to go through a lot to get where I am, and I find that I don't connect with people who haven't had hardships very well. I look at a lot of people my age and just don't understand how they can be the way they are and how they can be concerned with such trivial things.
- Shelly, Pediatric Cancer Survivor

Cancer Treatment and Infertility

Infertility is a commonly reported side effect of childhood cancer treatment, and risk for infertility is treatment specific [1]. Alkylating agents like cyclophosphamide and ifosfamide, or combined alkylator therapies like MOPP (Mechlorethamine, Oncovin, Procarbazine, and Prednisone), have a dose-related risk of infertility with higher cumulative dose and longer length of treatment conferring the greatest risk for fertility problems [2–4]. At 12 years post-diagnosis,

Kenney and colleagues found, for example, that only 12% of males treated with high dose cyclophosphamide for childhood sarcoma had normal sperm counts, whereas 59% were azoospermic, and 29% were oligospermic [5]. When cyclophosphamide is combined with ifosfamide, as in the treatment of Ewings sarcoma, or with ifosfamide and cisplatin, as in the treatment of osteosarcoma, azoospermia or oligospermia occurs in essentially all treated patients [6]. Young males receiving high dose melphalan or busulfan as part of hematopoietic stem cell transplantation preparation are also at high risk for infertility [7]. The dose-dependent relationship observed between chemotherapy and infertility is also observed in radiation therapy with higher doses to the testes translating to greater risk of gonadal dysfunction [8]. While oligospermia or azoospermia has been observed

J.L. Klosky (✉)
Department of Psychology, MS 740, St. Jude Children's Research Hospital, Memphis, TN 38105, USA
e-mail: james.klosky@stjude.org

G.P. Quinn, S.T. Vadaparampil (eds.), *Reproductive Health and Cancer in Adolescents and Young Adults*, Advances in Experimental Medicine and Biology 732,
DOI 10.1007/978-94-007-2492-1_12, © Springer Science+Business Media B.V. 2012

in males experiencing low dose testicular irradiation (100 cGy), the risk for permanent sterility significantly increases with radiation exposures of 1200–1500 cGy, as in the case of total body irradiation or pelvic/testicular irradiation [9–12]. Disruption to the hypothalamic-pituitary-gonadal axis as a result of cranial irradiation also places patients at significant risk for infertility due to gonadotropin insufficiencies.

Females treated for childhood cancer are also at increased risk for infertility [14, 25]. Treatments such as surgery, chemotherapy, and/or radiation therapy (RT) all have the potential to adversely affect fertility outcomes, with pelvic irradiation being implicated as one of the most damaging treatment factors. The adverse effects of pelvic RT on fertility appear to be mediated by several factors including RT dose, patient age at treatment, adjunctive use of alkylating agents, a diagnosis of Hodgkin's lymphoma, and RT exposure to the ovaries and uterus. Compared to childhood cancer patients who received abdominal RT alone, those whose radiation field extended to the pelvis were less likely to achieve pregnancy, live births, or spontaneous menstruation [15]. The RT-specific mechanisms responsible for poor reproductive outcomes are varied but primarily include acute ovarian failure or premature menopause (experienced by 6 and 8% of the population, respectively), or uterine dysfunction post-RT exposure including reduced volume, reduced elasticity, and vascular damage [14, 15, 25]. Offspring born to women post pelvic RT are at increased risk for preterm birth, low birth weight, and being small for gestational age [14, 16, 25].

Decisions Regarding Fertility Preservation and Reproduction

With the growing number of pediatric cancer patients who will survive into adulthood, the topic of fertility preservation becomes pertinent to address at the time of diagnosis. Not only does this give the family hope for a future beyond cancer diagnosis and treatment but it has been shown that discussion of fertility is related to the family's reports of increased positive emotions during the treatment period [17]. However, while oncologists have the potential to facilitate hope and positive emotions among these families, the majority acknowledge that they do not discuss fertility risks or preservation, in part because many have not received training related to approaching this topic. To date, several studies have investigated specific barriers to oncologist-patient communication regarding fertility risk and preservation options [18–22]. Findings indicated that the majority of oncologists did not know of resources available in the community for male or female patients to seek fertility preservation. Some physicians believed these conversations fall to the responsibility of those administering the chemotherapy or the patient's nurses. Furthermore, physicians reported feeling uncomfortable discussing fertility preservation with those patients who they deemed as having unfavorable diagnoses and prognoses.

Families have also reported a desire for more reproductive health information regardless of patient age, diagnosis, prognosis, or treatment plan [23, 24, 26–28]. In a focus group conducted by Nieman and colleagues [29], one parent stated, "It's about options. It just gives you another option. And the more options you have in life the better off you are" (p. 8). Oncologists typically agree that treatment should not be delayed in order to engage in fertility preservation, especially when prognoses are poor. However, given the growing emphasis on patient- and family-centered care, families need to be presented with information on fertility-related risks and afforded the opportunity to weigh options. Although families may be preoccupied with more immediate needs at diagnosis (i.e., initiating treatment, the child's survival), parents are also concerned with the possible negative effects of treatment, including fertility. If the possibility of infertility and options for preservation are not discussed, the patient and family may feel deceived by their medical team when this information is later addressed, typically after it is too late to engage in fertility preservation options. While physicians may feel they are only adding to a patient and family's pain by mentioning future infertility risk, Schover [110] stated that this news can be even more devastating for cancer survivors to hear after completing treatment in comparison to otherwise healthy individuals because it becomes "insult added to injury" (p. 55) [29]. Therefore, when making decisions that may impact future quality of life, fertility preservation is an important and timely decision for the family to consider. There is also familial distress associated with the financial burden a couple may encounter concerning medical appointments, fertility treatments, and the adoption process if they cannot conceive a biological child. Connolly and colleagues (2010) discussed the economics behind using assisted reproductive technologies and how the costs may affect families [13]. Because treatments are expensive, annual income and affordability are often related to whether a couple chooses infertility treatments. However, this study and others have examined discontinuation rates of treatments and found that psychological factors, such as "emotional strain", are more likely to be reasons to stop fertility treatments once they had begun [30].

For over 30 years, sperm cryopreservation has routinely been used to preserve male fertility and has become even more practical and effective with the development of in vitro fertilization with intracytoplasmic sperm injection. Banking sperm pre-cancer treatment has been associated with psychological relief, even if the sample is never used, and 96% of all men would or may recommend sperm banking to others [17]. Ginsberg and colleagues [38] recently reported that 55% of adolescents and 88% of their parents had favorable initial impressions of sperm banking when queried and that a majority of families felt the timing of sperm banking communications had been acceptable. One hundred percent of patients and parents responded "Yes" to the question "Did you make the right decision to attempt banking?" including those adolescents who attempted to bank but failed. Finally, 20% of the sample had to delay treatment in order to bank, but all of these families felt that banking was worth the delay. Yet, barriers to sperm banking among adolescents and young adults with cancer continue to persist.

Rates of sperm banking are significantly lower in the US as compared to many countries around the world. Among adult males for example, countries like Japan and Norway have a 50% sperm banking rate, whereas only 25% of American males bank sperm prior to cancer treatment [17, 31–33]. Assumptions have been made that these increased rates of banking are a function of national health care systems, which subsidize sperm banking costs, but the cost of sperm banking is rarely identified as a significant barrier within samples of young adult men [33, 34] (Among adolescent males, sperm banking rates reported from pediatric cancer centers in England, Denmark, and Israel range from 47 to 89%, whereas those in the US and Canada range from 18 to 26% [35–37]. The notable exception has been reported by Ginsberg and colleagues [38], who found that rates of adolescent sperm banking improved significantly following hospital initiatives to overcome barriers to sperm banking. These findings suggest that although sperm banking is significantly underutilized among adolescents diagnosed with cancer, rates can improve with intervention [38].

There has been a paucity of research examining the factors which predict adolescents' choices about banking sperm at cancer diagnosis. The studies which have been published are generally retrospective, qualitative in design and include few study participants. Furthermore, it has been difficult to apply the findings published in the adult literature to adolescents. Many of the factors that have been identified as positively associated with banking (e.g. younger age, more education, receiving treatment in a private oncology practice) and negatively associated (have all the children desired, previous history of infertility/vasectomy) with sperm banking in adults are less applicable to adolescents [31, 33]. More developmentally appropriate factors such as being past the early teens, greater knowledge of sperm banking procedures and demands, and parental support in decision making are associated with sperm banking among adolescents, whereas discomfort/embarrassment in talking about sex and fertility and having a parent accompany their child to the sperm banking clinic appear to make banking less likely.

Although lack of knowledge regarding infertility risk and absence of a physician recommendation to bank sperm have been associated with lower rates of sperm banking among both adolescents and young adults, adolescents also appear to be particularly vulnerable to anxiety at the time of diagnosis, which can result in a lower likelihood of sperm banking [41–43]. It may be that there is a multiplicative adverse effect when adolescent anxiety at diagnosis interacts with poor physician communication such that recommendations regarding the importance of banking sperm are never heard or processed. Inverse relationships between the amount of information recalled and anxiety level within a medical context have been well described, particularly among those younger in age [44, 45]. When adolescents are diagnosed with cancer, families often have an immediate preoccupation with initiating treatment and working toward cancer cure. As a result, issues related to preserving one's fertility may be perceived as secondary or less important.

Demographic, provider, and medical factors have also been identified as impacting the likelihood of banking sperm. Lower socioeconomic status has been related to not banking, whereas physician knowledge of treatment-related infertility-risk, physician recommendation to bank sperm, increased conviction when making this recommendation, presentation of sperm banking as standard care, and advising ambivalent adolescents that fatherhood will be important to them in the future have been associated with higher rates of banking among young adult males [33, 35, 42, 43]. Logistically, factors such as convenience or prompt availability of a sperm banking center or medical factors such as cancer diagnosis, urgency to begin treatment, and the timing of sperm banking messages have also been found to affect sperm banking outcomes. However, the contributions of developmental and parental/guardian factors have not yet been examined.

Both established and experimental options for preserving fertility are available for females diagnosed with pediatric cancer including embryo cryopreservation, ooctye cryopreservation, ovarian tissue freezing and grafting, immature ooctye preservation with in vitro maturation, and preventative efforts to protect ovarian function during treatment [46]. Embryo cryopreservation requires in vitro fertilization (IVF) with ovarian stimulation, ooctye retrieval, fertilization, and freezing the embryo for later implantation into the uterus. Although IVF has been utilized as a highly successful form of fertility preservation for nearly 40 years, there are significant drawbacks when considering this method of preservation among adolescent and young adult cancer patients. For example, this procedure typically requires hormone stimulation of the ovaries, which may increase risk for later cancers. Additionally, 10–14 days of follicular development is needed during which time treatment is delayed. As a result, this may not be a feasible option for patients requiring immediate intervention. In addition, there is often an immediate need for a male partner or donor sperm, which is frequently unavailable for adolescent patients. Oocyte cryopreservation raises many of the same concerns reported with embryo cryopreservation but does not require a male partner or sperm donor. Successful fertility preservation has also been demonstrated by excising ovarian tissue prior to the initiation of treatment, freezing the tissue, and then engrafting the tissue following treatment. This procedure minimizes delays in receiving therapy and increases the opportunity for follicles and ooctyes to be produced for future conception. Although there is significant variability regarding the success rates of these fertility preservation options, fertility preservation continues to be underutilized in this high risk group.

In addition to deciding whether or not to preserve fertility, a small subset of survivors will struggle with deciding to procreate due to an increased risk of passing on a cancer predisposition to their offspring. This is the case with survivors of bilateral retinoblastoma and in those with Li-Fraumeni syndrome. These patients are regularly counselled throughout their treatment course and into survivorship by their oncology team regarding their risk of transmitting a cancer predisposition should they pursue biological children [47]. Patients and families with familial cancer syndromes may experience psychological distress if these early message are not recalled or considered, particularly if the now-adult patient is sexually active and in a committed relationship with the intention of producing biological children. Although these survivors do not experience the time pressures associated with preservation decisions, these are difficult decisions to make and may have serious implications.

Psychological Distress Related to Infertility

Although 91% of oncologists agree that sperm banking should be offered to males of reproductive age at risk for treatment-related infertility, only 10% report discussing sperm banking with high-risk males routinely in their practices [48]. The majority of males surviving cancer are unaware of their fertility status and often become distressed when issues of infertility arise [27]. Male survivors who experience treatment-related infertility are at increased risk for emotional distress, particularly those who are younger, desire children, and were unaware of the problem [33, 34, 49, 50]. Although sadness has been reported among adult survivors of childhood cancer, anger is the primary expression of distress, particularly in regard to the previous withholding of information, denial of fathering choice, injustice of their plight, and lack of fertility control [25]. Lack of knowledge regarding one's fertility status has also been related to intimate relationship conflict, risky sexual behavior, and lower self-esteem [27]. Those who suspect infertility have significant concerns about being rejected by future partners [51].

Survivors of cancer place a high priority on fertility and report high levels of psychological distress associated with fertility loss [52]. Female adolescent cancer patients have been found to be concerned about fertility and interested in options to help preserve fertility during cancer treatments [53]. In a comprehensive review of the literature, Lee and colleagues (2006) found

that fertility preservation is extremely important to cancer survivors and that infertility resulting from cancer treatment has been associated with significant psychosocial distress [39]. In a broad sample of cancer survivors who were diagnosed before 35 years of age, younger cancer survivors expressed more concern than older survivors that cancer could adversely affect their fertility but were less likely to perceive themselves as infertile [34]. About half the sample as a whole perceived themselves as less fertile than their peer group. As a significant proportion of adults and adolescents do not recall being told about infertility risk as a side effect of cancer treatment it is important to determine what effect fertility expectations may have on subsequent psychological functioning, particularly in the case of unexpected infertility [54]. Furthermore, adolescent cancer patients often have misperceptions about their risk for infertility, so that those who are at low risk may suffer unnecessary anxiety about infertility and those at higher risk may not realize the importance of addressing fertility issues before or during their treatment [55].

Grief processes must also be considered within the context of infertility-related distress experienced by survivors of pediatric cancers. It has been demonstrated that couples facing infertility are often unable to "grieve adequately or to get empathy from family and friends, because they have lost a potential, rather than an actual child" [110, 111]. Similar findings were reported by Lukse and colleagues [56] who found that women undergoing infertility treatment endorsed significant levels of grief and depression. This study also found that some women undergoing such treatments felt abandoned by the team of doctors performing the in vitro fertilization and therefore did not feel a sense of control with their procedures [56]. Survivors of pediatric cancers facing reproductive health challenges report similar experiences, including inadequate support from medical team members, family, and friends, as they grieve the anticipated life experiences they may never have. Schover [111] also discussed society's perception of a cancer survivor's outlook on life, including fertility, stating that family, friends, and professionals may question their grief related to infertility. Survivors often receive the message that they should be grateful to be alive, which minimizes any late effects or perceived losses and regrets that exist. Commonly, survivors are held in high regard as heroes, role models, or people to admire because of their perceived persistence through difficult life experiences. However, through this portrayal, the ongoing struggles experienced by many survivors may be disregarded or diminished [57].

Identity Development: Roles as a Romantic Partner and Parent

While some survivors of pediatric cancers adjust relatively well to life during and following treatment, others face challenges in a variety of domains, including reproductive health [58–60]. Adolescent and emerging adult survivors of pediatric cancers may be especially vulnerable to experiencing difficulties in psychosocial adaptation as it relates to fertility and reproductive processes. This increased likelihood of difficulty is due, in part, to the already complex developmental changes occurring in these groups within social domains, which are further disrupted by having experienced cancer and/or being a cancer survivor [61, 62]. Reproductive health, for example, is closely tied to adolescents and emerging adults' developing identity as a romantic partner and parent. In industrialized countries, life expectations of what a person is to be working toward and accomplishing in his or her late teens and early twenties has shifted dramatically over the past 40 years [63–66]. While it was once common only for the elite and privileged to go through a stage of identity exploration and instability following adolescence, it is now typical for most young men and women in the United States to go through such a period. Research has indicated that marriage is no longer viewed as the quintessential marker of adulthood among the majority of American young people [63]. Rather, criteria for transitioning into adulthood, regardless of gender, are increasingly individualistic and include "accepting responsibility for one's self, making independent decisions" regarding beliefs and values and being financially independent [63]. For many, it has become less common for criteria such as marriage and parenthood to be viewed as necessary for the attainment of adulthood status. However, for survivors of pediatric cancers who are at high risk for infertility and other reproductive health concerns, typical identity development may be complicated and burdened by uncertainties about navigating otherwise typically anticipated outcomes that may no longer be feasible, such as having a biological child. Therefore, not being able to conceive can lead cancer survivors to feel damaged and uncertain of their role and identity when engaging in romantic relationships [67].

Pediatric cancer survivors face numerous potential challenges related to overall social skill development with research indicating that individuals growing up chronically ill are two to three times more likely to experience difficulties in social relationships [68]. Specifically, impaired romantic relationships among survivors have been reported as compared to healthy peers [69]. While many healthy adolescents and emerging adults also experience similar challenges, typical developmental processes may become magnified and result in a heightened propensity for social isolation among those coping with a cancer diagnosis and/or cancer survivorship [70, 71]. One study of emerging adult and adult pediatric cancer survivors reported survivors felt more mature than others their age, which led to challenges relating to potential romantic partners [72]. Others reported feeling that physical late effects, fear of relapse, and the risk of having a child diagnosed with cancer had interfered with their ability to form intimate romantic relationships [72, 73]. Some cited having already experienced a loss of social relationships due to their diagnosis and treatment and being fearful of developing new intimate relationships as young adults. However, it should be noted that not all responses cited difficulties with relationships with some participants reporting that they feel confident in their ability to develop and maintain relationships, suggesting that there may be protective factors that can interact with treatment-specific factors to promote positive social outcomes.

One challenge of particular interest to survivors of pediatric cancers is developing the self-efficacy to create and maintain romantic relationships. Romantic relationship self-efficacy is defined as the ability to develop and retain relationships and resolve interpersonal disputes specifically with romantic partners [74–77]. Not only is the existing literature regarding romantic relationship self-efficacy among adolescent and emerging adult pediatric cancer survivors sparse, almost no research has been identified examining these constructs among healthy adolescents and emerging adults. Moreover, the sole article identified within this area among healthy populations only briefly touches upon the triumphs and challenges faced with respect to building confidence and modifying perspectives in romantic relationships as adolescents approach adulthood [78]. This lack of information is unfortunate as social cognitive theory highlights the significance of distinguishing the individual's self-efficacy toward the completion of a social behaviors leading to a desired outcome from his or her evaluation of the outcome [79]. Put more simply, an individual must develop the necessary self-efficacy to complete a social behavior before being expected to successfully meet his or her relationship goals. In the case of romantic relationships, the individual needs to confidently believe or perceive that he or she is capable of developing and maintaining such relationships before these relationships can be formed and shaped successfully. However, as explained in both social cognitive theory and the Health Belief Model, perceived threats and susceptibilities may interfere with the ability to develop self-efficacy beliefs [79–81]. For example, child and adolescent cancer survivors have concerns regarding actual and perceived physical effects of cancer as they relate to engaging in romantic relationships, getting married, and having a family [52]. Many worry about infertility and have more negative outlooks on life. Potentially, these concerns may influence perceptions of attractiveness and developing the confidence to seek out and maintain romantic relationships. While no literature was identified specifically investigating romantic relationship self-efficacy among emerging adult survivors of pediatric cancers, adolescent survivors have reported having less positive self-images in terms of their social and sexual self in comparison to healthy peers, entering into marriage at slightly lower rates than the general population, and being less likely to have biological children [67, 82–85].

Among survivors of pediatric cancer, the threat of infertility and its potential negative impact on future relationships can be devastating. There is evidence that survivors of childhood cancer initiate lasting relationships at an older age than their peers. Approximately 20% of survivors report perceived limitations in their sexual life due to their cancer diagnosis [86]. Older survivors have reported feeling less experienced in terms of sexual encounters, and survivors, in general, have reported worse sexual quality of life than age-matched peers. Those receiving cancer treatment during adolescence have indicated feeling delayed with respect to psychosexual development including initiation of dating, establishing a longer term romantic relationship, masturbation, and sexual intercourse [86, 87]. Additionally, Puukko and colleagues [92] found that although women surviving childhood leukemia did not differ from controls in meeting several psychosexual milestones (with the exception of having experienced sexual intercourse), they reported a more negative subjective experience of sexuality. Schover [111] pointed out that whether it is a perceived or real threat, many cancer survivors feel that their disordered fertility may be a deterrent to finding a partner. They may feel fear of rejection following disclosure of their cancer history to potential partners. The survivor may feel shame in not being able to have a child, carry on the family name, or provide their parents with a grandchild. To this end, male survivors have reported choosing to use condoms in order to appear fertile and avoid having to disclose their infertility status [67]. Additionally, female survivors may feel pressured to enter into permanent relationships prematurely in order to increase opportunities for motherhood prior to experiencing premature ovarian failure. Therefore, in addition to struggles with adapting to potential infertility and other reproductive health problems, these findings suggest that survivors of childhood cancer may also experience differences in sexual development which may also impact transitioning to adulthood. Parents of cancer survivors may add to the stress by expressing disappointment at the possibility of not having biological grandchildren. Similar concerns have been reported by parents of survivors. These concerns were demonstrated in a qualitative study by Nieman and colleagues [29] in which a parent reported being worried no one would love her child if they knew she could not have children. Another parent was worried that with the threat of premature menopause, her daughter may hurry into marriage in order to have children at a young age.

Despite challenges reported with respect to identity development, those surviving childhood cancer often desire to have children and value parenting. Having children as a life goal among adolescents surviving cancer has been ranked above making money, owning a home or traveling in terms of priority [53]. Among adult males without children at diagnosis, 76% desire children and prefer biological offspring whenever possible [27, 33, 88]. Survivors view themselves as healthy enough to be good parents and believe that their cancer experience has enhanced (or will enhance) their parenting skills, desire for family closeness, and parent-child relationships [27, 33, 34]. Although some survivors worry about transmitting genetic risk of cancer to their children or having children with birth defects (both of which are generally unsubstantiated among those diagnosed with childhood cancer), the desire to parent children remains [27, 34].

Perceptions of Physical Attractiveness

Pediatric cancer survivors commonly encounter real and perceived challenges related to their physical development including delays in physical maturation (e.g., late onset of puberty, delayed physical growth), changes in physical appearance due to surgeries, chemotherapy, and radiation, and the risk of infertility due to certain cancer treatments [52, 62, 72, 89–91]. Many of these challenges continue to persist long after the cancer treatment is completed and influences perceptions of physical attractiveness [52, 92].

In a study of adolescent and emerging adult survivors of pediatric cancers who did not have obvious physical atypicalities (e.g., amputations, significant scars), participants reported their self-perceptions of physical attractiveness, body satisfaction, and personal sense of competence in several domains including self-worth, social acceptance, romantic appeal, and close friendships [93]. Objective ratings of attractiveness were made by research assistants as well. As compared to a healthy control group, cancer survivors reported engaging in more than 50% fewer social activities. Overall, using a blind rating system, cancer survivors were not rated by research assistants as less attractive, and survivors and healthy controls rated their own perceptions of physical attractiveness similarly. However, as time since treatment ended increased, cancer survivors reported lower perceptions of self-worth, higher levels of social anxiety, and more negative perceptions of physical attractiveness. Interpretation of these results suggests that additional difficulties with perceptions of physical attractiveness and social anxieties may not develop until survivors have been off treatment for a significant amount of time.

Consistent with the approach of Pendley and colleagues [93], Larouche and Chin-Peuckert (2006) investigated how perceptions of physical attractiveness change with a cancer diagnosis and how cancer patients maintain and/or re-establish social connections despite changes in their self-perceptions [40]. In their qualitative study, five adolescents (three males and two females, ages 14–17) were interviewed while receiving their cancer treatments. Interviews indicated that the participants no longer felt as though they looked "normal" (p. 204). Modified perceptions of physical attractiveness were reported to be a function of hair loss, scars, the presence of catheters, and changes in skin complexion. Changes in perceived physical attractiveness resulted in modified coping strategies. Some of the participants discussed tendencies to avoid social situations with both peers and romantic partners due to increased perceptions of vulnerability and loss of confidence. Others described using peers to shield them from others who may be negative about the physical changes that had occurred or opting to participate only in social situations in which the risk of negative outcomes was minimal.

Studies of healthy emerging adults consistently have shown that better perceptions of physical attractiveness are linked to perceiving oneself and others as more popular or acceptable among peer groups [94–96]. Those who have survived a pediatric cancer diagnosis are not immune to these perceptions. Emerging adult survivors of pediatric cancer often cite concerns surrounding romantic relationships [70]. Delayed physical maturation and alterations in physical appearance, which are correlated with poor body image, make adaptive socialization awkward [70, 72, 97]. In turn, poor social skills can lead to depression or anxiety, which may act to exacerbate the awareness and anxieties surrounding illness and physical delays thereby creating a cyclic effect of increased isolation and decreased peer and romantic relationship self-efficacy. Additionally, survivors may worry that relapse is likely or that cancer treatments have impacted their ability to procreate [52, 98, 99]. These anxieties then may lead a cancer survivor to feel that the pursuit of romantic relationships is a useless endeavor since others will not want to be involved in romantic relationships with someone who is ill and/or cannot have children [52, 99].

Psychosexual Functioning

Another, but understudied, outcome of cancer treatment relates to problems associated with psychosexual functioning. Depending on the treatment received, survivors may be at high risk for problems resulting from physical discomfort, poor body image, emotional distress, negative sexual self-concept, or structural abnormalities. Although difficulties with psychosexual functioning have been reported among adults post treatment of reproductive cancers, little research

exists substantiating psychosexual outcomes in those surviving childhood cancer, despite our clinical experience which suggests otherwise. Much like those adult women who have been treated for gynecologic cancer, females patients surviving childhood pelvic tumors (e.g., rhabdomyosarcoma of the genitourinary tract) may be at risk for sexual dissatisfaction and dysfunction, lower levels of sexual desire, and pain during vaginal intercourse [100, 101]. Pediatric cancer survivors experiencing psychosexual dysfunction may be at further risk for physical discomfort, emotional distress, and negative sexual self-concept. In a sample of long-term survivors of ovarian germ cell tumors, compared with controls, survivors had less sexual pleasure and lower total scores on a sexual activity scale [101]. Another study followed cancer survivors three years post bone marrow transplantation and found 52% of female survivors experienced increases in sexual problems in the areas of arousal and lubrication [102].

As is the case with infertility, pelvic irradiation has been implicated as one of the cancer treatments which have the most adverse effects on sexual functioning. A significant proportion of women experience sexual dysfunction following pelvic irradiation, and dysfunction typically results from distortion of the perineum and vagina. These structural problems adversely affect sexual activity, which in turn, leads to considerable psychological distress [103]. The physical late effects associated with pelvic irradiation may include vaginal dryness, atrophic vaginitis, vaginal/vulval ulceration or necrosis, vaginal stenosis, shortened vaginal canal, dyspareunia, and postcoital bleeding [104]. Furthermore, radiation induced ovarian failure may result in decreased vaginal lubrication and thinning of the vaginal epithelium. Reported changes in sexual function for those having received pelvic irradiation include decreases in sexual enjoyment, ability to attain orgasm, libido, sexual desire, coital opportunity, and frequency of intercourse [105, 106]. As a result, women receiving pelvic radiation are at risk for experiencing sexual problems, with up to 64% experiencing symptoms of severe sexual dysfunction [107, 108].

Psychosexual dysfunction, including erectile dysfunction, delay/absence of ejaculation, decreased sexual desire, difficulty reaching orgasm, and pain with ejaculation, is also an often reported consequence of cancer treatment among males [109]. For example, 47% of males treated for acute or chronic myelogenous leukemia report erectile dysfunction, with 38% experiencing delays or absence of orgasm/ejaculation [110]. Dysfunction continues three years post bone marrow transplantation in regard to erections (22%) and sexual arousal (20%) [102]. Although some relationships between cancer treatment and psychosexual dysfunction have been identified among males with adult onset cancer, there are essentially no reports in the literature which have tested these associations among males surviving childhood cancer.

Conclusion

Risks to reproductive health exist among survivors of pediatric cancer, and this adverse late effect is directly attributable to life saving cancer treatments. Options are available to preserve fertility among those at risk of infertility secondary to treatment; however, several barriers and risks exist which reduce the likelihood of fertility preservation engagement. These barriers are multifaceted and include oncologist/family communication of fertility threat, time limited decision-making at cancer diagnosis, unwillingness to delay treatment for preservation procedures, and the financial burden associated with preservation. Furthermore, patients and families often report increased psychological distress at the time of diagnosis which impairs familial understanding reproductive health risks which often results in anxiety and feelings of grief and loss associated with poor fertility outcomes. Identity development also appears to be vulnerable with respect to negotiating typical developmental tasks such as entering into longer term romantic relationships and parenthood. Threats to perceptions of physical attractiveness and psychosexual functioning have also been documented which may ultimately affect global quality of life outcomes.

Despite these concerns, survivors of pediatric cancers report strong desires to become parents and frequently tout the advantages of having survived cancer in that it provides excellent preparation for parenthood. These issues in combination exemplify the importance that survivors place on fertility and the promotion of normative developmental trajectories. As the number of survivors increase, so does the importance of quality of life outcomes in survivorship.

Provider Recommendations

1. One's risk of infertility secondary to cancer treatment should be discussed with patients and families prior to the initiation of cancer therapy. Even if the patient has no increased risk, this information should be provided and discussed so that unnecessary fertility-related distress is not experienced.

2. For patients who are at increased risk for infertility, risk-status should be communicated and options for fertility preservation provided. For adolescent males, cryopreservation of sperm should be recommended whenever possible. Among female patients, emphasis should be placed on the experimental nature of these procedures and its limited availability among select institutions with IRB-approved research protocols. Based on the family's receptivity, prompt referral to the fertility specialist (e.g. reproductive endocrinologist, urologist, OB/GYN) should be made. Patient assent is a critical feature which must considered.

3. Because families may experience difficulty adequately absorbing information regarding their child's fertility status in the context of a newly diagnosed cancer, assessment and re-assessment of the family's understanding should occur throughout the cancer care continuum, ranging from diagnosis to survivorship care. It is likely that multiple methods of communication (e.g., verbal discussion of risk, provision of written information, exposure to educational videos, etc.) may be needed over time in order to maximize the

likelihood of the patient's understanding and subsequent expectations of fertility outcome.

4. Although the discussion of cancer treatment-related risks can be difficult for family members and medical professionals alike, the vast majority of families prefer that this information be provided, regardless of potential discomforts associated with openly discussing this topic.

5. Medical professionals should seek out training and information regarding infertility and fertility preservation in the pediatric oncology context. Furthermore, these professionals should expect to provide logistical information to families including location of preservation clinic, estimated costs associated with preservation procedures and storage of materials, options for financial assistance, and the timeframe in which fertility preservation is an option. Discussion regarding the process by which materials will be collected should also occur. Being well-prepared to engage in such discussions with families can help alleviate the provider's hesitancy to talk about fertility and its associated risks secondary to cancer treatment.

6. Prognosis has often been reported as a determining factor associated with whether fertility preservation options are provided to a family. However, options need to be provided to families regardless of prognosis. In addition to the professional obligation that clinicians have of presenting families with pertinent information, research suggests that engaging in fertility preservation is associated with psychological relief regardless of whether the preserved material is ever used.

7. Discussion of fertility status needs to take place regardless of a family's cultural background, religious beliefs, sexual orientation, or socio-economic status. Although research suggests that these factors may play roles in a family's decision to engage in fertility preservation, all families need to be provided with adequate opportunities to make informed decisions.

8. Within each patient's medical team, it may be beneficial to appoint a specific team member to assume responsibility for initiating conversation with families surrounding fertility risk and fertility preservation. Doing so will not only decrease the chances that this discussion will be overlooked but will provide an identified "expert" that the family can consult with as fertility preservations decisions are being made.

References

1. Waring A, Wallace W (2000) Subfertility following treatment for childhood cancer. Hosp Med (Lond, Engl: 1998) 61(8):550–557
2. Bahadur G (2000) Fertility issues for cancer patients. Mol Cell Endocrinol 169(1–2):117–122
3. Mackie E, Radford M, Shalet SM (1996) Gonadal function following chemotherapy for childhood Hodgkin's disease. Med Pediatr Oncol 27(2):74–78
4. Meistrich M et al (1992) Impact of cyclophosphamide on long-term reduction in sperm count in men treated with combination chemotherapy for Ewing and soft tissue sarcomas. Cancer 70(11):2703–2712
5. Kenney LB et al (2001) High risk of infertility and long term gonadal damage in males treated with high dose cyclophosphamide for sarcoma during childhood. Cancer 91(3):613–621
6. Mansky P et al (2007) Treatment late effects in long-term survivors of pediatric sarcoma. Pediatr Blood Cancer 48(2):192–199
7. Critchley HOD, Wallace WHB (2005) Impact of cancer treatment on uterine function. JNCI Monogr 2005(34):64
8. Shalet SM et al (1989) Vulnerability of the human Leydig cell to radiation damage is dependent upon age. J Endocrinol 120(1):161–165
9. Leiper A, Grant D, Chessells J (1986) Gonadal function after testicular radiation for acute lymphoblastic leukaemia. Arch Dis Child 61:53–56
10. Oeffinger KC, Nathan PC, Kremer L (2008) Challenges after curative treatment for childhood cancer and long-term follow up of survivors. Pediatr Clin North Am 55:251–273
11. Rovo A et al (2006) Spermatogenesis in long-term survivors after allogeneic hematopoietic stem cell transplantation is associated with age, time interval since transplantation, and apparently absence of chronic GvHD. Blood 108(3):1100–1105
12. Speiser B, Rubin P, Casarett G (1973) Aspermia following lower truncal irradiation in Hodgkin's disease. Cancer 32(3):692–698
13. Connolly MP, Ledger W, Postma MJ (2010) Economics of assisted reproduction: access to

fertility treatments and valuing live births in economic terms. Hum Fertil 13:13–18

14. Green DM et al (2009) Fertility of female survivors of childhood cancer: a report from the childhood cancer survivor study. J Clin Oncol 27(16):2677–2685
15. Sudour H et al (2009) Fertility and pregnancy outcome after abdominal irradiation that included or excluded the pelvis in childhood tumor survivors. Int J Radiat Oncol Biol Phys 76(3):867–873
16. Signorello LB et al (2006) Female survivors of childhood cancer: preterm birth and low birth weight among their children. JNCI Cancer Spectrum 98(20):1453–1461
17. Saito K et al (2005) Sperm cryopreservation before cancer chemotherapy helps in the emotional battle against cancer. Cancer 104(3):521–524
18. Quinn GP, Vadaparampil ST (2009) Fertility preservation and adolescent/young adult cancer patients: physician communication challenges. J Adolesc Health 44(4):394–400
19. Quinn GP et al (2007) Discussion of fertility preservation with newly diagnosed patients: oncologists' views. J Cancer Survivorship 1(2):146–155
20. Quinn GP et al (2009) Impact of physicians' personal discomfort and patient prognosis on discussion of fertility preservation with young cancer patients. Patient Educ Couns 77(3):338–343
21. Vadaparampil S et al (2008) Barriers to fertility preservation among pediatric oncologists. Patient Educ Couns 72(3):402–410
22. Vadaparampil ST, Quinn GP, Clayton HB et al (2008) Institutional availability of fertility preservation. Clin Pediatr 47:302–305
23. Blacklay A, Eiser C, Ellis A (1998) Development and evaluation of an information booklet for adult survivors of cancer in childhood. Arch Dis Child 78(4):340–344
24. Davies H, Greenfield D, Ledger W (2003) Reproductive medicine in a late effects of cancer clinic. Hum Fertil 6(1):9–12
25. Green D, Galvin H, Horne B (2003) The psychosocial impact of infertility on young male cancer survivors: a qualitative investigation. Psycho Oncol 12(2):141–152
26. Weigers ME et al (1999) Self-reported worries among long-term survivors of childhood cancer and their peers. J Psychosoc Oncol 16(2):1–23
27. Zebrack BJ et al (2004) Fertility issues for young adult survivors of childhood cancer. Psycho Oncol 13(10):689–699
28. Zebrack BJ, Chesler M (2001) Health-related worries, self-image, and life outlooks of long-term survivors of childhood cancer. Health Soc Work 26(4):245–256
29. Nieman CL et al (2007) Fertility preservation and adolescent cancer patients: lessons from adult survivors of childhood cancer and their parents. Oncofertility Fertil Preserv Cancer Survivors 201–217
30. Goldfarb J et al (1997) Factors influencing patients' decision not to repeat IVF. J Assist Reprod Genet 14(7):381–384
31. Girasole CR et al (2007) Sperm banking: use and outcomes in patients treated for testicular cancer. BJU Int 99(1):33–36
32. Magelssen H et al (2005) Twenty years experience with semen cryopreservation in testicular cancer patients: who needs it? Eur Urol 48(5):779–785
33. Schover LR et al (2002) Knowledge and experience regarding cancer, infertility, and sperm banking in younger male survivors. J Clin Oncol 20(7):1880–1889
34. Schover LR et al (1999) Having children after cancer. Cancer 86(4):697–709
35. Klosky JL et al (2009) Sperm cryopreservation practices among adolescent cancer patients at risk for infertility. Pediatr Hematol Oncol 26(4):252–260
36. Nagel K, Neal M (2008) Discussions regarding sperm banking with adolescent and young adult males who have cancer. J Pediatr Oncol Nurs 25(2):102–106
37. Neal MS et al (2007) Effectiveness of sperm banking in adolescents and young adults with cancer. Cancer 110(5):1125–1129
38. Ginsberg JP et al (2008) Sperm banking for adolescent and young adult cancer patients: sperm quality, patient, and parent perspectives. Pediatr Blood Cancer 50(3):594–598
39. Lee SJ, Schover LR, Partridge AH et al (2006) American society of clinical oncology recommendations on fertility preservation in cancer patients. J Clin Oncol 24:2917–2931
40. Larouche SS, Chin-Peuckert L (2006) Changes in body image experienced by adolescent with cancer. J Pediatr Oncol Nurs 23:200–209
41. Edge B, Holmes D, Makin G (2006) Sperm banking in adolescent cancer patients. Arch Dis Child 91(2):149–152
42. Achille MA et al (2006) Facilitators and obstacles to sperm banking in young men receiving gonadotoxic chemotherapy for cancer: the perspective of survivors and health care professionals. Hum Reprod 21(12):3206–3216
43. Leonard M, Hammelef K, Smith GD (2004) Fertility considerations, counseling, and semen cryopreservation for males prior to the initiation of cancer therapy. Clin J Oncol Nurs 8(2):127–145
44. Ley P (1979) Memory for medical information. Br J Soc Clin Psychol 18(2):245–255
45. Millar MG, Millar K (1998) Processing messages about disease detection and health promotion behaviors: the effects of anxiety. Health Commun 10(3):211–226
46. Levine J, Canada A, Stern CJ (2010) Fertility preservation in adolescents and young adults with cancer. J Clin Oncol 28:4831–4841

47. Klosky JL, Spunt SL (2010) Sarcoma. In: Holland JC (ed) Psycho-oncology. Oxford University Press, New York, NY

48. Schover LR et al (2002) Oncologists' attitudes and practices regarding banking sperm before cancer treatment. J Clin Oncol 20(7):1890

49. Hartmann J et al (1999) Long-term effects on sexual function and fertility after treatment of testicular cancer. Br J Cancer 80(5/6):801

50. Rieker PP, Fitzgerald EM, Kalish LA (1990) Adaptive behavioral responses to potential infertility among survivors of testis cancer. J Clin Oncol 8(2):347

51. Chapple A et al (2007) Fertility issues: the perceptions and experiences of young men recently diagnosed and treated for cancer. J Adolesc Health 40(1):69

52. Langeveld N et al (2004) Quality of life, self esteem and worries in young adult survivors of childhood cancer. Psycho Oncol 13(12):867–881

53. Burns KC, Boudreau C, Panepinto JA (2006) Attitudes regarding fertility preservation in female adolescent cancer patients. J Pediatr Hematol Oncol 28(6):350

54. Zebrack BJ, Casillas J, Nohr L, Adams H, Zeltzer LK (2004) Fertility issues for young adult survivors of childhood cancer. Psycho Oncol 13:689–699

55. Oosterhuis BE et al (2008) Concerns about infertility risks among pediatric oncology patients and their parents. Pediatr Blood Cancer 50(1):85–89

56. Lukse MP, Vacc NA (1999) Grief, depression, and coping in women undergoing infertility treatment. Obstet Gynecol 93(2):245

57. Cella DF (1987) Cancer survival: psychosocial and public issues. Cancer Invest 5(1):59–67

58. Gortmaker SL et al (1993) An unexpected success story: transition to adulthood in youth with chronic physical health conditions. J Res Adolesc 3(3):317–336

59. Kazak AE (2005) Evidence-based interventions for survivors of childhood cancer and their families. J Pediatr Psychol 30(1):29

60. Patenaude AF, Kupst MJ (2005) Psychosocial functioning in pediatric cancer. J Pediatr Psychol 30(1):9

61. Ungerer JA et al (1988) Psychosocial functioning in children and young adults with juvenile arthritis. Pediatrics 81(2):195

62. Holmbeck GN (2002) A developmental perspective on adolescent health and illness: an introduction to the special issues. J Pediatr Psychol 27(5):409

63. Arnett JJ (2000) Emerging adulthood: a theory of development from the late teens through the twenties. Am Psychol 55:469–480

64. Arnett JJ (2000) High hopes in a grim world: emerging adults' views of their futures and "generation X." Youth Soc 31:267–286

65. Arnett JJ (2006) Emerging adulthood: understanding the new way of coming of age. In Arnett JJ, Tanner JL (eds) Emerging adults in America: coming of age in the 21st century. Washington, DC

66. Shulman S et al (2005) Emerging adulthood. J Adolesc Res 20(5):577

67. Crawshaw M, Sloper P (2010) 'Swimming against the tide'–the influence of fertility matters on the transition to adulthood or survivorship following adolescent cancer. Eur J Cancer Care 19(5):610–620

68. Creswell C, Christie D, Boylan J (2001) Ill or adolescent? Developing group work on an adolescent medicine unit. Clin Child Psychol Psychiatry 6(3):351

69. Hill J et al (2003) Adult psychosocial functioning following childhood cancer: the different roles of sons' and daughters' relationships with their fathers and mothers. J Child Psychol Psychiatry 44(5):752–762

70. Boice MM (1998) Chronic illness in adolescence. Adolescence 33(132):927–928

71. Maggiolini A et al (2000) Self-image of adolescent survivors of long-term childhood leukemia. J Pediatr Hematol Oncol 22(5):417

72. Forsbach T, Thompson A (2003) The impact of childhood cancer on adult survivors' interpersonal relationships. Child Care Pract 9(2):117–128

73. Carlson-Green B (2009) Brain tumor survivors speak out. J Pediatr Oncol Nurs 26(5):266

74. Bandura A et al (1996) Multifaceted impact of self-efficacy beliefs on academic functioning. Child Dev 67(3):1206–1222

75. Connolly J (1989) Social self-efficacy in adolescence: Relations with self-concept, social adjustment, and mental health. Can J Behav Sci 21(3):258–269

76. Wheeler VA, Ladd GW (1982) Assessment of children's self-efficacy for social interactions with peers. Dev Psychol 18(6):795–805

77. Shrauger JS, Schohn M (1995) Self-confidence in college students: conceptualization, measurement, and behavioral implications. Assessment 2(3):255

78. Schulenberg JE, Sameroff AJ, Cicchetti D (2004) The transition to adulthood as a critical juncture in the course of psychopathology and mental health. Dev Psychopathol 16(04):799–806

79. Bandura A, Adams NE, Beyer J (1977) Cognitive processes mediating behavioral change. J Pers Soc Psychol 35(3):125–139

80. Rosenstock I, Strecher V, Becker M (1988) Social learning theory and the health belief model. Health Educ Behav 2(15):175–183

81. Rosenstock IM (1974) Historical origins of the health belief model. Health Educ Monogr 2(4):328–335

82. Olivo E, Woolverton K (2001) Surviving childhood cancer: disruptions in the developmental

building blocks of sexuality. J Sex Educ Ther 26(3):172–181

83. Stern M, Norman SL, Zevon MA (1991) Career development of adolescent cancer patients: a comparative analysis. J Couns Psychol 38(4):431–439

84. Rauck AM et al (1999) Marriage in the survivors of childhood cancer: a preliminary description from the Childhood Cancer Survivor Study. Med Pediatr Oncol 33(1):60–63

85. Madanat LMS et al (2008) Probability of parenthood after early onset cancer: a population-based study. Int J Cancer 123(12):2891–2898

86. Van Dijk E et al (2008) Psychosexual functioning of childhood cancer survivors. Psycho Oncol 17(5):506–511

87. Stam H, Grootenhuis M, Last B (2005) The course of life of survivors of childhood cancer. Psycho Oncol 14(3):227–238

88. Reinmuth S et al (2008) Having children after surviving cancer in childhood or adolescence-results of a berlin survey. Eigene Kinder nach Krebserkrankung im Kindes-und Jugendalter-Ergebnisse einer Berliner Umfrage. Klin Padiatr 220:159–165

89. Kopel SJ et al (1998) Brief report: assessment of body image in survivors of childhood cancer. J Pediatr Psychol 23(2):141

90. Shaw S (2009) Endocrine late effects in survivors of pediatric brain tumors. J Pediatr Oncol Nurs 26(5):295

91. Canada AL, Schover LR, Li Y (2007) A pilot intervention to enhance psychosexual development in adolescents and young adults with cancer. Pediatr Blood Cancer 49:824–828

92. Puukko LR et al (1997) Childhood leukemia and body image: interview reveals impairment not found with a questionnaire. J Clin Psychol 53(2):133–137

93. Pendley JS, Dahlquist LM, Dreyer ZA (1997) Body image and psychosocial adjustment in adolescent cancer survivors. J Pediatr Psychol 22(1):29

94. Kennedy JH (1990) Determinants of peer social status: contributions of physical appearance, reputation, and behavior. J Youth Adolesc 19(3):233–244

95. LaFontana KM, Cillessen AHN (2002) Children's perceptions of popular and unpopular peers: a multimethod assessment. Dev Psychol 38(5):635–647

96. Urbaniak GC, Kilmann PR (2003) Physical attractiveness and the "nice guy paradox": do nice guys really finish last? Sex Roles 49(9):413–426

97. Brown RT, Boeving A, LaRosa A et al (2005) Health and chronic illness. In Wolfe D, Mash E (eds) Behavioral and emotional disorders in adolescents. New York, NY

98. Segrin C, Flora J (2000) Poor social skills are a vulnerability factor in the development of psychosocial problems. Hum Commun Res 26(3):489–514

99. Schwartz CL (1999) Long-term survivors of childhood cancer: the late effects of therapy. Oncologist 4(1):45

100. Carter J et al (2005) Gynecologic cancer treatment and the impact of cancer-related infertility. Gynecol Oncol 97(1):90–95

101. Gershenson DM et al (2007) Reproductive and sexual function after platinum-based chemotherapy in long-term ovarian germ cell tumor survivors: a gynecologic oncology group study. J Clin Oncol 25(19):2792

102. Syrjala KL et al (1998) Prevalence and predictors of sexual dysfunction in long-term survivors of marrow transplantation. J Clin Oncol 16(9):3148

103. Bergmark K et al (1999) Vaginal changes and sexuality in women with a history of cervical cancer. N Engl J Med 340(18):1383

104. Denton A, Maher E (2003) Interventions for the physical aspects of sexual dysfunction in women following pelvic radiotherapy. Cochrane Database Syst Rev 1:CD003750

105. Seibel M, Freeman, MG, Graves WL (1982) Sexual function after surgical and radiation therapy for cervical carcinoma. South Med J 75(10):1195

106. Seibel MM, Freeman, MG, Graves WL (1980) Carcinoma of the cervix and sexual function. Obstet Gynecol 55(4):484

107. Stead ML et al (2007) Psychosexual function and impact of gynaecological cancer. Baillière's Best Pract Res Clin Obstet Gynaecol 21(2):309–320

108. Carpenter KM et al (2009) Sexual self schema as a moderator of sexual and psychological outcomes for gynecologic cancer survivors. Arch Sex Behav 38(5):828–841

109. Schover LR (2005) Motivation for parenthood after cancer: a review. JNCI Cancer Spectrum 2005(34):2

110. Claessens J, Beerendonk C, Schattenberg A (2006) Quality of life, reproduction and sexuality after stem cell transplantation with partially T-cell-depleted grafts and after conditioning with a regimen including total body irradiation. Bone Marrow Transplant 37(9):831–836

111. Schover LR (1999) Psychosocial aspects of infertility and decisions about reproduction in young cancer survivors: a review. Med Pediatr Oncol 33:53–59

Institutional Approaches to Implementing Fertility Preservation for Cancer Patients

13

Joanne Frankel Kelvin, RN, MSN, AOCN and Joyce Reinecke, JD

When first diagnosed with cancer, patients suddenly face a million choices and are asked to make decisions that may have a life-long impact. That moment came for us in June 2006 when Ruth was diagnosed with Ewing's Sarcoma, a month before her 29th birthday. At our first appointment Ruth's oncologist told us that infertility was a possible side-effect of the chemotherapy regimen and asked if we needed to incorporate that concern into her treatment plan. Since we had hoped to start a family soon, we greatly appreciated the question and sensitivity.

We successfully banked embryos and Ruth was able to start treatment on schedule. We were fortunate. At every stage of the process our medical professionals were aware of options that could help us as a young couple facing cancer together. Over the past ten months of Ruth's treatment, we have met or heard of other young adults whose stories tell of how unique our fertility experience has been and how much work there still is to do.

We take real comfort in knowing that when we are ready to start a family, we still have options.
Parker, Husband of Adult Cancer Survivor

Introduction

With advances in cancer treatment, increasing numbers of patients are becoming long-term survivors. A concomitant interest in quality of life for cancer survivors has also developed. For patients of childbearing age, reproductive capacity and the ability to build a family is a significant survivorship concern [1–3]. Unfortunately, many cancer treatments compromise fertility, reducing the likelihood that these men and women will be able to conceive or carry children naturally. Infertility can impact self-esteem, identity, and body image; complicate intimate relationships;

J. Reinecke (✉)
Cancer & Fertility Advisor, LIVESTRONG, Lafayette,
California 94549, USA
e-mail: joyce@fertilehope.org

devastate plans for parenthood; and cause significant, on-going distress [3–6].

Several leading medical organizations, including the American Society of Reproductive Medicine, the American Society of Clinical Oncology, the American Academy of Pediatrics, and the European Society for Medical Oncology, have recognized the validity of these concerns and have issued guidelines to address them. They all highlight the need for oncology clinicians to inform patients about risks of infertility from treatment, discuss options for fertility preservation, and refer interested patients to reproductive specialists before treatment begins [7–10]. From the specific recommendations from the American Society of Clinical Oncology (see Table 13.1).

Contrary to the widely held assumption that newly diagnosed patients are too overwhelmed to handle this concern, patients do want to receive reproductive information [11–13].

G.P. Quinn, S.T. Vadaparampil (eds.), *Reproductive Health and Cancer in Adolescents and Young Adults*, Advances in Experimental Medicine and Biology 732,
DOI 10.1007/978-94-007-2492-1_13, © Springer Science+Business Media B.V. 2012

Table 13.1 American society of clinical oncology (ASCO) recommendations on fertility preservation in cancer patients

The (ASCO) panel recommends that oncologists discuss at the earliest opportunity the possibility of infertility as a risk of cancer treatment, recognizing that in many cases, adequate data are not available to provide accurate predictions for any one individual. For patients at risk for infertility who are interested in evaluating their options for fertility preservation, referral to appropriate specialists as early as possible is recommended.

Lee et al. [7]

However, oncologists and other oncology clinicians do not routinely address this topic with patients prior to treatment, and many patients do not recall being told about the impact of treatment on fertility [6]. In a recent survey of breast cancer survivors, only 11% felt they received adequate information about fertility preservation from their oncology care providers [14].

Patients are strongly influenced by the messages they receive from their health care providers and may be more likely to seek fertility preservation consultations and services if the provider introduces this topic as a legitimate concern [15, 16]. This chapter seeks to describe strategies for oncology care providers to integrate discussion of fertility preservation options and services into their practice.

Models for Developing a Cancer and Fertility Program

The Program at Memorial Sloan-Kettering Cancer Center

In 2003, Memorial Sloan-Kettering Cancer Center (MSKCC) established a Survivorship Initiative that included the development of programs and services to address the needs of patients who have completed treatment for adult-onset cancer and are free of disease. As part of the planning process to identify strategic goals for the initiative, patients were surveyed about services they wish had been provided to them at diagnosis and during treatment, but had not been offered. A number of patients stated that they had not received sufficient information about their fertility risks or about their fertility preservation options. Thus, establishing information and services related to reproductive health as well as access to specialists who offer fertility preservation became part of the initiative's strategic plan.

In January 2009, MSKCC hired a clinical nurse specialist (CNS) to direct its new program, *Fertility Preservation and Parenthood after Cancer Treatment*. The program is guided by an advisory committee, with clinical representatives from services that treat high volumes of patients of reproductive potential, as well as two former patients who underwent fertility preservation prior to their treatment.

The program goals are listed in Table 13.2. The program is built around seven key components, illustrated in Fig. 13.1 and described in detail in Table 13.3. The program provides clinicians with the information, resources, and assistance they need to inform their patients about the effects of treatment on fertility and the options available to them for fertility preservation, and to make referrals to reproductive specialists. In addition, the CNS is available to provide education and counseling to patients who want more

Table 13.2 Fertility preservation and parenthood after cancer treatment: goals of the MSKCC program

Provide *clinicians* caring for patients of reproductive potential with:

- Information about: effects of treatment on fertility, options for fertility preservation, and reproductive services where they can refer patients
- Resources to educate patients
- Assistance in referring patients interested in exploring fertility preservation options

Provide *patients* of reproductive potential with:

- Information about effects of treatment on fertility
- Information about options for fertility preservation
- Referrals to a reproductive specialist if they are interested in exploring these options
- Information about other options for parenthood if they are not able to have a biologic child

Kelvin, personal correspondence (2011)

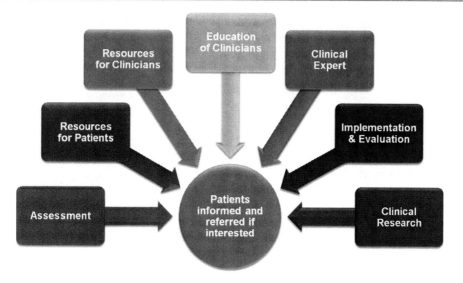

Fig. 13.1 Fertility preservation and parenthood after cancer treatment: components of the MSKCC program

Table 13.3 Fertility preservation and parenthood after cancer treatment: components of the MSKCC program

Assessment
- Patient volume
- Clinician survey
- Patient survey

Resources for Patients
- Booklets
- Internet
- Live and on-line classes
- Financial assistance

Resources for Clinicians
- Defined referral process
- Intranet
- Electronic orders

Education of Clinicians
- Instructional presentations
- Continuing education

Clinical Expertise
- Consultation
- Education and counseling
- Liaison with reproductive specialists and resources for financial assistance

Implementation and Evaluation
- Policies, procedures, guidelines
- Monitoring of referrals
- Monitoring use of resources

Clinical Research
- Multiple collaborative projects in development

Kelvin, personal correspondence, 2011

information than their oncologists are able to provide, facilitate referrals, and coordinate care between the oncology team and the reproductive specialist. The program infrastructure can be used as a model within any cancer setting seeking to improve how fertility is addressed with their patients.

Programs Based on Fertile Hope's Centers of Excellence Criteria

As the only national, nonprofit organization focused specifically on addressing the needs of cancer patients whose treatments presented the risk of infertility, Fertile Hope was aware of the persistent failure of the oncology community to provide their patients with adequate information about their reproductive risks and options. In 2004, the President's Cancer Panel (PCP) published its annual report, which was focused on survivorship, and recommended that written and verbal fertility-risk information be given to patients prior to the initiation of treatment [17]. This proved to be a catalyzing moment, and in 2005, Fertile Hope launched their Centers of Excellence (COE) Program in an attempt to highlight and reward cancer centers who were implementing these recommendations.

In designing the program, Fertile Hope sought to tackle the arbitrary way in which fertility information seemed to be dispensed. Published studies had shown, and survivors testifying to the PCP confirmed, that while some individual providers were routinely addressing fertility with their patients, others were silent on the issue. Therefore, the COE Program was developed to recognize cancer centers that had made an institutional commitment to meet their patients' reproductive needs in a deliberate, methodical way – by implementing systems to notify at-risk patients. The objective in showcasing excellence was to inspire emulation and wide-spread adoption of similar approaches.

To be recognized as a Fertile Hope COE, hospitals had to complete a simple application and submit a demonstration letter explaining how the institution's systems met the defined COE criteria. Fertile Hope regarded these criteria, listed in Table 13.4, to be the minimal components of a functioning cancer and fertility system.

Table 13.4 Criteria for Fertile Hope/LIVESTRONG's *Centers of Excellence Program*

Policy (as of 2009)	A hospital-wide policy stating the institution's commitment to addressing the cancer-related fertility needs of their patients
Notification Procedures	A systematic approach to ensure that all patients of (or under) reproductive age who are at risk are provided with complete information, both verbally and in writing, about their reproductive risks and options for preserving their fertility before potentially damaging therapy is initiated
Professional Education	Educational programs on the topic of cancer-related infertility and fertility preservation are conducted
Patient Education	Resources are available for patients, survivors and/or (when appropriate) family members
Referrals	Knowledge of and referral to appropriate reproductive specialists (internally or externally) for consultation, fertility preservation and/or parenthood after cancer for their patients
Research (Optional)	Research on cancer-related infertility, pregnancy after cancer and/or parenthood after cancer is being conducted

Reineke (personal communication, 2010)

Table 13.5 Examples of strategies used to meet COE criteria

Criteria	Examples of strategies used
Policy	• Issuance of formal hospital-wide policy • Description of fertility preservation discussions as part of "standard operating procedures" on hospital intranet
Notification Procedures	• Use of "best practice alerts" and mandatory fertility questions on electronic intake systems • Customized consent forms that require specific acknowledgment of reproductive risks • Use of designated "fertility navigator" for individualized discussions
Professional Education	• Live sessions at grand rounds, departmental meetings • Incorporation of topic into continuing nursing education
Patient Education	• Patient brochures • Printable patient education sheets linked to electronic intake system • Use of designated "fertility navigator" for individualized discussions
Referrals	• Referral form with fertility clinic information linked to intake system • Explicit agreements with fertility clinics and sperm banks to expedite cancer patients

While all of the criteria were mandatory, the means of satisfying the criteria were left up to the particular cancer centers, in deference to variations in resources, existing infrastructure, and institutional cultures. From the launch of the program in late 2005 until Fertile Hope's acquisition by LIVESTRONG in 2009, nine nationally-ranked cancer centers had attained the COE designation. Table 13.5 lists examples of how different centers have met the COE criteria.

Strategies for Developing a Program in Your Own Setting

These two models for establishing services to address cancer and fertility provide examples of strategies that can be used in any oncology setting.

Assessment

An important first step in developing a program is to collect baseline data about the organization, clinicians, and patients to guide efforts in building the program. Table 13.6 lists a number of

Table 13.6 Considerations for Assessment

Assessing the Heath Care Organization

Patient Population

- How many patients are seen annually in this age group?
- What are the most common diagnoses and stages?
- Are there special needs, for example socioeconomic, language, cultural, or religious?

Institutional & Clinical Culture

- Is shared-decision making the norm, or is the structure more hierarchical?
- Is there wide variation in practice between individual oncologists/clinics or are there centralized efforts to reduce variation?
- What providers (physicians, nurses, social workers) see patients prior to treatment and what role does each provider play in regard to counseling the patient? How much time does each provider spend with the patient?
- Are electronic systems used for intake, entering orders, or documenting clinical care?

Existing Resources

- Are reproductive specialists on staff to provide consultation/services? Are these providers available in the community?
- Are there existing patient or professional resources available?

Assessing Clinicians

- What is the current level of knowledge about fertility among physicians, nurses, and social workers?
- What are their attitudes about discussing risks and preservation options?
- What are their current practices in regard to discussion of risks and preservation options and in making referrals?
- What barriers currently exist?

Assessing Patients

- What fertility information do they recall receiving?
- What is their satisfaction with the information that they received?
- What is their satisfaction about how and when the information was delivered, and by whom?
- What would they have changed about the content and/or the process?

issues to consider as you assess your health care organization, clinicians, and patients.

Referral Process

For oncology clinicians to initiate discussions about fertility with their patients, they need to know where and how to refer interested patients to reproductive specialists. Identify sperm banks, reproductive urologists, and reproductive endocrinologists in the region. Table 13.7 lists internet resources to assist with this. There may be reproductive specialists affiliated with your hospital system, making referrals and collaboration relatively easy. Meet with the staff at each of the center to discuss about the services the center can provide. Establish a simple method for referring patients to and outline a process to ensure that patients are seen quickly, relevant medical information is shared, and fertility preservation efforts are coordinated with the planned timing for initiation of the patient's cancer treatment.

Resources for Patients

To ensure patients are adequately informed, it is important to have educational materials available

Table 13.7 Resources for identifying local reproductive specialists

Sperm banks

- American Association of Tissue Banks (www.aatb.org)
- Sperm Center (www.spermcenter.com)

Reproductive urologists

- Society for Male Reproduction and Urology (www.smru.org)

Reproductive endocrinologists

- American Society for Reproductive Medicine (www.asrm.org)
- Society for Assisted Reproductive Technology (www.sart.org)

For all reproductive services

- FertileHope/LIVE**STRONG**'s *Fertility Resource Guide* (www.fertilehope.org/tool-bar/referral-guide.cfm)

that provide more in-depth information than oncology clinicians might have the knowledge or time to discuss. Materials should address such topics as the effects of treatment on fertility and options for fertility preservation; how to select a sperm bank or reproductive endocrinologist; early menopause due to cancer treatment; and options for parenthood after completing treatment. However, while you may want to consider developing customized resources for your institution that include contact or referral information, it is not essential to develop new materials. Free downloadable brochures, fact sheets and other patient tools are available from organizations focused on cancer and fertility. Table 13.8 lists internet resources with relevant information.

In addition to providing informational resources for your patients, resources for financial assistance are also important. The costs of

Table 13.8 Internet resources on cancer and fertility

Sites on Fertility for Patients with Cancer

● Fertile Hope (www.fertilehope.org)
A nonprofit organization, incorporated as a **LIVESTRONG** initiative, dedicated to providing reproductive information, support and hope to cancer patients and survivors whose medical treatments present the risk of infertility.

● MyOncoFertility (myoncofertility.org)
An informational resource, developed by the Oncofertility consortium, a national, interdisciplinary initiative to explore the reproductive options for patients diagnosed with cancer or other serious diseases.

● LIVESTRONG (www.livestrong.org)
A nonprofit organization dedicated to inspiring and empowering people affected by cancer. [Search *Male Infertility* or *Female Infertility*]

Sites on Fertility for Teens with Cancer

● Cancer Net (www.cancer.net)
An informational resource for patients and families, developed by the American Society of Clinical Oncology (ASCO) [Search *Fertility and Teens*]

● Center for Young Women's Health (www.youngwomenshealth.org)
An informational resource for teen girls and young women, developed by Children's Hospital Boston [search *Cancer and Fertility*]

● Cure Search (www.curesearch.org)
A professional organization of the Children's Oncology Group and the National Childhood Cancer Foundation with health information resources for patients [Search *Male Fertility* or *Female Fertility*]

Sites on Fertility as a General Issue

● American Society for Reproductive Medicine (www.asrm.org)
A professional organization for specialists in reproductive medicine with information for patients on a variety of topics. [Patients > Patient Resources > Patient Fact Sheets and Booklets > Scroll to find Assisted Reproductive Technologies]

● Resolve (www.resolve.org)
A community offering information and support to women and men with infertility, developed by The National Infertility Association.

● Society for Assisted Reproductive Technology (www.sart.org)
A professional organization for specialists in assisted reproductive technologies (ART) which provides information on IVF success rates of fertility centers throughout the United States.

● International Council on Infertility Information and Dissemination (www.inciid.org)
A nonprofit organization that helps individuals and couples explore their family-building options.

Sites on Menopause

● The North American Menopause Society (www.menopause.org)
A nonprofit organization devoted to promoting women's health and quality of life through an understanding of menopause.

● The National Women's Health Information Center (www.womenshealth.gov/menopause)
An office in the US Department of Health and Human Services devoted to provide information on women's health.

fertility preservation present a significant barrier for many patients, and insurance coverage is rarely available. LIVESTRONG's Sharing Hope program provides financial assistance to eligible patients undertaking fertility preservation at a participating center. Providing clinicians access to this program will facilitate fertility preservation for many patients who would not otherwise be able to afford these services.

Resources and Education for Clinicians

Clinicians should be provided with access to resources at the time they encounter patients who need fertility-related information and referrals. Create paper packets, or if the organization or practice has an internal web site, create fertility-related web pages with relevant information, including steps for making referrals, printable resources for patients, references, clinical algorithms, and other related tools. The benefit of creating a web site is that it is accessible from any workstation, at any location throughout the organization, and documents can be updated in real time, without worrying about having outdated materials stocked in the clinical setting. The home page of the MSKCC site is illustrated in Fig. 13.2.

If the organization or practice has computerized order entry, create fertility-related order sets for such services as sperm banking, semen analysis, or referral to a reproductive endocrinologist. Depending on the system, these can generate direct referrals or can generate referral prescriptions.

Educational presentations should be planned about the effects of treatment on fertility and options for fertility preservation. Schedule these during grand rounds, staff orientations, medical service conferences and meetings, journal clubs, or case presentations. Include nurses, residents, fellows, and social workers in all educational efforts. Consider inviting local reproductive specialists to present updates on the current technology to help oncology clinicians stay abreast of all of the advances and choices available for their patients.

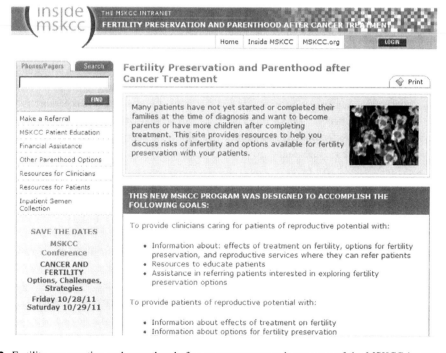

Fig. 13.2 Fertility preservation and parenthood after cancer treatment: home page of the MSKCC intranet site with resources for clinicians

Implementation and Evaluation

The active involvement of clinicians who will be served by the program is essential as resources and services are developed and refined. Bring together clinicians with a shared interest and commitment to the issue of fertility. Reach out to colleagues in medical, surgical, and radiation oncology; survivorship; general gynecology and urology; and reproductive medicine. This is a key group as the program is rolled out. Having individuals champion this day-to-day in the clinical setting and provide feedback on improvements and enhancements needed is essential to successful implementation.

The commitment of a handful of enthusiastic practitioners to implement the above-discussed strategies will probably not be sufficient to change practice. Instituting a policy "standard" or guideline mandating or recommending that clinicians discuss fertility with all patients and refer those interested in fertility preservation when "appropriate" makes a strong statement about the organization's dedication to this issue. This can lay the foundation for subsequent practice change.

Once your resources are in place, use a systematic approach to implementing the program. It may be best to roll out the program gradually, focusing first where there is a high volume of young adult patients and where there is interest. Consider strategies to remind or prompt clinicians prior to scheduling procedures or ordering treatments that may affect fertility, for example, inserting fertility reminders into standard processes or workflows. These can be in the form of paper checklists or can be computer-based alerts or hard stops if a required step is not followed. If the organization or practice has computerized documentation, consider embedding a field for clinicians to document fertility discussions and referrals.

If feasible, establish a role for a designated clinician to focus on fertility issues. For example, MSKCC has a full time CNS responsible for building and maintaining the infrastructure required. She is available to "navigate" patients through the system, providing individualized education and counseling to patients who want more information than their oncologist is able to provide. In addition, she also serves as a liaison with the reproductive specialists to coordinate care and direct patients to additional resources.

Evaluation of the program can be challenging. If the workflow requires electronic documentation or order entry for most clinical activity, work with the systems staff to create reports indicating what percentage of all patients of reproductive potential is receiving information about fertility. Alternatively, perform chart audits, although this can be very labor intensive. Examples of other strategies to evaluate the program include monitoring the number of educational materials distributed, the number of clinicians trained, the number of referrals made to reproductive specialists, or utilization of internal or external web sites. If a formal survey of clinicians or patients was conducted as part of your initial assessment, repeat the survey at intervals after the program has launched to monitor the impact of the program – the reach and satisfaction with the information provided.

Conclusion

Neither the publication of professional guidelines nor documented evidence citing the value of future fertility to cancer survivors has been sufficient to substantially alter clinicians' practice around reproductive disclosure. While the question as to how to increase the frequency and the substance of these discussions remains open, the development of resources and a comprehensive approach is surely a significant advance. While no single approach is right for every center, these key strategies can enhance the likelihood that patients will receive the risk and options information that they desire and deserve.

Provider Recommendations

1. Oncology clinicians have the responsibility to initiate discussion about potential risks to fertility from planned cancer treatment.

2. As per the ASCO recommendations, fertility should be discussed as early in treatment planning as feasible, to afford patients the chance to access fertility preservation if desired.
3. For patients interested in future parenting, they should also discuss options for fertility preservation, and make referrals to reproductive specialists when indicated.
4. Providing education, resources, and assistance will enable oncology clinicians to do this more effectively.
5. Strategies can be customized based on the clinical setting.

References

1. Schover LR, Rybicki LA, Martin BA, Bringelsen KA (1999) Having children after cancer. A pilot survey of survivors' attitudes and experiences. Cancer 86(4):697–709
2. Schover LR (2005) Motivation for parenthood after cancer: a review. J Natl Cancer Inst Monogr (34):2–5
3. Schover LR, Brey K, Lichtin A, Lipshultz LI, Jeha S (2002) Knowledge and experience regarding cancer, infertility, and sperm banking in younger male survivors. J Clin Oncol 20(7):1880–1889
4. Schover LR (1999) Psychosocial aspects of infertility and decisions about reproduction in young cancer survivors: a review. Med Pediatr Oncol 33(1):53–59
5. Crawshaw M, Sloper P (2010) 'Swimming against the tide'– the influence of fertility matters on the transition to adulthood or survivorship following adolescent cancer. Eur J Cancer Care 19(5):610–620
6. Tschudin S, Bitzer J (2009) Psychological aspects of fertility preservation in men and women affected by cancer and other life-threatening diseases. Hum Reprod Update 15(5):587–597
7. Lee SJ, Schover LR, Partridge AH, Patrizio P, Wallace WH, Hagerty K et al (2006) American Society of clinical oncology recommendations on fertility preservation in cancer patients. J Clin Oncol 24(18):2917–2931

8. Pentheroudakis G, Orecchia R, Hoekstra HJ, Pavlidis N, Group ObotEG W (2010) Cancer, fertility and pregnancy: ESMO Clinical Practice Guidelines for diagnosis, treatment and follow-up. Ann Oncol 21(Suppl 5):v266–v73
9. ASRM (2005) Fertility preservation and reproduction in cancer patients. Fertil Steril 83(6):1622–1628. doi: 10.1016/j.fertnstert.2005.03.013
10. Fallat ME, Hutter J, the Committee on Bioethics SoHO, Section on Surgery (2008) Preservation of fertility in pediatric and adolescent patients with cancer. Pediatrics 121(5):e1461–9
11. Crawshaw MA, Glaser AW, Hale JP, Sloper P (2009) Male and female experiences of having fertility matters raised alongside a cancer diagnosis during the teenage and young adult years. Eur J Cancer Care 18(4):381–390
12. Thewes B, Meiser B, Taylor A, Phillips KA, Pendlebury S, Capp A et al (2005) Fertility- and menopause-related information needs of younger women with a diagnosis of early breast cancer. J Clin Oncol 23(22):5155–5165
13. Peate M, Meiser B, Hickey M, Friedlander M (2009) The fertility-related concerns, needs and preferences of younger women with breast cancer: a systematic review. Breast Cancer Res Treat 116(2):215–223
14. Meneses K, McNees P, Azuero A, Jukkala A (2010) Development of the fertility and cancer project: an internet approach to help young cancer survivors. Oncol Nurs Forum 37(2):191–197. doi: 10.1188/10.ONF.191–197
15. Achille MA, Rosberger Z, Robitaille R, Lebel S, Gouin J-P, Bultz BD et al (2006) Facilitators and obstacles to sperm banking in young men receiving gonadotoxic chemotherapy for cancer: the perspective of survivors and health care professionals. Hum Reprod 21(12):3206–3216
16. Crawshaw M, Glaser A, Hale J, Sloper P (2009) Male and female experiences of having fertility matters raised alongside a cancer diagnosis during the teenage and young adult years. Eur J Cancer Care 18(4):381–390
17. President's Cancer Panel (2003–2004) Annual report: living beyond cancer: finding a new balance. Bethesda, MD.: U.S. Department of Health and Human Services, National Institutes of Health, National Cancer Institute, p vi, 87 p

Patient Provider Communication and Reproductive Health

14

Caprice A. Knapp, PhD, Gwendolyn
P. Quinn, PhD, Deborah Rapalo, MPH,
and Lindsey Woodworth, MA

It's difficult to talk about sex with my patients. I wasn't trained to have these discussions; I was trained to treat cancer. It's even more difficult when the patient has his or her parents in the room. The shock of the cancer diagnosis is still hanging in the air and everyone is focused on survival. Parents often don't want to think about their child as a sexually active person. I've had plenty of mothers assure me their son or daughter is a virgin, even when the kid is twenty-five years old. I usually catch a glimpse of the patient with a sly smile. It may be the only time anyone smiles during the whole conversation.
Dr. K, Pediatric Oncologist

I was afraid to ask about having a child in the future. I was afraid it was too much to ask for to survive cancer and have a child too. My doctor didn't mention it except to tell me I would likely be sterile after my treatment. I regret not asking about it. I don't know if I would have done anything but at least I would have explored my options. I am a five year survivor now and grateful for every day, but every time I hear about a friend having a baby or see a pregnant woman I wish I could go back in time and ask my doctor if there was something I could have done to preserve my options. I have a great guy in my life, he would have made a great dad, but now he won't have that chance, at least not with me.
Janice, 35 year old Non- Hodgkin's Lymphoma Survivor

I know it's important to talk about fertility with my patients but it makes me uncomfortable. Some patients can't afford the bus fare to get to clinic and I'm going to talk to them about an expensive procedure that is not imperative to their survival? And some patients are getting really bad news. . . . their chance of survival is low; so I'm going to tell them they have a less than 10% chance of long-term survival and then say have you ever thought about having kids? It seems insensitive and like a double slap in the face.
Dr. C, Oncologist

The prevalence among youth aged 15–19 ever having sexual intercourse has decreased from 1991–2007. However, the 2007 Youth Risk Behavior Surveillance Survey (YRBS) of AYA in the United States reports 48% of this population has had sexual intercourse [1]. Along with these rates of sexual activity, 28% of adolescents who have requested pregnancy tests at local health departments had already used a home pregnancy test [2]. Considering these high rates of sexual activity in teens in conjunction with the public health risk of adolescent pregnancies [3] and sexually transmitted infections (STIs) [4], the American Academy of Pediatrics (AAP) and the American Congress of Obstetricians and Gynecologists (ACOG)

C.A. Knapp (✉)
Department of Health Outcomes and Policy, University
of Florida, Gainesville, FL 32608, USA
e-mail: caprice1@ufl.edu

G.P. Quinn, S.T. Vadaparampil (eds.), *Reproductive Health and Cancer in Adolescents and Young Adults*, Advances in Experimental Medicine and Biology 732,
DOI 10.1007/978-94-007-2492-1_14, © Springer Science+Business Media B.V. 2012

provide professional guidelines stressing the responsibility of health professionals to offer comprehensive reproductive health services such as sex education, counseling, and contraceptive awareness [5, 6]. These guidelines are consistent with research that sex education results in lower rates of sexual activity, increased contraceptive use, and fewer adolescent pregnancies [7, 8].

The rate of cancer in AYA is on the rise, with an annual incidence rate of 202.2 per million young adults [9]. While the need to protect and preserve fertility in this population is of high importance for quality cancer care and improved survivorship, one aspect of protection often overlooked in this population is contraception and sex education, specifically unintended pregnancy and the prevention of STIs. Advancements in cancer therapies allow young adults to carry on similar lives to their peers, calling attention to the risk associated with sexual activity during and after treatment. Oncologists and other members of the health care team are often relied upon by patients and their families to recommend appropriate lifestyle choices during treatment, including the unique risks associated with sexual activity. However, an overshadowing focus on survival, misperceptions of views regarding asexuality among cancer patients [10], and opinions from family and partners, and cultural taboos of sexuality may present barriers to conveying medically imperative information to cancer patients regarding sexual behavior and contraception.

However, available data indicates that AYA populations with a chronic illness are at least as sexually active as their healthy counterparts, if not more [11–13]. Furthermore, chronically ill AYA patients may be at an increased risk to engage in unsafe sexual practices such as not using contraceptives due to psychological issues associated with impending mortality and beliefs that cancer treatment renders one infertile [13]. Though no study to date measures the sexual activity of AYA cancer patients specifically, research on older adult cancer patients indicates sexual activity remains a component of day-to-day life both during and after treatment [14, 15]. Thus, there are three main areas related

to sexual activity among AYA cancer patients that should be discussed by health care providers: (1) pregnancy prevention; (2) prevention of sexually transmitted infections (STI); (3) implications of cancer treatment on future fertility; and (4) fertility preservation options. Although the majority of these topics are covered in detail in other chapters, we will provide a brief summary of the key points relevant to AYA populations.

Pregnancy Prevention

Many cancer treatments are unlikely to influence reproductive potential immediately. The risk of infertility following cancer treatments for pediatric cancer patients is between 40 and 90% for females and 30–70% for males, though it is dependent on many factors including gender, age, and treatment modality [16]. In fact, many AYA undergoing cancer treatments are indeed fertile [16]. However, some cancer patients may be aware of their risk of infertility due to treatments and presume a false sense of security thereby electing not to use contraceptives. This may be coupled with other factors that have been cited by chronically ill teens with similar experiences who engage in early/risky sexual behavior as compensation for poor body image, and a desire to experience fulfilling sexual relationships before death [17]. Furthermore, symptoms of pregnancy such as fatigue and nausea may be confused for the similar common side effects from chemotherapy (Fig. 14.1).

Unintended pregnancy in the cancer patient has significant social consequences as well as

Common Symptoms of Pregnancy	Common Side Effects from Chemotherapy
Fatigue	Fatigue
Disruption in Menses	Disruption in Menses
Changes in Weight	Changes in Weight
Body Aches	Body Aches
Changes in Mood	Changes in Mood
Changes in Skin/Hair	Hair Loss
Nausea	Nausea

Fig. 14.1 Pregnancy vs chemotherapy side effects

physiological effects for the patient. Cancer patients face additional potential risks including transmission of chemotherapy and radiation agents to partners and have greater physiological susceptibility to acquiring STIs due to compromised immune systems [18]. Furthermore, the concern of pregnancy is amplified in this group (patients on active treatment) considering the substantial risks to the mother as well as the fetus. Cancer treatments including chemotherapy, antimetabolites, and alkylating agents have known teratogenic risks to the developing fetus ranging from spontaneous abortion to severe congenital malformations [19–21]. Considering these risks, cancer treatment would be specifically modified or delayed in the event of a pregnancy [22].

Sexually Transmitted Infection (STI) Prevention

The primary approach to prevention of both pregnancy and STI among sexually active AYA is focused on the use of contraceptive methods. Chapter 4 provides a detailed table of various contraceptive methods, as well as their associated advantages and disadvantages. In the context of the current issues, there are clearly methods that may be effective at preventing pregnancy (e.g., oral contraception) but not reducing STI risk.

Contraceptive Discussions Barriers

Perceived irrelevance and misconceptions regarding the sexuality of cancer patients may inhibit transmitting important information regarding contraceptive use in cancer patients. These practices are of concern as patients may engage in more frequent unprotected sexual behavior if they misconstrue treatment or the risk of infertility as conferring similar protection to contraception. Importantly, even young patients that have not begun their menstrual cycles are still at risk of pregnancy if sexually active [23]. Professional guidelines from AAP and ACOG recognize the health care provider's important

role in conveying contraceptive use to young cancer patients but no research has examined the actual rates of recommendation or content of discussions about contraceptive use prior to cancer treatments among AYA. Many institutions have no formal guidelines in place despite recommendations [18, 24]. ACOG as well as the National Cancer Institute have available educational pamphlets regarding contraceptive use during cancer treatment however they are not specific to any populations [25, 26].

Some studies have investigated the use of contraceptives among adult cancer patients. A study by Valle of adult women found that 21% undergoing treatment for breast cancer received contraceptive advice prior to chemotherapy treatment, wherein 15% were provided educational material [14]. This study also showed that participants demonstrated confusion concerning the importance of contraceptive use during chemotherapy. 74% reported using some form of contraceptive during treatment [14]. Only one previous research study identifies the relevance of having guidelines for contraception discussions among physicians and AYA cancer patients. In a qualitative study of pediatric oncologists, Vadaparampil and colleagues note a physician's personal concern of treating teen patients who become pregnant during treatments [27]. Barriers to contraception recommendation likely parallel barriers to discussing issues of fertility and preservation methods with patients including a perception that the priority focus is on survival, personal discomfort with the topic, and a lack of training on the topic [27]. In an earlier study, a questionnaire administered to 15 pediatric oncology units in the United Kingdom found that *no facility* had a policy on contraceptive discussions for teenage patients [18]. Although The National Comprehensive Cancer Network (NCCN) has established clinical practice guidelines related to recommendation of contraception in the adult oncology setting, there are currently no parallel guidelines for pediatric oncology. Of special note, due to the risk of congenital anomalies from isotretinoin, a medication prescribed for acne, guidelines for pregnancy prevention have already been established from the U.S. Food and

Common chemotherapy brands	Recommendations from manufacturer website
CARBOPLATIN *Ovarian and non-small cell lung cancer, sometimes for testicular, stomach, and bladder cancers, as well as other carcinomas.*	Investigational or post-marketing data show risk to fetus. Nevertheless, potential benefits may outweigh the risk. Do not take this medicine if you are pregnant or nursing. Use a birth control you trust to not get pregnant. If you are a male and sexually active, protect your partner from pregnancy.
EMEND *Anti-emetic used with primarily cisplatin based chemotherapy like osteosarcoma or germ cell tumors*	The efficacy of hormonal contraceptives may be reduced during co-administration with EMEND and for 28 days after the last dose of EMEND. Alternative or backup methods of contraception should be used during treatment with EMEND and for 1 month after the last dose of EMEND.
TEMODAR *Brain tumors. Generic brand is temozolomide.*	It is not advisable to become pregnant or father a child while taking temozolomide as it may harm the developing fetus. However, <u>do not use oral contraceptives ("the pill") without checking with your doctor</u>. If you are pregnant, breast feeding or planning children in the future, inform your doctor of this before treatment. Many chemotherapy drugs can cause sterility.
AVASTIN *Brain tumors but has been used in neuroblastoma and researched in other sarcomas as therapy in multiply relapsed patients. Generic brand is bevacizumab.*	This medication may affect a baby's development in the womb and should not be used during pregnancy. It is strongly recommended that women who may become pregnant take proper contraceptive measures (e.g., use of a condom) for at least 6 months after the last dose of bevacizumab. If sexually active, pts will take contraceptive measures for duration of treatments
ELSPAR *ALL/AML, non-Hodgkin lymphoma. Generic brand is asparaginase*	For both men and women: Do not conceive a child (get pregnant) while taking asparaginase. Barrier methods of contraception, such as condoms, are recommended. Discuss with your doctor when you may safely become pregnant or conceive a child after therapy.
CYTOXAN *ALL, neuroblastoma, Ewing sarcoma, rhabdomyosarcoma, other sarcoma, Wilms tumor, BMT preps, aplastic anemia, some brain tumors, Hodgkin lymphoma, non-Hodgkin lymphoma. Generic brand is cyclophosphamide.*	If you are pregnant or plan to become pregnant, inform your doctor immediately. When taken during pregnancy, Cytoxan can cause birth defects. Women taking Cytoxan should use effective contraception. Do not breastfeed while you are taking Cytoxan.
VINCRISTINE *ALL, Hodgkin lymphoma, non-Hodgkin lymphoma, Wilms tumor, brain tumors, rhabdomyosarcoma, Ewing sarcoma*	For both men and women: Do not conceive a child (get pregnant) while taking. Barrier methods of contraception, such as condoms, are recommended. Discuss with your doctor when you may safely become pregnant or conceive a child after therapy. Do not breast feed while taking Vincristine.
DACTINOMYCIN *Wilms tumor, sarcomas*	Contraception It is not advisable to become pregnant or father a child while taking, as the developing foetus may be harmed. It is important to use effective contraception while taking this drug, and for at least a few months afterwards. Again, discuss this with your doctor.
THIOTEPA *Brain tumors*	Effective contraception should be used during thiotepa therapy if either the patient or the partner is of childbearing potential.
HYDREA *Sickle cell patients, CML. Generic brand is hydroxyurea.*	Hydroxyurea may harm your unborn baby. You should contact your prescriber immediately if you believe or suspect you or your partner has become pregnant while you are taking hydroxyrea. Both men and women must use effective birth control continuously while taking hydroxyurea. It is recommended that you use 2 reliable forms of contraception together.
MYLOTARG *CD33+ acute myeloid leukemia*	must not be used during pregnancy and in women of childbearing potential not using effective contraception, unless the potential benefits outweigh the potential risks.

Fig. 14.2 Chemotherapy brand and recommendations regarding pregnancy

Drug Administration since 1998 [28]. Despite the known effects from chemotherapy and radiation, similar guidelines for discussing pregnancy and contraception among AYA treated for cancer are absent.

Schover's review of clinician counseling strategies for cancer patients regarding changing sexual function describes a common failure to address the sexual health concerns of cancer patients such as assessments of sexual functioning or concerns [29]. However, sexual health and contraception have not been well studied in populations of young cancer patients. Patients will seldom directly express sexual concerns to their health care provider, either prior to or after cancer treatment, and therefore it is a key quality of life issue for these topics to be addressed [29]. Current research in healthy young adult populations has highlighted the relevance and necessity of contraception recommendation.

Further research is necessary to identify oncologist contraception recommendation practice behaviors to determine best practices and gaps in knowledge. This will lead to improved provider education and interventions to enhance the consistency and quality of care for a population with unique, emerging needs that begin during the treatment phase and continue through survivorship. Although there are existing CME opportunities for health care providers to learn more about contraception recommendation and reproductive health among AYA populations there are limits to many of them. It is important and useful for health care providers to know what their colleagues are doing and to identify evidence-based best practices of the profession.

Communication Barriers to Fertility Preservation

With the release of the ASCO guidelines in 2006, the role of the oncologist in discussing potential infertility due to cancer treatments and fertility preservation options has been clearly defined. Despite these guidelines, to date, rates of discussion and referrals to reproductive endocrinologists have been sub-optimal. Several studies have identified significant barriers to this important communication process. These barriers can be categorized into three groups: health care system, health care provider, and patient.

System Barriers

In some cancer hospitals or clinics, there are no institutional guidelines for fertility discussions or places to refer patients for fertility preservation. Although national guidelines exist they may be out of sync with hospital policies and practices. There can also be communication gaps between various clinics within the hospital, for example, the pharmacy may assume the physician writing the orders for chemo has discussed the potential for infertility with the patient, while the physician may assume this discussion is covered by the nurse or pharmacist who will administer the chemo.

Some states have an abundance of infertility clinics and reproductive endocrinologists (RE) to whom patients can be referred. Some states, such as Wyoming, do not have any clinics or board certified RE's. Other states, such as New York, have so many RE's it can be difficult for a hospital to form an affiliation.

One of the most important factors that can influence the adaption of medical interventions or medical procedures is the creation of guidelines by professional organizations. Several professional organizations have published position statements and recommended guidelines for fertility preservation. In 2006 the American Society for Clinical Oncology (ASCO) published recommendations on fertility preservation for cancer patients of childbearing age. These guidelines were developed by a panel of experts representing oncology, obstetrics and gynecology, infertility, reproductive endocrinology, health services research, and bioethics. Guidelines were developed based on the existing evidence although they do not address assisted reproduction techniques or interventions aimed at restoring fertility after the completion of treatment. In regard to recommendations for oncologist in the role they should play in the decision making process of patients to preserve fertility, the guidelines state that physicians should

Answer specific questions about whether fertility preservation options decrease the chance of successful cancer treatment, increase the risk of maternal or perinatal complications, or compromise the health of offspring, and as needed, refer patients to reproductive specialists and psychosocial providers.

Similarly the British Fertility Society published recommendations for oncology units, assisted conception units, representative bodies, and the government. The guidelines state that all patients should have the opportunity to discuss fertility preservation, that protocols should be in place, that research on ovarian tissue retrieval and storage should be developed, that consortiums should be established, and that the courts should address matters of consent for young persons [30]. The European Society of Human Reproduction and Embryology Task Force have released similar consensus statements and guidelines on medically assisted reproduction [31]. The Ethics Committee of the American Society for Reproductive Medicine (ASRM) released its own guidelines for fertility preservation and reproduction in cancer patients in 2005. ASRM guidelines include the following seven points:

- Physicians should inform cancer patients about options for fertility preservation and future reproduction prior to treatment.
- The only established methods of fertility preservation are sperm and embryo cryopreservation.
- Experimental procedures such as ovarian tissue cryopreservation should only be offered in research institutions with Institutional Review Board approval.
- Concerns for the welfare of potential offspring should not prevent cancer patients from assistance in reproduction.
- Parents may provide consent to preserve a minor's fertility if the minor assents and the intervention is likely to provide benefits to the minor.
- Precise instructions in regard to disposal of tissue should be given in the event of death, unavailability, or other contingency.
- Preimplantaion genetic diagnosis to avoid the birth of offspring with a high risk of inherited cancer is ethically acceptable.

Beyond professional organizations, many advocacy groups such as the Lance Armstrong Foundation (http://www. fertilehope.org/), the American Cancer Society (http://www.cancer.org/Treatment/ TreatmentsandSideEffects/PhysicalSideEffects/ FertilityandCancerWhatAreMyOptions/index? sitearea=&level=), and the Susan G. Komen Foundation all support fertility preservation efforts for cancer patients (http://ww5.komen. org/uploadedFiles/Content_Binaries/806-352a. pdf).

Several studies have assessed the frequency of fertility preservation discussions and the endorsement of those discussions by oncologists [32–34]. Yet, these studies were conducted before the ASCO and ASRM guidelines were published. Few studies have been conducted to specifically determine the impact of these published guidelines on the attitudes and actions towards fertility preservation of heath care providers, and these studies are summarized below.

Clayton and colleagues conducted surveys with 210 pediatric oncology nurses to determine trends in their attitudes towards and awareness of the ASCO guidelines [35]. Surveys, were administered and completed at the annual meetings of the Florida Association of Pediatric Tumor Programs in 2005 and 2006. When asked if they were aware of the ASCO guidelines, 96% of nurses in 2006 reported they were not. Clearly the dissemination of information is not instantaneous. However in this sample of nurses, who were highly likely to be affected by the guidelines in their clinical practice, knowledge of the guidelines was minimal.

In 2008, Quinn and colleagues conducted a national study to examine the current trends in physician discussions and referrals of adult oncology patients for fertility preservation [36]. They administered a 53-question survey to measure (i) fertility preservation knowledge, (ii) practice behaviors, (iii) barriers to fertility preservation, (iv) fertility preservation attitudes and perceptions, and (v) demographic, medical training, and practice information. Using the American Medical Association Physician database, nearly 2,000 eligible physicians were identified and invited to participate in the survey. Over 600 of these physicians returned surveys, and in total, 516 completed surveys were used to generate the report's findings. The focus of the survey was on adult cancer patients. Based on physicians' responses, female physicians were almost twice as likely to refer their patients for fertility preservation, as were those that indicated that their patients frequently ask them about the effects of cancer treatment on their fertility. Furthermore, physicians with unfavorable views towards fertility preservation were less inclined to refer their patients. The results suggest that although the ASCO guidelines explicitly state that physicians should discuss fertility preservation with all patients, this is not occurring.

Several studies have been conducted that can shed light on how the guidelines have affected fertility preservation, specifically for adolescent and pediatric cancer patients. A recent (2010) study by Kohler and colleagues surveyed pediatric oncology specialists' attitudes towards fertility preservation. Results from the study suggest that while pediatric oncologists acknowledge and understand the importance of addressing fertility preservation, less than one-half reported that they refer male patients and 12% reported that they refer female patients to a fertility specialist prior to treatment. In regard to the ASCO guidelines, 44% noted that they were familiar with them.

Another study by Vadaparampil et al considered barriers to fertility preservation among pediatric oncologists. Qualitative semi-structured interviews were conducted with pediatric hematologist/oncologists practicing in Florida. Face-to-face interviews were held with four oncologists, and an additional eighteen oncologists participated in over-the-phone interviews. Responses were organized according to knowledge of, attitudes towards, and barriers to fertility preservation. Physician factors were related to lack of formal training in discussing fertility preservation. Parent and patient factors included extreme sensitivity and care with which fertility preservation must be discussed. Fertility preservation is simply not a top priority for many patients and their families. Moreover, the discussion of reproductive concerns may create an even greater burden for patients and their parents. Finally, half of the pediatric oncologists expressed a desire for fertility preservation institutional guidelines.

As demonstrated by these studies, many providers are simply unaware of current guidelines. Physicians are in favor of structured methods for introducing, discussing, and providing fertility preservation services, yet they continue to face much difficulty in addressing these concerns. There is general agreement among practitioners that the reproductive health of their adolescent cancer patients is of great importance, and clear professional guidance encourages delivery.

Insurance

Fertility Preservation

Fertility preservation for cancer treatment is currently an expensive procedure typically not covered by most health insurance companies. The costs involved in most preservation procedures are not only prohibitive for cancer patients, but often serve as a barrier for health care professionals to discuss loss of fertility and associated options with patients who they believe will be unable to afford these costs. In the United States, insurance is the primary gatekeeper to receiving health care. The U.S. has a private-public health insurance system. Private health insurance can be purchased by individuals and the majority of Americans purchase this insurance through their employer. For individuals who are below specific poverty levels, public health insurance programs such as Medicaid and the State Children's Health Insurance Program are available in each state. Public insurance programs have a shared financing structure whereby the state pays for a portion of the expenses and the federal government pays the remaining. Each state's cost-sharing portion is decided by a formula that accounts for a number of socioeconomic indicators. Through various insurance types, approximately 84% of Americans were covered by health insurance in 2009. While in aggregate this is a strong majority, insurance rates across demographic groups are not consistent. For example, according to one Gallup poll, an estimated 42% of Hispanic citizens do not have health insurance. Likewise, individuals earning less than $36,000, or who are between the ages of 18–29, have significantly lower coverage rates than the national average. On March 23, 2010, the Obama Administration enacted federal Health Care Reform legislation, which was designed in part, to provide insurance coverage to the 16% of Americans who were previously not covered.

Obtaining insurance is just one step in accessing reproductive health care for cancer patients. Beyond federal mandates to provide a core of health care services, insurance companies are oftentimes within their purview to decide which optional benefits they wish to cover. Sometimes these optional benefits can be affected by state legislation which mandates their coverage and sometimes they are voluntarily added and present a comparative advantage over competitors. Coverage of in vitro fertilization (IVF) is a good example of how state mandates can affect coverage. A 2010 study by Quinn et al. examined state insurance mandates of insurance coverage for IVF and infertility in general. After examining codified mandates from all 50 states and the District of Columbia, the authors found that nine states mandate coverage of infertility treatments, one mandates offer of coverage for infertility treatments (California), seven mandate coverage of IVF, and two specifically exclude coverage of IVF (California and Maryland). In regard to cancer patients, the authors found that no states mandated coverage for fertility preservation for cancer patients prior to treatment. Moreover, the state definitions of infertility are problematic for cancer patients. For example, many states define infertility as the attempt to become pregnant through unprotected intercourse for at least one year. For cancer patients who need to quickly bank sperm, eggs, or embryos prior to chemotherapy or radiation, these definitions would hinder reimbursement. These definitions are also not equitable to cancer patients without a partner who wish to become parents.

Health Policy

Fertility Preservation

Given that no states currently mandate coverage for reproduction or fertility preservation for cancer patients, the question becomes what health policies could be proposed, and ultimately enacted, to advance the recognition of this issue and subsequently lead to insurance coverage. Two potential health policies could lead to reproductive or fertility preservation coverage for cancer patients. First, states could choose to revise their coverage clauses for IVF and definitions of infertility. The definition of infertility could be broadened from those who have been unable to conceive in existing timeframes as imposed by the state law, to include those who face sterilization more immediate reduction in fertility due to medical treatment. For cancer patients, evidence suggests that approximately 60% of cancer patients of childbearing age will face reduced fertility or even sterility after the completion of treatment [37]. Illinois has already implemented this strategy whereby the one-year waiting period has been waived for cancer patients under 50 III. Adm. Code 2015.30 enacted September 2, 2004. The statue defines infertility as, "...the ability to conceive after one year of unprotected sexual intercourse or the ability to sustain a successful pregnancy. In the event a physician determines a medical condition exists that renders conception impossible through unprotected sexual intercourse, including but not limited to congenital absence of the uterus or ovaries, absence of the uterus or ovaries due to surgical removal due to a medical condition, or involuntary sterilization due to chemotherapy or radiation treatment, the one year requirement shall be waived." Under this health policy approach where the definition of infertility is altered, current IVF mandates would also cover patients whose loss in fertility is directly related to treatment for cancer. It cannot be assumed that changing the definition of infertility will directly increase coverage of procedures such as IVF that may be needed to complete the parenting project; however, this would at least be recognition by governing bodies that the present definition is exclusive and inequitable to cancer patients and cancer survivors.

A second health policy approach is to incentivize organizations and providers to promote fertility preservation. An example is ASCO's Quality Oncology Practice Initiative. Practices submit data related to core cancer indicators, symptom management, and care at the end of life. Fertility preservation is included in the symptom management measures [38]. Practices benefit from participating in the program by receiving recognition for high quality care, being able to use their data for maintenance of certification, and the receipt of CME credits. The Lance Armstrong Foundation (LAF) has a similar program to recognize leaders across the country in fertility preservation for cancer patients called the Centers for Excellence. All of the centers provide essential and effective care to cancer survivors including addressing fertility preservation and reproduction [39]. Although neither of these programs are health policies per se, they provide a framework for more formal policies. Recognizing fertility preservation and adherence to guidelines could be quality indicators for cancer centers in the United States. For example, the National Cancer Institutes could include access to fertility preservation services (e.g., egg, sperm, and embryo cryopreservation) as one of its benchmark metrics in achieving comprehensive cancer center status. This may solidify the importance of fertility preservation across the leading cancer centers and other cancer centers might follow.

Patient Communication Barriers

Many patients like Janice are often too overwhelmed with their cancer diagnosis to think about anything else. Some physicians have reported that during attempts to discuss cancer related infertility and preservation options a patient has held up his or hand and said "I don't want to hear about it, just get rid of the cancer." A patient's unwillingness to discuss fertility at the time of diagnosis is not uncommon, however, multiple studies show patients experience remorse and regret later on when the shock of the diagnosis has softened or treatment is complete [40].

Another patient-physician communication barrier is timing. There is a narrow window for men and women to consider most fertility preservation options. However, some patients learn about potential loss of fertility from cancer treatment and believe they will "worry about it later." These patients are often the most remorseful and even resentful when they realize they

have reduced opportunities for future biological children. Still other patients believe that they will consider adoption if they are rendered sterile. While adoption is certainly an option, cancer survivors face unique challenges with some adoption attempts due to medical qualifications (see Chapter 9 on Family Building).

Another barrier for considering fertility preservation related to timing is the potential for delay of treatment to pursue preservation options. Several studies of physician barriers to fertility preservation note a patient's inability to delay treatment as one of the top barriers. Although male patients may need only a day or two to bank sperm, some oncologists, and particularly pediatric oncologists believe their patients are best served by immediate commencement of cancer treatment. Female patients typically need two to six week to pursue most preservation options, and in the case of some patients, may be able to pursue fertility preservation during a break in treatment or immediately after completion (see Chapter 2).

Multiple studies with survivors, particularly adult survivors of pediatric or young adult cancer, suggest patients do not recall having a discussion about loss of fertility. It is not known if these discussions did in fact occur for the majority of patients but resulted in patients not remembering them or if the conversations did not take place at all. What is known is that the ability to parent a biological child is of great importance to cancer survivors. Several studies suggest that as many as 75% of childless patients who are diagnosed with cancer wish to have a child in the future. Studies conducted among survivors of pediatric cancer indicate a strong fear that they will be rejected by future partners due to their inability to have a child. In the case of pediatric patients, discussion of infertility and fertility preservation options is fraught with emotional and potentially uncomfortable discussions. As with discussion of contraception, this may be an uncomfortable topic for a health care provider, and the presence of parents may intensify the situation. However it is important to verbally address this information with patients and to follow up with educational materials that patients may review and refer to.

Provider Recommendations

There are several reproductive health messages that are essential to relay to patients:

1. Pregnancy Prevention
   - Your cancer treatment is not a form of pregnancy protection. It is not advisable to become pregnant during cancer treatment. If you are sexually active you should use contraception. Condoms are the most effective and least likely to interfere with your other medical treatments or conditions.
2. STI Prevention
   - Not all contraception works to prevent STI. You may be at increased risk for a sexually transmitted infection during or after your cancer treatment because your immune system is compromised. It is important to reduce/prevent your exposure to STI.
3. Future Fertility
   - Currently, we can not say with precision whether or not you will be temporarily or permanently infertile from your cancer treatments. For women, some cancer treatments may not immediately affect fertility however, ovarian failure (premature menopause) may occur about five years after treatment has been completed.
4. Fertility Preservation
   - Have you ever thought about having a child or more children? How do you think you might feel if having a biological child were not an option for you? How you feel about wanting a family today may not be how you feel in 10 years. I can discuss options with your for preserving fertility/or I can refer you to a specialist who can discuss fertility preservation options with you.

References

1. Center for Disease Control and Prevention (2008) Youth risk behavior surveillance – United States, 2007. Surveill Summ MMWR (57):NO.SS-4
2. Zabin LS, Emerson MR, Ringers PA, Sedivy V (1996) Adolescents with negative pregnancy test results: an accessible at-risk group. J Am Med Assoc 275(2):113–117
3. Committee on Adolescence (1998) Adolescent pregnancy–current trends and issues. Pediatrics 103(2):516–520
4. Bunnell RebeccaÂ E, Dahlberg L, Rolfs R et al (1999) High Prevalence And Incidence Of Sexually Transmitted Diseases In Urban Adolescent Females Despite Moderate Risk Behaviors. J Infect Dis 180(5):1624–1631
5. American College of Obstetricians and Gynecologists (ACOG) (2006) Use of hormonal contraception in women with coexisting medical conditions. American College of Obstetricians and Gynecologists (ACOG), Washington, DC, 20 p. (ACOG practice bulletin; no. 73).
6. Committee on Adolescence (2007) Contraception and adolescents. Pediatrics 120(5):1135–1148
7. Kirby DB, Laris BA, Rolleri LA (2007) Sex and HIV education programs: their impact on sexual behaviors of young people throughout the world. J Adolesc Health 40(3):206–217
8. Kohler R, Manhart L, Lafferty W (2008) Abstinence-only and comprehensive sex education and the initiation of sexual activity and teen pregnancy. J Adolesc Health 42:344–351
9. Ries LAG, Smith MA, Gurney JG, Linet M, Tamra T, Young JL, Bunin GR (eds) (1999) Cancer incidence and survival among children and adolescents: United States SEER Program 1975–1995, National Cancer Institute, SEER Program. NIH Pub. No. 99-4649. Bethesda, MD, pp 157–164.
10. Tyc VL, Hadley W, Crockett G (2001) Prediction of health behaviors in pediatric cancer survivors. Med Pediatr Oncol 37(1):42–46
11. Alderman EM, Lauby J, Coupey SM (1992) High risk behaviors in urban adolescents with chronic illness. J Adolesc Health 13(1):55–55
12. Surís J-C, Resnick MD, Cassuto N, Blum RWM (1996) Sexual behavior of adolescents with chronic disease and disability. J Adolesc Health 19(2):124–131
13. Choquet M, Du Pasquier Fediaevsky L, Manfredi R (1997) Sexual behavior among adolescents reporting chronic conditions: a French national survey. J Adolesc Health 20(1):62–67
14. Valle J, Clemons M, Hayes S, Fallowfield L, Howell A (1998) Contraceptive use by women receiving chemotherapy for breast cancer. Breast 7(3):143–149
15. Thranov I, Klee M (1994) Sexuality among gynecologic cancer patients–a cross-sectional study. Gynecol Oncol 52(1):14–19
16. Byrne J, Mulvihill J, Myers M et al (1987) Effects of treatment on fertility in long-term survivors of childhood or adolescent cancer. N Engl J Med 317(21):1315–1321
17. Grinyer A (2002) Sexuality and fertility: confronting the taboo. In: Clarke D (ed) Cancer in young adults: through parent's eyes. Open University Press, Buckingham-Philadelphia, pp 61–75
18. Laurence V, Gbolade BA, Morgan SJ, Glaser A (2004) Contraception for teenagers and

young adults with cancer. Eur J Cancer 40(18): 2705–2716

19. Chapman R (1992) Gonadal toxicity and teratogenicity. In: Perry MC (ed) The chemotherapy soource book. Williams & Wilkins, Baltimore

20. Doll D, Ringenberg Q, Yarbro J (1989) Antineoplastic agents and pregnancy. Semin Oncol 16:337–346

21. Kalter H, Warkany J (1983) Congenital malformations. N Engl J Med 308(424–431):491–497

22. Doll DC, Ringenberg QS, Yarbro JW (1988) Management of cancer during pregnancy. Arch Intern Med 148(9):2058–2064

23. Polaneczky M, O'Connor K (1999) Pregnancy in the adolescent patient: screening, diagnosis, and initial management. Pediatr Clin North Am 46(4):649–670

24. Heiney SP (1989) Adolescents with cancer: sexual and reproductive issues. Cancer Nurs 12(2):95–101

25. American Congress of Obstetrics and Gynecology: Birth Control Especially for Teens. 2007: Committee on Patient Education of the American College of Obstetricians and Gynecologists; Washington DC [Brochure]. http://www.acog.org/publications/ patient_education/bp112.cfm; %20http://www. acog.org/publications/patient_education/bp112.cfm. Accessed 15 Apr 2010

26. National Cancer Institute: Sexual and Fertility Changes in Women (2008) Managing chemotherapy side effects; [Brochure]. http://www.cancer.gov/ cancertopics/chemo-side-effects/womenfertility. Accessed 15 Apr 2010

27. Quinn GP, Vadaparampil ST (2009) Fertility preservation and adolescent/young adult cancer patients: physician communication challenges. J Adolesc Health 44(4):394–400

28. Mitchell AA, Van Bennekom CM, Louik C (1995) A pregnancy-prevention program in women of childbearing age receiving isotretinoin. N Engl J Med 333(2):101–106

29. Schover L (1999) Counseling cancer patients about changes in sexual function. Oncology 13(11): 1585–1591

30. Multidisciplinary working group British Fertility Society. A strategy for fertility service for survivors of childhood cancer. Accessed from http:// www.britishfertilitysociety.org.uk/practicepolicy/ documents/fccpaper.pdf

31. European Society of Human Reproduction and Embryology (2011) Medically assisted reproduction within families: a position paper by the European Society of Human Reproduction and Embryology. Accessed from http://www.eshre.eu/ ESHRE/English/Press-Room/Press-Releases/2011- Press-Releases/IMAR/page.aspx/1206.

32. Goodwin T, Elizabeth Oosterhuis B, Kiernan M, Hudson MM, Dahl GV (2007) Attitudes and practices of pediatric oncology providers regarding fertility issues. Pediatr Blood Cancer 48:80–85. doi:10.1002/pbc.20814

33. Zapzalka DM, Redmon JB, Pryor JL (1999) A survey of oncologists regarding sperm cryopreservation and assisted reproductive techniques for male cancer patients. Cancer 86:1812–1817

34. Schover LR, Brey K, Lichtin A et al (2002) Oncologists' attitudes and practices regarding banking sperm before cancer treatment. J Clin Oncol 20:1890–1897

35. Clayton H, Quinn G, Lee J-H et al (2008) Trends in clinical practice and nurses' attitudes about fertility preservation for pediatric patients with cancer. Oncol Nurs Forum 35(2):249–255

36. Quinn GP, Vadaparampil ST, Lee J-H et al (2009) Physician referral for fertility preservation in oncology patients: a national study of practice behaviors. J Clin Oncol 27(35):5952–5957

37. Lee SJ, Schrover SR, Patridge AH et al (2006) American Society of clinical oncology recommendations on fertility preservation in cancer patients. J Clin Oncol 24(18):2917–2831

38. American Society of Clinical Oncology (2010) The quality of oncology practice initiative summary of measures, Fall 2010. Accessed from http://qopi.asco. org/Documents/QOPIFall2010MeasuresSummary. pdf

39. Livestrong Survivorship Centers of Excellence. Accessed from http://www.livestrong.org/What-We-Do/Our-Actions/Programs-Partnerships/ LIVESTRONG-Survivorship-Centers-of-Excellence

40. Tschudin S, Bitzer J (2009) Pyschological aspects of fertility preservation in men and women affected by cancer and other life threatening diseases. Hum Reprod 15(5):587–597

Fertility Preservation in Cancer Patients: Ethical Considerations

15

Bethanne Bower, BA and Gwendolyn
P. Quinn, PhD

It was an endless series of bad news, good news – an emotional rollercoaster. The day the doctors told me my six year old daughter had cancer was the darkest day of my life. Then they told me her chances of survival were good but she would never have children and she may have other permanent damage like hearing loss and heart problems. I thought about how much having children meant to me, how being a mother was what I had dreamed of when I was a little girl. My little girl seemed to have the same dream. She mothered her dolls, mothered the cat, she liked to dress up in my high heels and purse and say she was going to the store to buy food for her baby dolls. Now she was going to be robbed of this experience. The good news was she was likely to survive but the bad news was she was never going to have the life we wanted for her and we thought she wanted for herself. I asked her doctor if there was anything we could do to prevent the sterility. He told me there was an experimental procedure we could consider where they froze some tissue from her ovaries. He said there were no guarantees and it was expensive and not likely to be covered by our insurance. I thought about it for a long time and weighed the pros and cons. If I didn't do this procedure for her would she be angry at me when she was older? If I allowed her to have the procedure would the extra time and money be worth it? Would my daughter feel compelled to have a child because I had stored her tissue for her? Would this experimental procedure lead to a baby for her one day? I had a lot of questions but no answers. I asked the doctors if there was another parent I could talk to who was faced with the same decisions as me. I felt very alone, and even selfish when they told me that most parents were grateful if their child had a good survival prognosis and didn't worry about fertility. I didn't have a lot of time to make a decision either – they wanted to start treatment right away. I did some searching on the Internet and found a national organization. I started to read about how other parents were in the same quandary as me – I was not alone but most parents didn't express their concerns to their child's oncology team because they were waiting for the team to bring it up. In the end I decided to have my daughter's ovarian tissue frozen. Was it the right thing to do? I don't know and won't know for a long time. But I thought about how we saved for college for her, so she would have that option. This seemed like another type of savings plan. Time will tell if I made the right decision.
Emma, Mother of Pediatric Cancer Survivor

Introduction

Ethical consideration has a strong history and is of prime importance in the field medicine. Starting from the birth of Western medical ethics, the Hippocratic Oath, to the modern framework set forth by the Principalist approach [1] which

G.P. Quinn (✉)
Moffitt Cancer Center, College of Medicine, University
of South Florida, Tampa, FL 33612, USA
e-mail: gwen.quinn@moffitt.org

G.P. Quinn, S.T. Vadaparampil (eds.), *Reproductive Health and Cancer in Adolescents
and Young Adults*, Advances in Experimental Medicine and Biology 732,
DOI 10.1007/978-94-007-2492-1_15, © Springer Science+Business Media B.V. 2012

187

involves the consideration of four principles – autonomy, beneficence, non-malfeasance, and justice. These four principles are not rigid mandates. Rather, these principles are meant to provide a useful framework to help health care providers make decisions when reflecting on moral issues as they arise. Although these principles are useful for many medical encounters, certain situations may present conflict between two or more principles and ethical dilemmas may arise.

The burgeoning field of reproductive medical technology is ripe with ethical dilemmas and suggests a need for on-going ethical analysis as the sensitive topics of human life and reproductive rights are addressed. One of the most recent medical advances in reproductive medicine, attracting ethical consideration, is the practice of fertility preservation in cancer patients. The reproductive technologies allowing fertility preservation in cancer patients were born out of a recognized need to address the reported psychological distressed caused by infertility [2–7] in the increasing population of cancer survivors with impaired fertility [8]. The ethical endorsement of the practice of offering fertility preservation to cancer patients stems from the ethical principle of autonomy, referring to self-government and free choice, which promotes the individual right to reproduce and beneficence, to do good to patients by relieving distress associated with infertility. However, the competing ethical concerns of non-maleficence, meaning "doing no harm", raise concerns about the health of the cancer patient and wellbeing of the offspring. Further, concerns with the ethical concern of justice, referring to the quality of being right or fair, raise questions of equal access for all patients. The high cost of these procedures may mean only the wealthy are able to pursue fertility preservation. The ethical concerns of equal access to fertility preservation for all cancer patients speak to both the principles of autonomy of reproductive rights and justice. Two main barriers to fertility preservation in cancer patients are lack of knowledge about preservation options and inability to pay for procedures [3, 9, 10].

The purpose of this chapter is to present a brief review of the ethical considerations regarding the practice of fertility preservation in cancer patients.

Lack of Knowledge Regarding Fertility Preservation Options: Oncologist's Role

Patients may be unable to use fertility preservation options in the limited time frame which they will benefit because they are not aware of fertility preservation options. In fact, many patients are not even aware that their fertility was adversely affective my cancer treatments. Considering oncologist role in treatment decisions and communication of treatment side effects, both the American Society of Clinical Oncology (ASCO) and the American Society for Reproductive Medicine (ASRM) have guidelines which highlight the importance of patients education and recognizing the oncologists as the main communicator of fertility related information [11, 12]. ASCO guidelines state that "as part of the informed consent before cancer therapy, oncologists should address the possibility of infertility with patients treated during their reproductive years and be prepared to discuss possible fertility preservation options or refer appropriate and interested patients to reproductive specialist [11]." ASRM similarly states that physicians should inform cancer patients about future fertility and fertility preservation options prior to treatment [12]. In sum, these guidelines stress that addressing this issue with patients is an important aspect of quality cancer care and that health care providers must provide timely information [11, 12]. Despite these guidelines, recent research suggests that oncologists are not always providing or referring for fertility information to their patients [13]. Many factors may contribute to the lack of discussion of fertility issues between patients and physicians, including oncologist's screening, perceived inability to pay, patients with a poor prognosis, and perceived effectiveness [14–17].

Oncologist's Screening

Health care providers may selectively discuss fertility preservation with a choice group of patients based on the perception that parenthood is only acceptable for a subgroup of patients. For instance, research demonstrates oncologists view of who should pursue fertility preservation influences rate of referral to sperm banking with reports of lower referral to men who were homosexual and HIV-positive [3]. Other patient considerations may be age, marital status, and number of children [18, 19]. Yet, other health care providers may feel that the practice of fertility preservation is generally wrong based on concerns with the ethics of the procedure and may not discuss with all patients. This type of screening does not allow equal access to fertility preservation technologies to all cancer patients.

Cost

The physician's perception of a patient's ability to afford the procedure including the patient's insurance status, availability of resources, and cost of procedures may also serve as barriers. Equal access is squelched by costly ART procedures that are often not covered by insurance and therefore, must be paid out-of-pocket by patients. Patients who undergo many cycles of treatment hoping to achieve pregnancy face daunting expenses. The current dilemma for cancer patients regarding lack of insurance coverage comes from both insufficient insurance coverage for infertility treatments and the definition of infertility itself. In general, infertility treatments are generally not covered by insurance companies because they are not considered a medical necessity. Only 15 states have laws related to insurance cover for infertility or in vitro fertilization (IVF) [20]; however, these policies all limit fertility treatments to patients that demonstrate an inability to conceive a child after 1 year of unprotected sexual intercourse. Clearly this definition was developed for the general population and is not responsive to patients with a cancer diagnosis or cancer survivors [12]. Consistent

with this definition, no state laws or regulations address insurance cover for fertility preservation specific to cancer patients [20]. In sum, physicians' concern regarding cost is not unfounded, as the financially disadvantaged do not have equal access to this medical procedure. Still, some programs such as Sharing Hope may be able to assist by working with companies and clinics to arrange for discounted services and donated medications for some patients.

Poor Prognosis

Oncologists' reluctance to discuss fertility issue in patients with a poor prognosis has been reported in multiple studies with the general consensus being that fertility preservation is not important at a time when the patient is fighting for survival [21]. Treating the cancer is the highest priority. Further, these patients with a poor prognosis may not have time to delay treatment to pursue fertility preservation. Even if the physician presents the fertility information, the patient may be overwhelmed with the diagnosis and want to focus on surviving and physician may not want to push this issue on a patient who is focused on survival. Further, physicians may be also be concerned with or disagree with enabling cancer patients with a poor prognosis to reproduce and, possibly, posthumous reproduction because of concerns regarding the welfare of the children.

Are the Odds of Successful Pregnancy Great Enough to Consider?

Oncologist may not discuss fertility preservation options with their patients because they may have uncertainty about the success of fertility preservation methods. Oncologists may not be aware of recent medical advances and thus, underestimate the effectiveness of fertility preservation methods. For instance, one study showed that oncologists overestimated the number of sperm samples needed to make cryopreservation worthwhile [3]. Consistent with this survey, most oncologists surveyed were unaware of recent advances in reproductive technology in which only a few sperm are needed for successful IVF with intracytoplasmic sperm injection (ICSI) [19]. This lack of awareness may be contributing to underutilization of sperm cryopreservation by male cancer patients. Currently, all male cancer patients of reproductive age who will have treatment that may affect reproductive function and who may desire children in the future should cryopreserve sperm before the initiation of treatment [19].

Posthumous Assisted Reproduction

Posthumous assisted reproduction (PAR) refers o the posthumous conception of a child with the use of ART [22]. This is particularly the case in cancer patients such that cancer treatments may not be effective and the patient may die prior to the use of stored gametes or gonadal tissue leading to the posthumous use and subsequent posthumous reproduction by spouse or family of the deceased. The likeliness of PAR is much higher in cancer patients compared to the general population considering the life threatening and unpredictable nature of cancer. Although survival rates have steadily increased and most patients expect to live long post cancer lives, many patients die prior to use of reproductive materials. Ethical concerns of PAR can be grouped into three major principles: classification of reproductive material, autonomy of the patient, and welfare of future posthumously conceived children.

Classification and Rights to Unused Materials

One main ethical issue concerning PAR is who has authority to decide the fate of unused embryos and gametes subsequent to the death of a cancer patient. The ASRM guidelines state that "Precise instructions should be given about the disposition of stored gametes, embryos, or gonadal tissue in the event of the patient's death, unavailability, or other contingency" [12]. However, these guidelines are not always followed, resulting in legal debate of who has the

authority to decide the disposition of unused embryos and gametes following the death of the intended parent. This is further complicated by the obscure categorization of reproductive materials. In regards to PAR, the prevailing view is that embryos and gametes are neither person nor property, but a unique category, over which progenitors have the authority to decide the fate [23]. The lack of legislation and adherence to consenting policies result in debate and ethical dilemmas concerning the disposition of reproductive materials.

Autonomy of the Patient

Another important ethical consideration is respecting patient's autonomous decision to pursue fertility preservation and posthumously reproduce. Though this does not imply unconditional acceptance of the patient's wishes, consistent with the principle of autonomy, personal reserves on the physicians' part should not impede transmission of fertility preservation options to the patient. The concept of respecting patient wishes may seem straightforward; however, patient wishes are not always clearly evident in the instance of posthumous reproductive cases. A major challenge to posthumous use of reproductive material in determining the deceased wishes regarding disposition of unused genetic materials subsequent their death.

Consent

A key question is determining if a reliable indicator of consent was in place in the form of an advanced directive or will before death. If consent is not in place, the main legal dilemma of PAR involve determining what should become of the fertility preservation materials and who has the authority to decide what should happen to this material in instance of death prior to use. These decisions are often complicated by the lack of written consent and variations in the interpretation of unwritten consent. There have been many legal cases concerning whether the deceased would have wanted posthumous use of fertility preservation material when written consent was not in place [24]. Implied consent, bias interpretations of the deceased intent, is the determining factor. In these instances, the general consensus is that use of materials must only be sought when considering if the patient would have wanted to still be a parent after death.

Desire to Reproduce after Death

Though the use of fertility preservation may be a presumed indicator of cancer patients desires to procreate it is unclear if they desired to be a biological parent or if preservation efforts were intended for the upbringing of their children [25]. Few people discuss if they still want biological children if they were not alive to raise them [25]. The concept of posthumously conceived children challenges the concept of parenthood. PAR suggest that parenthood is a purely a biological construct. Conversely, opponents of PAR claim parenting has strong roots in upbringing and are concerned about the implications of PAR to the family structure [25].

The current view maintains that the deceased wishes prior to death control reproductive material use or disposal [12]. Physicians have leverage to impose their own sense of what they feel is appropriate consent [25]. However, both the AMA and the ASRM have expressed concern for more complete ART informed consent including patients intentions for preserving [12]. Specifically, the ASRM states that a spouse's request for sperm harvest of terminally ill or deceased person "need not be honored" if the "consent is unclear" [12].

Welfare of Posthumous Offspring

Another ethical consideration is the welfare of the posthumously conceived child on the belief that children should not suffer physically, economically, or emotionally for choices they had no influence in making. Because of the small number of posthumous cases, psychosocial and

other risks cannot be adequately estimated at this time [22]. ASRM guidelines regarding physician's role in transmitting fertility information states that "Concerns about the welfare of resulting offspring should not be cause for denying cancer patients assistance in reproducing" [12].

Potential Economic Harm

The obscurity of the legal status of posthumously conceived child has financial implications such that posthumous offspring may not have rights to inheritance or may not be entitlement to government benefits [24, 25]. This means that posthumously conceived children may be more likely to me economically disadvantaged.

Potential Emotional Harm

When considering fertility preservation in general for cancer patients, a number of concerns for the emotional welfare of potential offspring are evident. Though little is known about the psychological detriment of PAR, psychological consequences are a concern in posthumously conceived children left bereft of a parent [23, 26]. However, though two parents are desirable, there is not sufficient evidence to support that single parenthood causes great enough harm to make it unethical for a single parent to reproduce [24].

Progeny's Wellbeing

Assisted reproduction in cancer patients may raise ethical issues about the impact of their reproduction on physical and psychological wellbeing of future children. Both the treating physician and the patients may be concerned about compromised health of offspring because of previous treatment or the effects of reproductive technologies. Indeed, research with survivors indicate that the health of future offspring is a major concern including concerns with potential birth defects and cancer [2, 27]. Further, some health care providers may question whether it is ethical to enable reproduction of an individual whose poor health and possible early death would likely impair parental ability and in turn, adversely affect offspring. This concern is particularly an ethical dilemma for those that consider the embryo to be human because this would require the physician to apply the four principles of ethics to the embryo. Therefore, such individual is likely to be very concerned about ethical considerations that involve the wellbeing of potential offspring.

Ability to Care for the Child

Concerns with the ability of the cancer patient to raise the child may raise the ethical question of whether a physician is acting responsibly by enabling reproduction in cancer patients if the child is likely to suffer neglect or grief in the instance the parent may die prematurely or be unable to care for the child because of the disease. This dilemma forces the odd consideration that the child might be better off if they were never born. However, further consideration makes this proposal unlikely. For instance, many children are currently raised by only one or neither parent; yet if you were to query these children on their hardships, it is unlikely that they are so great that they wish they were never born. Further, alternative caregivers may fill this void. Although physicians concern with the wellbeing of future offspring may be considered an ethical reason to refer certain cancer patients for fertility preservation, ASRM recommends physicians not deny patients fertility preservation information based on concern for the welfare [12]. In sum, protecting children by preventing birth does not seem like reasonable grounds to deny cancer survivors the chance to reproduce.

Poor Obstetric Outcome

ART increases the likeliness of multiple births, low birth rate, prematurely, cerebral palsy, mental retardation, and perinatal mortality [28, 29]. Recent research comparing the obstetric outcomes of singleton IVF babies compared to multiple gestations suggest that most of these adverse outcomes are due to the high incidence of multiple births. The routine IVF protocol in the past involved the implantation of three or more embryos because transferring fewer embryos resulted in low live birth rates and multiple pregnancies were not viewed as on adverse outcome [30]. In hopes of improving health of IVF children, researchers, especially in Europe have focused on reducing multiple birth rates by decreasing the number of embryos transferred. Consequently, voluntary and, in some countries, legislative guidelines targeted at limiting the number of embryos transferred have been promulgated in an effort to reduce the incidence of multiple gestations after ART. In most European countries, single embryo transfer is now recommended because of higher success rates, lower risk of multiples, and subsequently improved health of IVF children [31]. Despite widespread use of single embryo transfer in much of Europe, adoption of this approach has been slow in the United States. Though the ASRM and the Society for Assisted Reproductive Technology (SART) published guidelines discouraging the implantation of more than two embryos for women under 35, touting the benefits of single embryo transfer for women under 35 who have a good chance of achieving a pregnancy, no laws in the United States to date address the practice of multiple embryo transfer [32]. With single embryo transfer, it can be expected that obstetric outcomes of IVF children should be comparable to children conceived naturally [33]. In light of these findings, it is essential that physicians be updated on current research so they are able to provide the best care with minimal risk to both the mother and the offspring.

Increased Risk for Genetic Defects and Cancer Risk

Another concern is the possibility that offspring of both ART patients and cancer patients are at a risk for congenital anomalies and chromosomal defects [34]. Though there have been conflicting reports regarding defects and ART, one study reported that children conceived through ART have up to two times the risk of birth defects compared to natural birth [35]. Still, there is no evidence that cryopreserved embryos or sperm have a deleterious effect on the offspring and the number of children born from oocytes and ovarian tissue are too small to determine negative effects [22]. A recent study conducted in Denmark concluded there was no significant evidence of risk of transmission of cancer (nonhereditary) to offspring of cancer survivors conceived naturally or through assisted reproductive technology [36]. However, patients with heritable cancer risk passing genetic predisposition of cancer to their offspring (see Chapter 8).

Wellbeing and Health of Cancer Patient

The principle of non-maleficence questions the ethics of fertility preservation in cancer patients in light of concerns with the wellbeing of the cancer patient health and the potential emotional and physical obstacles to undergo treatment that may be ineffective and therefore, give false hope. Many of these ethical concerns have been met with scientific advancements to ensure no harm to cancer patients or to dispel inaccurate information with scientific data to allay these concerned, but physicians may be unaware of such information. Therefore, they may base their ethical decisions on inaccurate information or outdated technologies.

The diagnosis of cancer is itself is a life crisis, and dealing with the additional possibility of infertility compounds the cancer patient's distress. In order to preserve fertility, a patient has many decisions to make in a limited timeframe including altering treatment plan and taking the necessary steps to preserve their reproductive materials which may involve their own sets of risks and uncertainties. Some men find producing sperm highly stressful under such circumstances and may need medical intervention to retrieve sperm. Fertility preservation for women is more complex and intrusive involving a serious of

injections to stimulate ovaries and medical procedure to retrieve oocytes all at a time the vulnerable timeframe immediately following diagnosis and before cancer treatment. Further, the chemical hormones used to harvest eggs may induce multiple complications such as ovarian hyperstimulation syndrome, bleeding, infection, and cysts. Some physicians may questions whether it is ethical to suggest such treatment that involves such emotional and potential physical harm.

Contraindication of Fertility Preservation in Cancer Patients?

The hormone injections required to stimulate follicle production may be contradictive for some cancer patients. Consistent with the principle of non-maleficence, a physician would recommend that women with hormone sensitive cancers not use ovarian stimulation because of concerns over possible exacerbation of hormone sensitive cancers from the elevation of estrogen, which accompanies ovarian stimulation. In response to this concern, alternative methods are available to allay some of the concerns of harm. One option is "natural cycle-IVF" which involves monitoring the natural reproductive cycle without stimulating ovulation; however, not many embryos are yielded with this method [11]. Other options are aromatase inhibitors which blunt the rise of estrogen resulting from ovarian stimulation and use of an estrogen receptor blocker, such as Tamoxifen, to block the estrogen receptor. These new, safer, technologies have been proven to have similar efficacy as traditional ovarian stimulation methods [37].

More Harm Than Good?

Consistent with the principles of non-maleficence, we must consider the additional psychological and physical risk of fertility preservation options available to pediatric patients, especially in the context of limited efficacy of these treatments. The pursuit of fertility preservation decreases the likelihood that child will suffer from the mental anguish of infertility [38] and be deprived of the opportunity of biological parenthood. Thus, the act of the offering fertility preservation is "good", the intended effect is also "good." However, there are additional hardships to consider for prepubertal patients to because of the limited medical options available. Currently, there are no established options to preserve fertility in prepubertal populations. The only option for prepubertal children is the, removal and subsequent storage of gonadal tissue. This, is considered experimental and there is lack of research on the safety and efficacy [39]. Although studies are limited, ASCO concludes there is no medical evidence to suggest fertility preservation techniques will adversely affect the health of a survivor nor interfere with cancer treatment [11]. Thus, these procedural risk are generally regarded as minimal and are generally considered to be outweighed by the potential good.

Cost Barriers

An additional concern of these experimental preservation options are the high costs of the medical procedures deemed "exorbitant" by some opponents [40]. For instance, the current estimates on the costs of ovarian tissue cryopreservation range from $5,000 to $12,000 [20, 41]. These high costs are calling to the ethical principle of justice in the sense that financial reality may serve as a barrier to equal access for all patients.

Child's Best Interest

Fertility preservation in pediatric cancer patients presents additional concerns with the child's ability to contribute to the complex decisions related to making an autonomous decision regarding fertility preservation treatment and future disposition of unused reproductive materials. Autonomy in the decision making process differs by child's age. Young children are obviously unable to contribute to the decision making process while older

children take a very active role in the informed decision making process. Regardless, both health care providers and guardians have major roles in the decision making process.

Consistent with the principle of beneficence, just as the development of technologies to preserve fertility in children was indeed created with the ethical obligation to act in the good intentions, guardians and health care providers role in the decision making process is to ensure that children are protected and to ensure the best choice is made in regards to making a decision that is in the best interest of the child.

Conclusion

In sum, fertility preservation in cancer patients is a new concept that raises multiple ethical considerations. These issues often require health care professionals to examine their own value and, on a case-by-case basis, provider recommendations and referrals. A health care provider's personal ethics may interfere with the patient's right to reproduce as these issues may pose barriers to the discussion of or assistance with the use of ART by cancer patients. Consistent with the principles of autonomy, the health care provider has the duty to be compassionate to patients whose desire to reproduce may conflict with their own moral values. Yet, as demonstrated by this review, there are multiple ethical dilemmas involving the other ethical principles – beneficence, non-maleficence, and justice, which makes reaching conclusion regarding ethical practice behavior less straightforward. In light of these murky conclusions, it is evident that future action is needed to elucidate appropriate practice behavior which will allow the best outcome for patients without compromising the value of human life.

Provider Recommendations

1. Health care providers should be cognizant of medical advances and options as they become available.

2. Inaccurate or outdated information may lead providers to reach inaccurate ethical conclusions regarding the use of fertility preservation in patients.

3. Future policy analyses should consider these ethical dilemmas to provide guidance on the limits of these technologies. Such guidelines may allay some of these ethical concerns.

4. Both ASCO and ASRM medical guidelines clearly state the role of the health care provider to provide fertility information to their patients. The prospect of future policy or legislation to enforce this behavior is favorable and may alleviate providers from the daunting task of pondering ethical dilemmas.

References

1. Beauchamp TL, Childress JF (1994) Principles of biomedical ethics, 4th edn. Oxford University Press, Oxford

2. Schover LR, Rybicki LA, Martin BA, Bringelsen KA (1999) Having children after cancer. Cancer 86(4):697–709

3. Schover LR, Brey K, Lichtin A, Lipshultz LI, Jeha S (2002) Knowledge and experience regarding cancer, infertility, and sperm banking in younger male survivors. J Clin Oncol 20(7):1880–1889

4. Carter J, Rowland K, Chi D, Brown C, Abu-Rustum N, Castiel M et al (2005) Gynecologic cancer treatment and the impact of cancer-related infertility. Gynecol Oncol 97(1):90–95

5. Hartmann JT, Albrecht C, Schmoll HJ, Kuczyk MA, Kollmannsberger C, Bokemeyer C (1999) Long-term effects on sexual function and fertility after treatment of testicular cancer. Br J Cancer 80(5–6):801–807

6. Partridge AH, Gelber S, Peppercorn J, Sampson E, Knudsen K, Laufer M et al (2004) Web-based survey of fertility issues in young women with breast cancer. J Clin Oncol 22(20):4174–4183

7. Rieker P, Fitzgerald E, Kalish L (1990) Adaptive behavioral responses to potential infertility among survivors of testis cancer. J Clin Oncol 8(2):347–355

8. American Cancer Society (2007) Global cancer facts and figures. American Cancer Society, Atlanta, GA, p 7

9. Tschudin S, Bitzer J (2009) Psychological aspects of fertility preservation in men and women affected by cancer and other life-threatening diseases. Hum Reprod Update 15(5):587–597

10. Coyne KD, Kader A, Agarwal A (2010) Creating a standard of care for fertility preservation. Curr Women's Health Rev 6:261–266

11. Lee S, Schover L, Partridge A, Patrizio P, Wallace W, Hagerty K et al (2006) American Society of Clinical Oncology recommendations on fertility preservation in cancer patients. J Clin Oncol 24:2917–2931

12. The Ethics Committee of the American Society for Reproductive (2005) Medicine fertility preservation and reproduction in cancer patients. Fertil Steril 83(6):1622–1628

13. Quinn GP, Vadaparampil ST, Lee J-H, Jacobsen PB, Bepler G, Lancaster J et al (2009) Physician referral for fertility preservation in oncology patients: a national study of practice behaviors. J Clin Oncol 27(35):5952–5957

14. Quinn GP, Vadaparampil ST (2008) Fertility preservation and adolescent/young adult cancer patients: physician communication challenges. J Adolesc Health 44(4):394–400

15. Quinn G, Vadaparampil S, Gwede C, Miree C, King L, Clayton H et al (2007) Discussion of fertility preservation with newly diagnosed patients: oncologists' views. J Cancer Survivorship 1(2): 146–155

16. Schover LR, Brey K, Lichtin A, Lipshultz LI, Jeha S (2002) Oncologists' attitudes and practices regarding banking sperm before cancer treatment. J Clin Oncol 20(7):1890–1897

17. Quinn GP, Vadaparampil ST, Bell-Ellison BA, Gwede CK, Albrecht TL (2008) Patient-physician communication barriers regarding fertility preservation among newly diagnosed cancer patients. Soc Sci Med 66(3):784–789

18. Fraietta R, Spaine DM, Bertolla RP, Ortiz V, Cedenho AP Individual and seminal characteristics of patients with testicular germ cell tumors. Fertil Steril 94(6):2107–2112

19. Zapzalka DM, Redmon JB, Pryor JL (1999) A survey of oncologists regarding sperm cryopreservation and assisted reproductive techniques for male cancer patients. Cancer 86(9):1812–1817

20. Quinn GP, Vadaparampil ST, McGowan Lowrey K, Eidson S, Knapp C, Bukulmez O. State laws and regulations addressing third-party reimbursement for infertility treatment: implications for cancer survivors. Fertil Steril 95(1):72–78

21. Debono DJ, Kohnke JM, Helft PR (2009) Addressing fertility in patients with advanced cancer: how the quality oncology practice initiative standards and ASCO guidelines facilitate ethical communication. J Oncol Pract 5(6):298–300

22. Pennings G, de Wert G, Shenfield F, Cohen J, Devroey P et al (2006) ESHRE task force on ethics and law 11: posthumous assisted reproduction. Hum Reprod 21(12):3050–3053

23. Bahadur G (2004) Ethical challenges in reproductive medicine: posthumous reproduction. Int Congr Series 1266:295–302

24. Robertson JA (2005) Cancer and fertility: ethical and legal challenges. J Natl Cancer Inst Monogr 34: 104–106

25. Kramer A (2009) Sperm retrieval from terminally ill or recently deceased patients: a review. Can J Urol 16(3):4627–4631
26. Aziza-Shuster E (1994) Ethics and society: a child at all costs: posthumous reproduction and the meaning of parenthood. Hum Reprod 9(11):2182–2185
27. Schover LR (2005) Motivation for parenthood after cancer: a review. J Natl Cancer Inst Monogr 2005(34):2–5
28. Ericson A, Kallen B (2001) Congenital malformations in infants born after IVF: a population-based study. Hum Reprod 16(3):504–509
29. Strömberg B, Dahlquist G, Ericson A, Finnström O, Köster M, Stjernqvist K (2002) Neurological sequelae in children born after in-vitro fertilisation: a population-based study. Lancet 359(9305):461–465
30. Reynolds MA, Schieve LA (2006) Trends in embryo transfer practices and multiple gestation for IVF procedures in the USA, 1996–2002. Hum Reprod 21(3):694–700
31. Maheshwari A, Griffiths S, Bhattacharya S (2011) Global variations in the uptake of single embryo transfer. Hum Reprod Update 17(1):107–120
32. American Society for Reproductive Medicine (2008) Guidelines on number of embryos transferred. American Society for Reproductive Medicine, Birmingham, AL
33. Vilska S, Tiitinen A, Hydén-Granskog C, Hovatta O (1999) Elective transfer of one embryo results in an acceptable pregnancy rate and eliminates the risk of multiple birth. Hum Reprod 14(9):2392–2395
34. Lyerly AD, Steinhauser K, Voils C, Namey E, Alexander C, Bankowski B et al (2010) Fertility patients' views about frozen embryo disposition: results of a multi-institutional U.S. survey. Fertil Steril 93(2):499–509
35. Kurinczuk JJ, Hansen Ml, Bower C (2004) The risk of birth defects in children born after assisted reproductive technologies. Curr Opin Obstet Gynecol 16(3):201–209
36. Sankila R, Olsen JH, Anderson H, Garwicz S et al (2010) Risk of cancer among offspring of childhood cancer survivors. New Engl J Med 338: 1339–1344
37. Casper RF, Mitwally MFM (2006) Aromatase inhibitors for ovulation induction. J Clin Endocrinol Metab 91(3):760–771
38. Schover LR (1999) Psychosocial aspects of infertility and decisions about reproduction in young cancer survivors: a review. Med Pediatr Oncol 33: 53–59
39. Levine J, Canada A, Stern C (2010) Fertility preservation in adolescents and young adults with cancer. J Clin Oncol 22:1–11
40. Cohen CB (2008) Some perils of "waiting to be born": fertility preservation in girls facing certain treatments for cancer. Am J Bioeth 8:30–35
41. Livestrong (2011) Fertilehope.org.

The Legal Issue and of Assisted Reproductive Technologies

16

Diana Brock, Esq

Three years ago I had breast cancer. Faced with this news and knowing my husband and I wanted children I decided to go through IVF and freeze my embryos. Fortunately, I recovered from breast cancer and I now have two beautiful children. The problem is that I have five frozen embryos left over from my IVF treatment. My husband wishes to donate the extra embryos to research. However, I am deeply torn by this decision as I feel this would be murdering my unborn children. I believe the better decision is to donate their remaining five embryos to another couple. My husband, however, does not like the idea of having children genetically related to him raised by someone else. Sadly, this issue among others, has torn our family apart and my husband and I are now divorced. I filed a lawsuit to determine who gets the embryos but litigation has been slow. Even more tragic, during this process my husband was suddenly killed in a car accident. I have since implanted the frozen embryos and have a healthy beautiful boy, Aiden. Because of my husband's tragic death and other financial hardships I am struggling to get by as a single mom. I filed for social security benefits for my children including Aiden. The government however, is now saying that Aiden is not entitled to social security since he was conceived after his father's death. I wish I had known of the legal repercussions of IVF and freezing my embryos. While I have three beautiful children life is hard and I feel much of my hardship could have been avoided if I had been aware of the law in my state.
- Stacy, Adult Cancer Survivor

Introduction

Couples or women diagnosed with cancer, often rush to take advantage of technology as they are under duress from their diagnosis and the threat of infertility. It is important future patients of these procedures be warned that ART often produce more embryos than will be needed for implantation. The extra embryos are often cryopreserved. Consequently, decisions regarding the fate of these embryos will need to be made in the future. Generally speaking there are three options for extra cryopreserved embryos: (1) to dispose or let the embryo thaw out and cease to grow, (2) to donate to research; or (3) to donate to an infertile couple for implantation/adoption [1]. However, not all of these options are viable when taking into account the controlling law in the jurisdiction or the religious views of the particular patients. If one partner has strong religious views and wishes to have all embryos implanted while the other partner wishes to donate the excess embryos to research, a legal battle may ensue as to the appropriate disposition. Therefore, in order to avoid conflict in the future, it is important future patients of ART are informed and knowledgeable of their options.

D. Brock (✉)
Adjunct Legal Studies Professor, Hodges University,
2655 Northbrooke Drive, Naples, FL 34119
e-mail: djzink@gmail.com

G.P. Quinn, S.T. Vadaparampil (eds.), *Reproductive Health and Cancer in Adolescents and Young Adults*, Advances in Experimental Medicine and Biology 732,
DOI 10.1007/978-94-007-2492-1_16, © Springer Science+Business Media B.V. 2012

Disputes regarding the disposition of cryopreserved embryos often turn on how that particular jurisdiction legally defines the cryopreserved embryos. Thus it is important that women, couples, and particularly women who are not married or who are relying on a partner or friend for sperm, understand the legal ramifications of their actions. The below example is illustrative.

Imagine, for example, Mike and Robyn a couple who created eighteen embryos through IVF after discovering Robyn had cancer. They live and used the services of a fertility clinic in Louisiana. After having three children from the embryos created, the couple divorces. While Mike wishes to donate the extra embryos to research, Robyn wishes to donate their remaining six embryos to another couple, Bill and Susan, who live in Georgia. Should Mike or Robyn's wishes prevail? If the embryos are donated to Bill and Susan what law governs this disposition? Is it adoption law or property law or contract law? If Georgia and Louisiana law differs, which state controls? Unfortunately the law surrounding these questions is unsettled and those states that do touch on some of these issues have differing outcomes.

The legal issues surrounding ART do not end here. The advancements in ART have also led to problems surrounding Social Security benefits and intestacy rights[1] of posthumously conceived children. The issue occurs for example when a mother conceives using the sperm previously deposited from a deceased husband/partner. Some states do not recognize the child being that of the deceased husband/partner and therefore not entitled to social security, while other states require proof of paternity and more before granting social security benefits to the child.

Because the law on these issues is so unsettled, it is important for health care professionals to be aware of and warn patients of the many legal dilemmas that may arise when dealing with IVF and other ART's. This chapter will take a look at some of the legal issues surrounding ART. It will begin with a discussion on the legal status of cryopreserved embryos and finish with a discussion on the inheritance rights and social security issues of posthumously conceived births.

The Disposition of Excess Cryopreserved Embryos

As a result of IVF and the routine practice of extracting extra embryos there are currently an estimated 500,000 cryopreserved embryos stored in fertility clinics in the United States today [2].[2] The issue some survivors face is what to do with these excess cryopreserved embryos. The arguments over the best most appropriate means of disposing the embryos are deeply rooted within political, emotional, moral, and religious beliefs [3].[3]

When couples/families do not agree on the proper disposition of an embryo they sometimes look to the courts for resolution. Unfortunately the law is anything but clear [4].[4] When a couple freezes embryos one could argue they do so with the intent to use them in the future. When an unforeseen event such as divorce, death of one or of the parties, financial reversals, or simple disenchantment with the IVF process occurs before the embryos are implanted, the issue of what to do with them arises. A couple facing this problem generally has three options, (1) to dispose or let the embryo thaw out and cease to grow, (2) to donate to research; and (3) to donate to an infertile couple for implantation/adoption [1].[5] However, each party may have a different opinion as to how to discard the embryos. For example, the sperm donor may wish to let the embryo thaw out, while the egg donor may wish to donate to an infertile couple. Another factor that can complicate this scenario is if the fertility clinic refuses to give up custody of the embryos. When these issues arise the courts often look to how that particular jurisdiction legally defines the embryos; for example as property, or person, or special/interim status. The three options above may not be available depending on how the particular jurisdiction legally defines the cryopreserved embryos. The next section discusses how the legal classification of cryopreserved embryos effects the viability these three options.

Legal Status of Cryopreserved Embryos

The problem of how to deal with these excess embryos originates from the fact the law is unclear how they are to be legally classified [1].[6] For example, if classified as *Property* then all the above options are viable [1].[7] However, if viewed as a *Person* than thawing and discarding the cryopreserved embryo would be viewed, to some, as murder and not a viable option [1].[8] Moreover, some jurisdictions believe these embryos should not be given the same legal status as a *person* or *property* but should be given an interim, *special* status [1].[9] Thus, the solution of how to dispose of these cryopreserved embryos is related to how they are classified. It is important for patients to be aware of their states legal classifications given to cryopreserved embryos. This can help survivors become more knowledgeable about their rights and help better prepare and plan for how they will possibly dispose of the excess cryopreserved embryos left over from IVF.

Once the cryopreserved embryo is given a legal status, one must determine what rights that legal status grants. For example, if the cryopreserved embryos are legally recognized persons should they then be afforded the same basic human rights? If so, what is the state's interest in protecting the rights of these cryopreserved embryos? The Louisiana and New Mexico Legislatures are two legislatures that ascribe to this *person* designation [1].[10]

Legal Status: Person

Those that believe embryos should be entitled to legal status as a *person* further believe that donating them to research or letting them thaw out and cease to grow are not viable options [3].[11] Thus, they believe embryo adoption is the only workable solution [3].[12] Generally speaking, those that believe life begins with conception vehemently adhere to this designation as they fear that if the embryos are donated to research or thawed out without implantation the soul will not be granted salvation [3].[13]

Louisiana takes the most protective approach of any American state, expressly declaring a human embryo to be a "biological human being" which is not the property of the physician which acts as an agent of fertilization, or the facility which employs him, or the donors of the sperm and ovum [1].[14] An in vitro fertilized human ovum is recognized as a separate entity [5].[15] The legislature defines "human embryo" as "composed of one or more living cells and human genetic material so unified and organized that it will develop in utero into an unborn child [6]."[16] The statute prohibits intentionally destroying or creating human embryos for the sole purpose of research [6].[17] Further, the "best interest" standard, taken from family law principles, governs custody disputes of the embryos between male and female donor.[18] Moreover, Louisiana allows IVF patients to relinquish their parental rights to the embryo as long as another married couple implants the embryos.[19]

New Mexico's statute falls short of defining an embryo as a judicial person, however it encompasses embryo within the definition of fetus ensuring its safety by prohibiting procedures unless the purpose is "to meet the health needs of the particular fetus [7]".[20] New Mexico further mandates those who undergo IVF to either implant all excess embryos or indefinite cryopreservation [7].[21]

Critics of these statutes and the designation of *person* status to embryos argue that the so-called embryo is merely a cluster of cells and carries only the potential for life [8].[22] Therefore, the state's interest cannot be as great as that of a fully developed human being or even of a developing fetus at certain stages, in the womb [8].[23]

The flaws in the *person* legal status have not gone unnoticed by other jurisdictions. In fact, the majority of states have rejected New Mexico and Louisiana's approaches [1].[24] Colorado and Montana are two such states where voters rejected the person designation.

Legal Status: Property

If not person, some believe cryopreserved embryos are best treated as property and therefore are able to be thrown away, donated to research or donated for implantation [9].[25] This would deem the biological creators of the frozen embryos to have sole decision making authority

[9].[26] Hence, the biological creators would be entitled to own, sell, bequeath, and destroy them as they wish [9].[27] Advocates of this approach look at the stages of development that take place and distinguish pre-embryos from embryos that have undergone biological changes and cellular division [9].[28] They argue that cryopreserved embryos should be called pre-embryo's because they have not gone through a certain biological transformation [9].[29]

Advocates of the *property* designation distinguish between that which should be considered an embryo or "tiny human being" from a group of cells more closely related to the physiologic interaction with the mother; giving the former *person* designation and the latter, known as a pre-embryo, *property* designation. Upon classifying cryopreserved embryo/frozen pre-embryo as *property*, courts tend to assign property law principles to resolve issues regarding the transferring or disposing of these frozen pre-embryos. For example, courts tend to find that a bailor/bailee relationship exists between the biological creators and the clinic holding the frozen pre-embryos. A bailment is created when a party obtains lawful possession along with a duty to account for the thing as the property of another. The essential nature of a bailment relationship imposes on a bailee (one taking lawful possession) an absolute obligation to return the subject matter of the bailment to the bailor (owner of the subject matter) upon termination of the bailment.

This approach was implicitly adopted in *York v. Jones* where the Federal District Court for the Eastern District of Virginia relied on property law principles to decide a case between a couple and a fertility clinic over control of disputed embryos [10].[30] The couple sought to transfer their embryos to another clinic, but was denied by the clinic where the embryos were currently stored [10].[31] The court held that property law principles apply and a bailor-bailee relationship was present between the couple and the fertility clinic [8].[32]

Another example of the treatment of cryopreserved embryos as property is exhibited in the Florida Statute [1].[33] There, the statute codified a genetic donor's property interest in his other embryos, granting the sperm and egg donor joint decision making authority regarding their embryos' disposition [1].[34] The Florida legislature bolstered its property position by declaring that "control" and decisional authority always remains with the genetic donors; if one donor dies, the living donor immediately assumes full decisional authority [1].[35]

Michigan followed Florida's lead, categorizing embryos as property, allowing Michigan researchers to create new embryonic stem-cell lines from embryos created solely for fertility treatment purposes [1].[36] The embryos affected by this amendment are those that would have been destroyed if not used for medical research [1].[37]

While many argue this model to be most practical, others fervently disagree as religious and social views come into play [11].[38] The underlying question behind this entire issue is when one believes life begins [11].[39] Those that believe conception is the starting point of life would be hard-pressed to allow cryopreserved embryos be treated as property and the only viable option would be that of adoption/donation for implantation in other infertile couples [11].[40]

Because many people that undergo IVF have strong religious views it is important for healthcare professionals to take their time explaining the options for the disposition of the potential excess cryopreserved embryos. It is important that both sperm and egg donors are on the same page regarding this decision. If one partner has strong religious views and wishes to have all embryos implanted while the other partner wishes to donate the excess embryos to research, a legal battle may ensue as to the appropriate disposition. And the options regarding such disposition may be limited depending on the legal classification of the embryos in that particular jurisdiction.

Legal Status: Interim, Special Status

In the middle of the *person* versus *property* debate is an interim *special* status [9].[41] This view appears to be superior as it provides interim protection and acknowledges the frozen embryos unique capability to give rise to new human life.

Because it avoids categorizing the cryopreserved embryo as a person, it is still philosophically possible to transfer/donate these embryos to other infertile couples wishing to have children. This categorization was discussed in *Davis*, where the Tennessee court rejected the notion that embryos are either *persons* or *property* and instead held that they "occupy an interim category that entitles them to special respect because of their potential for human life [9]."[42]

In *Davis,* the court looked at current state and federal law and found that a *person* designation would contradict the present status of those laws [9].[43] In particular, the *person* designation would be in direct conflict with state statutes governing wrongful death, abortion, murder, and assault.[44] The court thus adopted the "special respect" approach [9].[45]

This interim *special* status is also followed by Arizona [12].[46] The Arizona Court of Appeals in *Jeter v. Mayo Clinic* held that the embryo was something more than human tissue but not yet a person [12].[47] Therefore, the Court of Appeals held the embryo to hold an interim *special* status [12].[48] The court further urged its Legislatures to determine the legal status of a cryopreserved embryo.[49] The Massachusetts court in *A.Z v. B.Z.* also followed this interim status designation as set forth in *Davis* [13].[50]

Further, Pennsylvania follows the interim special interests designation by protecting a woman's constitutional right to reproduce while criminalizing the creation of embryos solely for research purposes [1].[51] Other states following this approach are Maine and North Dakota [1].[52] These states refuse to treat embryos as mere property by prohibiting the sale of embryos for research [1].[53]

The problem with this designation is it lacks a clear definition as to what protections the embryo should receive. Furthermore, the same critics who believe life begins at conception will still argue for a *person* designation while the critics on the opposite end of the spectrum will argue for *property* designation as they believe cryopreserved embryos are nothing more than a group of cells. The heart of the conflict revolves around two very disparate philosophical views.

The interim status however serves as a buffer between the two opposite ends of the spectrum. This status takes both views into account. It reflects the fact that a cryopreserved embryo is not just a group of cells as it has the potential for human life. On the other hand these embryos will not develop further without a gestational carrier. Therefore it should not be afforded more rights than that of a fetus in gestation. For these reasons, it appears this *special* interim status is superior to both the *person* and *property* designations.

Options for Excess Cryopreserved Embryos: What Law Governs?

Even assuming cryopreserved embryos are given the interim legal status, the issue of what law governs their disposition still exists. Only a handful of states have adopted legislation aimed at regulating the disposition of embryos. Moreover, those limited statutes are not helpful in resolving disputes that may arise between a recipient couple as to the fate of excess embryos remaining at their divorce [1].[54]

Cryopreserved Embryos: Should Adoption Law Govern

Those who believe life begins at conception and that embryos are legally recognized persons urge state legislatures to apply adoption law to the disposition of excess cryopreserved embryos [11].[55] This means that embryo donation would be based on the overall goal of protecting the best interests of the embryo [1].[56] Under the legal protections of adoption law, all fertility clinics offering embryo adoption would execute a home study prior to implantation to ensure the prospective adoptive parents' fitness and the safety of their home [1].[57] Inquiry into the prospective parents' relationship, criminal record, and physical health would be likely [1].[58]

While Catholic theologians and philosophers have expressed their opposition for ART, several have supported embryo adoption because of the belief that these embryos are human life

[11].[59] Philosophers such as Grisez, Surtees and Watt proclaim embryo adoption should be distinguished from acts of IVF, surrogacy, or other forms of ART that the church repudiates [11].[60] This is so as adoption involves a child that is already conceived but rejected.[61] Surtees states, "though the embryo's first adoptive 'home' . . . would be the womb of his new mother, I can see no reason why such a 'home' should not be made available [11]."[62]

One issue with the adoption model is whether the biological creator's parental rights would terminate at implantation, birth (as is the case in a typical adoption), or some other point [14].[63] Another issue is whether the unused embryos should be returned to the original biological creators [14].[64] Some advocate the biological creators should be required to terminate their parental rights once the home study is complete [14].[65] This would deny the genetic creators a post implantation period during which time consent to the embryo adoption could be revoked [14].[66] These issues show the adoption model is not a perfect fit, however aspects of adoption law such as the inquiry process for prospective parents seems appropriate for those wishing to donate their embryos for future implantation.

Cryopreserved Embryos: Contract Law Prevails

Most fertility clinics require patients to sign an agreement addressing the issues which may arise as consequence to IVF [1].[67] These agreements often establish how any unused frozen embryos should be treated or disposed [1].[68] The issue of whether these contracts should be enforced often arises in the context of divorce [1].[69] Where the dispute over disposition arises from divorce, courts have generally voiced support for treating the agreements as presumptively valid, binding contracts [1].[70] This is the case when the contract provides the cryopreserved embryo (a) remain frozen, (b) thawed and thrown away, or (c) donated to medical research [15].[71] However, results to the contrary effect occur when the agreement provides the excess embryos be used

for subsequent implantation [15].[72] Up to date no court has enforced a contract forcing parenthood on the objecting parent [15].[73] It is argued public policy does not give states a strong enough interest in protecting potential life to force parenthood [11, 15].[74]

Dispositional agreements signed prior to initiating IVF services are both useful and necessary [8, 15].[75] While most fertility clinics provide dispositional agreements, not all do, and they are certainly not required to do so. These agreements are beneficial to the IVF process as they encourage parties to consider the consequences of this type of treatment thoroughly [8, 15].[76] They allow parties to specify their intentions in advance [8, 15].[77] Further, they prevent costly litigation, define the roles of the parties, and provide certainty [8, 15].[78]

Those that advocate a contractual approach generally view the cryopreserved embryos as *property* [16].[79] Proponents of this view analogize the cryopreserved embryos to that of human organs, blood, tissues, and semen [16].[80] As mentioned previously, the problem with this comparison is that it does not take into account the fact cryopreserved embryos have the potential for human life [16].[81] Because of this potential, the contract controlling disposition has been subject to criticism [8].[82]

Courts differ on how to treat contracts that control the disposition of the cryopreserved embryo [15].[83] While agreements providing that upon divorce the cryopreserved embryos remain frozen, thawed and thrown away, or donated to medical research have been generally upheld by courts [15],[84] agreements which provide the cryopreserved embryos be implanted or donated for implanation have not received the same support [15, 17].[85] Some courts are not willing to uphold these agreements entered into at the time IVF is commenced, arguing that it is against public policy to force an individual to have a child [17].[86]

A variation of the contract approach is the Mutual Consent Theory which seeks to enforce the agreement entered into at the time IVF is undergone, subject to the right of *either* party to change his or her mind about disposition up to the point of use or destruction of any stored embryos [18].[87] The Supreme Court of Iowa adopted this mutual consent approach in the case of *In re Marriage of Witten* [18].[88] There, the court held that should one or both parties change his or her mind as to the terms of the contract, the frozen embryos may not be used, destroyed, or donated unless both donors give their written consent. If a mutually agreeable result cannot be reached, the embryos will remain frozen [18].[89]

This variation of the contract theory undermines the finality of the contract and implies the frozen embryos are not just property of the biological creators but something more [18].[90] Under contract law it is particularly important that courts seek to honor the parties' expressions of choice, before disputes erupt [18].[91] Knowing that advance agreements will not be enforced underscores the seriousness and integrity of the consent process [18].[92] Advance agreements as to disposition would have little purpose if they were enforceable only in the event the parties continued to agree [18].[93] To the extent possible, it should be the biological creators, not the state or courts, which make this deeply personal life choice [19].[94]

While the mutual consent theory allows the parties to reach an agreement at a later time enabling the decision to continue in the hands of the biological creators, in reality this approach allows the vetoing party who wishes to let the embryos remain frozen, prevail [19].[95] In practice it is unknown how long frozen embryos remain viable. Scientific data only shows live births from embryos which have been frozen for a period of time no longer than 12–13 years. Furthermore, the success rates for frozen embryo transfers are typically lower than those for embryos that have not been frozen [19].[96] In a scenario where one wishes to donate the frozen embryo to an infertile couple or use for implanting the embryo in the female biological creator, while the other wishes it destroyed, the party wishing it destroyed prevails. It logically follows that at some point maintaining status quo allows the frozen embryo to become no longer viable and thus the vetoing party wishing to destroy the frozen embryo prevails [19].[97]

As we have seen the law is very unclear on how to legally define and subsequently dispose of excess cryopreserved embryos which leads us to the real question: is there a solution to his ever present dilemma?

Is There a Solution to the Problem?

There may not be a quick fix to the issues surrounding excess cryopreserved embryos. However, here are some suggestions as to how these issues may be improved.

First, legislatures could start recognizing cryopreserved embryos for what they are; cellular matter containing the potential for human life. Thus, neither *person* nor *property*, these cryopreserved embryos would be afforded the interim *special* status as it would be the most appropriate designation. From here, it is incumbent on legislatures to clearly define the scope of this designation. A combination of both contract law and adoption law could be used in defining the scope of this *special* status.

Second, it is up to healthcare professionals to take on the responsibility of preparing newly diagnosed patients for the consequences they will face following IVF and other ART's that they may use as survivors. Healthcare professionals should explain to patients the importance of preparing a contractual plan and being cautioned of the law of the patient's particular jurisdiction. It is important that both egg and sperm donors are on the same page when it comes to the issue of how to dispose of the possible extra cryopreserved embryos because, as we have seen, the law may not provide a clear outcome.

Couples going through IVF are often so eager to start treatment that they may not have thoroughly considered the consequences. It is important to discuss with patients specifications as to disposition under a divorce or death scenario. Discussion as to what the parties will do with any excess embryos and if cryopreserved the number of years or length of time to which the cryopreserved embryos will be stored. Both the female and male parties should be advised to consult individual legal advice. A waiting period between the time the contract is signed and the time when IVF takes place is also a good mechanism for ensuring both parties fully grasp and understand the decisions they have made. Another useful safeguard might be a choice of law clause which specifies what law governs a dispute arising under the contract. The contract could then be brought before court and given a judicial decree of enforceability. At this point, a judge, by declaratory judgment could decide whether the contract was enforceable; thus limiting uncertainty as to a future dispute.

Another legal battle taking place as consequence to ART's is that of intestacy and social security rights of posthumously conceived children.

Posthumously Conceived Children and Intestacy/Social Security Issues

As mentioned at the beginning of this chapter the issues concerning excess embryos due to IVF are not the only legal issues arising from ART's. Another legal battle is that concerning intestacy and social security rights of posthumously conceived children. A posthumously conceived child differs from the posthumously born child in that the former is both born and conceived after the death of one or both of the child's genetic parents. Hence a posthumously conceived child is by definition, a non marital child even though the child's parent might have been married prior to the child's conception.

Historically, children of unmarried parents were treated harshly. A child born out of wedlock could inherit from neither father nor mother. Only the child's spouse and descendants could inherit from the child. If the child died intestate (without will) and left neither spouse nor descendants, the child's property passed to the king or other overlord. Today most states have loosened intestacy laws for non marital children. Most permit paternity to be established with proof of certain evidence. In most states, if not all, paternity may be established by the subsequent marriage of the parents, acknowledgement by the father by adjudication during the life of the father

or by clear and convincing proof after his death. These statutes are not of much help, however, for that of a posthumously conceived child. Whether the government has to pay benefits is predominantly dependent upon the particular state of the posthumously conceived child.

It appears the underlying issues and policies concerning intestacy rights of posthumously conceived children concern that of the state and families interests in finality of the administration of estates, the human right to bear children, as well as, those rights of the children born as a result of ART's.

One of the latest cases concerning social security rights of posthumously conceived children has made it to Utah's Supreme Court [20].[98] At the center of the case is a 38-year-old widow, Gayle Burns of Utah. In December 2003, she gave birth to a son, Ian, using sperm that her husband, Michael, had deposited in a sperm bank the year prior to his death. The agreement Michael signed made numerous references to use of the semen to achieve pregnancy and specifically asked that his specimen be kept in storage for "future donation" to Gayle if Michael died. Michael died in 2001 of complications from Non-Hodgkin's Lymphoma.

Ian received a total of about $35,000 in Social Security survivor benefits. Last August, however, the agency decided that Ms. Burns had failed to show Ian was her dead husband's child, as defined under the federal Social Security Act. Utah law requires that a person must have consented "in a record" to become a parent through assisted reproduction before death but doesn't define what qualifies as a record [21].[99] Utah is among 11 states that have addressed posthumously conceived children through its probate and parentage laws as of 2006. Those states require a written record of consent or, in one instance, provision in the deceased's will. But the type of record isn't specified [21].[100] In response to the agency's demands to return the money, Ms. Burns was forced to file for personal bankruptcy.

A couple of months later, Ms. Burns sued the agency and the case ended up in the state's Supreme Court in June of 2010. The issue for the Supreme Court will be whether a signed sperm donor agreement is evidence of a man's desire to become a father, even after his death.; And, whether the child becomes his legal heir. More specifically, the issue will be whether a semen storage agreement is evidence of his record of consent.

The Massachusetts case of *Woodward v. Commissioner of Social Security* is illustrative of how the Utah Supreme Court may decide the case [22].[101]

In the 2002 case of *Woodward*, Lauren and Warren, a married couple, decided to deposit sperm at a sperm bank after receiving news that Warren would have to undergo radiation treatment due to cancer. Unfortunately, Warren lost his battle to cancer and 2 years *after* his death Lauren gave birth to his two kids through artificial insemination. Lauren subsequently filed for social security but was denied. Under federal law a child of a deceased father is eligible for Social Security survivor's benefits only if the child would inherit from the father under state law. Under state law the children were not eligible to inherit from their father. The court concluded that the fact the husband was the genetic father of the wife's children was insufficient in and of it to establish the husband was the children's legal father for purposes of distribution of his intestate estate. The court went on to state, however, that limited circumstances exist which allow posthumously conceived children to enjoy the same inheritance rights of our intestacy law. These limited circumstances occurred when the surviving parent or the child's other legal representative confirmed a genetic relationship between the child and the decedent and the survivor or representative demonstrates both that the decedent affirmatively approved of posthumous conception and to wished to provide for any resulting child. Furthermore, even where such circumstances exist, time limitations may preclude commencing a claim for inheritance rights on behalf of a posthumously conceived child. Finally, any action brought to establish such rights; notice must be given to all interested parties.

Attempting to answer the issues faced in *Woodard*, Eleven state legislatures responded by explicitly recognizing a parent-child relationship that begins with posthumous conception. For example under Cal. Prob. Code § 249.5 (2008), "a child of the decedent conceived after the death of the decedent shall be deemed to have been born in the lifetime of the decedent" if (a) the decedent consented in a signed and dated writing; (b) within four months of the decedent's death, notice of the possibility of posthumous conception is served upon "a person who has the power to control the distribution" of the decedent's property; and (c) the child "was in utero within two years of the decedent's death and the child is not a clone of the decedent." The laws of most states, however, define the parent-child relationship more traditionally. For the relationship to exist, a parent must be alive at the time of conception. Other state statutes recognizing this issue is Louisiana. La. Rev. Stat. 9:391.1 (2008) which grants posthumously conceived children inheritance rights if born to the surviving spouse within three years of the decedent's death. Overall, the majority of states limit parenthood to only parents that are alive at the time of conception. Among the states whose courts recognized social security benefits to posthumously conceived children include Massachusetts, New Jersey, Arizona, and Iowa. Florida, New Hampshire, and Arkansas however, have concluded that such children are not entitled to social security benefits.

If there is a trend, however, it is to allow intestacy rights to posthumously conceived children if (1) there is written consent to posthumous conception, and (2) a time frame to which they are born is provided and consented to in writing. For example, UPC 2-120 provides that a posthumously conceived child inherits from the deceased parent if (1) during life the parent consented to posthumous conception in a signed writing or consent is otherwise proved by clear and convincing evidence, and (2) the child is in utero not later than 36 months or is born not later than 45 months after the parent's death. Furthermore, the Restatement (third) of Property Wills and Other Donative Transfers § 2.5, cmt. 1 (1999) takes the stance that to inherit from the decedent, a child produced from genetic material of the decedent by assisted reproductive technology must born within a reasonable time after the decedent's death in circumstances indicating that the decedent would have approved of the child's right to inherit.

The case of *Woodard* should be compared with that of *In Re Martin B* [5].[102] In this NY case the court was asked whether the terms "issue" and "descendants", used in the trust instruments include children conceived by means of in vitro fertilization with the cryopreserved semen of the Grantor's son, James, who had died several years prior to such conception. After being diagnosed with Hodgkin's Lymphoma James deposited a sample of semen at a laboratory with instructions that it be cryopreserved and that, in the event of his death, it be held subject to the directions of his wife, Nancy. Subsequently following both Grantor's death and James's death Nancy gave birth to two boys. In holding that the posthumously conceived children were issue and descendants for all purposes of the trust, the court distinguished this case from that of Woodard. In the former, the administrative concern is nonexistent as the case concerns the administration of trust benefits. The court looked to interpret the trust to achieve Grantor's intent and not James' intent.

As this chapter has shown, the advancements in ART have led to a new legal frontier. Ambiguities in the law surrounding the legal rights of a child born posthumously are increasingly leading to lawsuits. The law will only get murkier if state legislatures do not act. Healthcare professionals however can help patients make more informed decisions regarding these very personal life choices. By becoming aware of the law of one's jurisdiction lawsuits like that of Ms. Burns' can be prevented.

Conclusion

Many of the issues that patients of ARTs are facing are preventable through research and discussions made by healthcare professionals with their patients. A well informed patient can better protect herself/himself against some of the pitfalls that ART's have produced. It is important for patients and healthcare professionals working in the area of ART to know the law of their jurisdiction and to be aware of what rights of the frozen pre-embryo,

patient, and doctor/fertility clinic as to avoid conflict in the future as to the cryopreserved embryos disposition. The laws dealing with ART and posthumous children are in constant evolution. For this reason it is incumbent that patients of ART and healthcare professionals to do their research prior to embarking on such procedures.

Provider Recommendations

1. As a result of IVF and the routine practice of extracting extra embryos there are currently an estimated 500,000 cryopreserved embryos stored in fertility clinics in the United States today.
2. The problem of how to deal with these excess embryos originates from the fact the law is unclear how they are to be legally classified; whether it be person, property or an interim status.
3. It is important for patients and healthcare professionals working in the area of ART to know the law of their jurisdiction and to be aware of what rights of the frozen pre-embryo, patient, and doctor/fertility clinic as to avoid conflict in the future as to the cryopreserved embryos disposition.
4. IVF and other reproductive procedures have also caused issues in the United States Social Security laws.
5. In terms of awarding social security benefits, the majority of states limit parenthood to only parents that are alive at the time of conception.

Notes

1. *Intestacy law* refers to the body of law that determines who is entitled to the property of one who dies without a will or other binding declaration.
2. Elizabeth E. Swire Falker, Esq., The Disposition of Cryopreserved Embryos: Why Embryo Adoption is an Inapposite Model for Application to Third-Party Assisted Reproduction, 35 WMLR 489, 493, fn 15 (2009); www.youtube.com/watch?v=TqqtErMzfCQ&feature=related.
3. Moral Challenges, supra note i at 115-121.
4. Ann Marie Noonan, The Uncertainty of Embryo Disposition Law: How Alterations to Roe Could

Change Everything, 40 Suffolk U.L. Rev. 485, 487-487 nn. 12-13 (2007).

5. Alexia M. Baiman, Cryopreserved Embryos as America's Prospective Adoptees: Are Couples Truly "Adopting" or Merely Transferring Property Rights?, 16 Wm. & Mary J. Women & L. 133, 137 n. 25 (2009).

6. Alexia M. Baiman, Cryopreserved Embryos as America's Prospective Adoptees: Are Couples Truly "Adopting" or Merely Transferring Property Rights?, 16 Wm. & Mary J. Women & L. 133, 142-143 (2009). ii

7. Id.

8. Id.

9. Id. at 143-145.

10. Id. at 140 n. 49; La. Stat. Ann. §§ 121-133 (2009); N.M. Stat. § 24-9A-3 (2008).

11. Moral Challenges, supra note i at 115-121.

12. Id.

13. Id.

14. Id. at 111; Alexia M. Baiman, Cryopreserved Embryos as America's Prospective Adoptees: Are Couples Truly "Adopting" or Merely Transferring Property Rights?, 16 Wm. & Mary J. Women & L. 133, 140-141 (2009).

15. La. Stat. Ann. § 125.

16. La. Stat. Ann. §§ 121-133.

17. Id.

18. Id; The Best Interest standard is used by most courts to determine a wide range of issues relating to the well-being of children. It is often used in disputes regarding custody, visitation, and guardianship of the child. The court will consider a number of factors revolving around the well being of the child to determine the outcome of the dispute. footnote

19. Id.

20. N.M. Stat. § 24-9A-3 (2008).

21. Id.

22. Jessica L. Lambert, Boston College Law Review Developing a Legal Framework for Resolving Disputes Between "Adoptive Parents" of Frozen Embryos: A comparison to Resolutions of Divorce Disputes between Progenitors, 529, 537-538; nn. 59-71.

23. Id.

24. Alexia M. Baiman, Cryopreserved Embryos as America's Prospective Adoptees: Are Couples Truly "Adopting" or Merely Transferring Property Rights?, 16 Wm. & Mary J. Women & L. 133, 141 (2009).

25. Davis v. Davis, 842 S.W.2d 588, 594-597 (Tenn. 1992).

26. Id.

27. Id.

28. Id.

29. Id.

30. York v. Jones, 717 F. Supp. 421, 425-27 (E.D. Va. 1989).

31. Id.

32. Id.; see also Jessica L. Lambert, Boston College Law Review Developing a Legal Framework for Resolving Disputes Between "Adoptive Parents" of Frozen Embryos: A comparison to Resolutions of Divorce Disputes between Progenitors, 529, 538-539 n. 73-76.

33. Alexia M. Baiman, Cryopreserved Embryos as America's Prospective Adoptees: Are Couples Truly "Adopting" or Merely Transferring Property Rights?, 16 Wm. & Mary J. Women & L. 133, 143 (2009).

34. Id.

35. Id.

36. Id.

37. Id.

38. Supra note i.

39. Id.

40. Id.

41. Davis v. Davis, 842 S.W.2d 588, 594-597 (Tenn. 1992).

42. Id.

43. Id.

44. Id.

45. Id.

46. Jeter v. Mayo 121 P.3d 1256 (Ariz. Ct. App. 2005); Alexia M. Baiman, Cryopreserved Embryos as America's Prospective Adoptees: Are Couples Truly "Adopting" or Merely Transferring Property Rights?, 16 Wm. & Mary J. Women & L. 133, 137 n. 98 (2009).

47. Id.

48. Id.

49. Id.

50. A.Z. v. B.Z., 431 mass. 150, 725 N.E.2d 1051, 1056-1059 (2000).

51. 18 Pa. Cons. Stat. § 3216(a) (2009). Alexia M. Baiman, Cryopreserved Embryos as America's Prospective Adoptees: Are Couples Truly "Adopting" or Merely Transferring Property Rights?, 16 Wm. & Mary J. Women & L. 133, 137 n. 104 (2009).

52. Alexia M. Baiman, Cryopreserved Embryos as America's Prospective Adoptees: Are Couples Truly "Adopting" or Merely Transferring Property Rights?, 16 Wm. & Mary J. Women & L. 133, 137 n. 105 (2009).

53. Id.

54. Id.

55. Supra note i.

56. Alexia M. Baiman, Cryopreserved Embryos as America's Prospective Adoptees: Are Couples Truly "Adopting" or Merely Transferring Property Rights?, 16 Wm. & Mary J. Women & L. 133, 146-148 (2009).

57. Id.

58. Id.

59. Supra note i at 190.

60. Id.

61. Id.

62. Id.
63. Charles P. Kindregan, Jr., Maureen McBrien, Embryo Donation: Unresolved Legal Issues in the Transfer of Surplus Cryopreserved Embryos, 49 Vill. L. Rev. 169, 173-177 (2004).
64. Id.
65. Id.
66. Id.
67. Alexia M. Baiman, Cryopreserved Embryos as America's Prospective Adoptees: Are Couples Truly "Adopting" or Merely Transferring Property Rights?, 16 Wm. & Mary J. Women & L. 133, 148-151 (2009).
68. Id.
69. Id.
70. Id.
71. Id. see *Kass v. Kass*, 696 N.E.2d 174 (N.Y. 1998)(Court of Appeals of New York held that an informed consent agreement signed by a couple which states the embryos would be donated to research was upheld and binding even though wife sought to use the embryos for implantation); *LItowitz v. Litowitz*, 10 P.3d 1086, 948-949 (Wash. Ct. App. 2000) (where the supreme court enforced an agreement between a couple that stated the cryopreserved embryos would be destroyed, even though the wife wished to have embryos implanted in a surrogate and the husband wanted to donate the embryos to another couple.); *Roman v. Roman*, 193 S.W.3d 40, 55 (Tx. 1st Dist. Ct App. 2006) (where the court of appeals held that an informed consent agreement signed by the former husband and wife what provided for their frozen embryos to be discarded in the event of divorce was valid and enforceable.
72. Id.
73. Id.
74. Supra note i at 151 n. 165; see also *Kass*, 696 N.E.2d 174; *A.Z. v. B.Z.*, 431 mass. 150, 725 N.E.2d 1051, 1056-1059 (2000).
75. *Kass*, 696 N.E.2d 174; Jessica L. Lambert, Boston College Law Review Developing a Legal Framework for Resolving Disputes Between "Adoptive Parents" of Frozen Embryos: A comparison to Resolutions of Divorce Disputes between Progenitors, 529, 558-559.
76. Id.
77. Id.
78. Id.
79. Embryo Donation, Facts about Embryos, http://www.miracleswaiting.org/factsembryos.html#q17; supra note i.
80. Id.
81. Id.
82. Jessica L. Lambert, Boston College Law Review Developing a Legal Framework for Resolving Disputes Between "Adoptive Parents" of Frozen Embryos: A comparison to Resolutions of Divorce Disputes between Progenitors, 529, 558-559.
83. *Kass v. Kass*, 696 N.E.2d 174,182 (holding the agreements signed by a couple prior to undergoing IVF treatments should presumptively be valid, binding, and enforceable, subject to the couples mutual change of mind) but see *In re Marriage of Witten*, 672 N.W.2d (2003) 768, 778; see *A.Z. v. B.Z.*, 431 mass. 150, 725 N.E.2d 1051, 1056-1059 (2000) (holding as a matter of public policy forced procreation is not an area amenable to judicial enforcement citing the unfairness of the contractual approach and in favor of a mutual consent theory); *J.B. v. M.B.* 783 A.2d. 707 (N.J. 2001) (Evaluating relative interests of parties in disposition of embryos, concluding husband should not be able to use embryos over wife's objection); *Davis v. Davis*, 842 S.W.2d 588, 594-597 (holding that ordinarily the party wishing to avoid procreation should prevail under a balancing approach) Susan B. Apel, Disposition of Frozen Embryos: Are Contracts the Solution?, Vermont Bar Journal, March 2001, at 31 (Some argue that the party seeking to avoid procreation should prevail, and indeed, this appears to be the one harmonizing rationale of the four reported case."
84. *Kass v. Kass*, 696 N.E.2d 174, 182.
85. *J.B. v M.B.* 783 A.2d. 707, 717-718.
86. Id.
87. 672 N.W.2d at 782.
88. Id.
89. Id. at 783.
90. Supra note xci.
91. Id.
92. Id.
93. Id.
94. *In re Marriage of Witten*, 672 N.W.2d 768, 778 (2003).
95. See Id.
96. Id.
97. Id.
98. *Burns v. Astrue*, 2:2009cv00926 Utah District Court (2009)
99. Brooke Adams, Should boy born 3 years after dad's death get social security?, The Salt Lake Tribune (2010); http://www.sltrib.com/csp/cms/sites/sltrib/pages/printerfriendly.csp?id=49775477
100. Brooke Adams, Should boy born 3 years after dad's death get social security?, The Salt Lake Tribune (2010); http://www.sltrib.c
101. 760 N.E.2d 257, (Mass 2002).
102. 6. *La. Stat. Ann. § 125*.2008).

References

1. Baiman AM (2009) Cryopreserved embryos as America's prospective adoptees: are couples truly "adopting" or merely transferring property rights? Wm & Mary J Women & L 16:133–205

2. Falker EES, Elizabeth E (2009) The disposition of cryopreserved embryos: why embryo adoption is an inapposite model for application to third-party assisted reproduction. Wm Mitchell L Rev 35:489, 493
3. Moral Challenges
4. Noonan AM (2007) The uncertainty of embryo disposition law: how alterations to roe could change everything. Suffolk UL Rev 40:485–1049
5. La. Stat. Ann. § 125
6. La. Stat. Ann. §§ 121-133
7. N.M. Stat. § 24-9A-3. 2008
8. Lambert JL (2008) Developing a legal framework for resolving disputes between "adoptive parents" of frozen embryos: a comparison to resolutions of divorce disputes between progenitors. BCL Rev 49:529–1431
9. Davis v. Davis 1992, Supreme Court of Tennesee
10. York v. Jones. 1989
11. Moore KA (2007) Embryo adoption: the legal and moral challenges. U St Thomas JL & Pub Pol'y 1:100
12. Jeter v. Mayo Clinic Arizona. 2005, Arizona Court of Appeals
13. A.Z. v. B.Z 2000, Supreme Court of Massachusetts
14. Kindregan CP Jr, McBrien M (2004) Embryo donation: unresolved legal issues in the transfer of surplus cryopreserved embryos. Villanova Law Rev 49:169
15. Kass v. Kass. 1998, New York State Court of Appeals
16. Facts about Embryos. Available from: http://www.miracleswaiting.org/factsembryos.html.
17. J.B. v. M. B. 2000, Superior Court of New Jersey Appellate Division
18. 672 N.W.2d at 782
19. In re Marriage of Witten, 672 N.W.2d 768, 788. 2003
20. Burns v. Astrue. 2009, Utah District Court
21. Adams B (2010) Should boy born 3 years after dad's death get social security? The Salt Lake City Tribune. http://www.atheistnexus.org/forum/topics/should-boy-born-3-years-after?xg_source=activity
22. 760 N.E.2d 257 Mass 2002

Appendix

Table A.1 Types and definitions of assisted reproductive technology (ART)[a]

ART type	Definition
In vitro fertilization (IVF)	A woman's eggs are extracted, fertilized in the laboratory, and the resulting embryos are transferred into the woman's uterus through the cervix.
Intracytoplasmic sperm injection (ICSI)	A single sperm is injected directly into the woman's egg. This is used with some IVF procedures to overcome low sperm count, motility, or antisperm antibodies.
Gamete intrafallopian transfer (GIFT)	A laparoscope is used to guide the transfer of unfertilized eggs and sperm (gametes) into the woman's fallopian tubes through small incisions in her abdomen.
Zygote intrafallopian transfer (ZIFT)	A woman's eggs are fertilized in the laboratory then a laparoscope is used to guide the transfer of the fertilized eggs (zygotes) into her fallopian tubes.
Embryo biopsy	When an embryo reaches the 8 cell stage, a hole is made in the zona pellucida and one or two blastomeres containing a nucleus are gently aspirated through the opening and examined for genetic and chromosomal abnormalities.
Preimplantation genetic diagnosis	A procedure used in conjunction with IVF to screen for specific genetic or chromosomal abnormalities before transferring the fertilized eggs into the woman. One or two cells are removed 3 days after fertilization, then examined for chromosomal and genetic abnormalities
Oocyte or embryo donation	Donor eggs and embryos can be used if a woman's ovaries have been removed or if she doesn't have any healthy eggs. Donor eggs are often fertilized in the lab with partner or donor sperm to create embryos. Donor embryos are cryopreserved embryos that come from couples who created embryos but have completed their families. These donor embryos are transferred to the woman's uterus. The embryos may also be transferred to a surrogate if a woman cannot carry a pregnancy for medical reasons.
Gestational surrogacy	Surrogacy is when one woman carries a baby for another woman. This can be an option for women for whom a pregnancy is not medically safe or who are physically unable to carry a child due to a hysterectomy. Surrogates typically carry the biological child of the requester; however, donor eggs or embryos can also be used. Surrogacy laws vary from state to state.

[a] Assisted Reproductive Technology (ART) consists of clinical treatments and laboratory procedures that include the handling of human oocytes, sperm, or embryos, with the intent of establishing a pregnancy. This includes, but is not limited to, the techniques listed in this table [1]

G.P. Quinn, S.T. Vadaparampil (eds.), *Reproductive Health and Cancer in Adolescents and Young Adults*, Advances in Experimental Medicine and Biology 732,
DOI 10.1007/978-94-007-2492-1, © Springer Science+Business Media B.V. 2012

Table A.2 Assisted reproductive technologies estimated cost

Assisted reproductive technologies and preservation procedures	Cost
In vitro fertilization (IVF)	$8,000–18,000 including office visits and medications
Intrauterine insemination (IUI)	$300–$700 per cycle. Monitoring and medications can be an additional $1,500–$4,000
Intracytoplasmic sperm injection (ICSI)	$2,500 per cycle.
Gamete Intrafallopian Transfer (GIFT)	$15,000–20,000
Zygote Intrafallopian Transfer (ZIFT)	$15,000–20,000
Sperm cryopreservation (S) after masturbation	$1,500 for three samples stored for 3 years
Embryo cryopreservation (S)	Approximately $8,000 per cycle, $350 per year storage fees
Oocyte cryopreservation (I)	Approximately $8,000 per cycle, $350/yr storage fees
Gonadal shielding during radiation therapy (S)	Generally included in the cost of radiation treatments
Ovarian suppression with gonadotropin releasing hormone (GnRH) analogs or antagonists (I)	Approximately $500/mo

Costs are average estimates (without insurance) from Fertile Hope Parenthood Options and American Society of Clinical Oncology Recommendations on Fertility Preservation in Cancer Patients [1–4]
S Standard, *I* investigational

Table A.3 Fertility preservation options in females

Intervention	Definition	Comment	Considerations
Embryo cryopreservation (S)	Harvesting eggs, in vitro fertilization, and freezing of embryos for later implantation	The most established technique for fertility preservation in women	Requires 10–14 days of ovarian stimulation from the beginning of menstrual cycle Outpatient surgical procedure Requires partner or donor sperm
Oocyte cryopreservation (I)	Harvesting and freezing of unfertilized eggs	Small case series and case reports; as of 2005, 120 deliveries reported, approximately 2% live births per thawed oocyte (3–4 times lower than standard IVF)	Requires 10–14 days of ovarian stimulation from the beginning of menstrual cycle Outpatient surgical procedure
Ovarian cryopreservation and transplantation (I)	Freezing of ovarian tissue and reimplantation after cancer treatment	Case reports; as of 2005, two live births reported	Not suitable when risk of ovarian involvement is high Same day outpatient surgical procedure
Gonadal shielding during radiation therapy (S)	Use of shielding to reduce the dose of radiation delivered to the reproductive organs	Case series	Only possible with selected radiation fields and anatomy Expertise is required to ensure shielding does not increase dose delivered to the reproductive organs
Ovarian transposition (oophoropexy) (S)	Surgical repositioning of ovaries away from the radiation field	Large cohort studies and case series suggest approximately 50% chance of success due to altered ovarian blood flow and scattered radiation	Same day outpatient surgical procedure Transposition should be performed just before radiation therapy to prevent return of ovaries to former position May need repositioning or in vitro fertilization (IVF) to conceive

Table A.3 (continued)

Intervention	Definition	Comment	Considerations
Trachelectomy (S)	Surgical removal of the cervix while preserving the uterus	Large case series and case reports	Inpatient surgical procedure Limited to early stage cervical cancer; no evidence of higher cancer relapse rate in appropriate candidates Expertise may not be widely available
Other conservative gynecologic surgery (S/I)	Minimization of normal tissue resection	Large case series and case reports	Expertise may not be widely available
Ovarian suppression with gonadotropin releasing hormone (GnRH) analogs or antagonists (I)	Use of hormonal therapies to protect ovarian tissue during chemotherapy or radiation therapy	Small randomized studies and case series. Larger randomized trials in progress	Medication given before and during treatment with chemotherapy

S Standard, *I* Investigational
Lee et al. [1]

Table A.4 Fertility preservation options in males

Intervention	Definition	Comment	Considerations
Sperm cryopreservation (S) after masturbation	Freezing sperm obtained through masturbation	The most established technique for fertility preservation in men; large cohort studies in men with cancer	Outpatient procedure
Sperm cryopreservation (S) after alternative methods of sperm collection	Freezing sperm obtained through testicular aspiration or extraction, electroejaculation under sedation, or from a post-masturbation urine sample	Small case series and case reports	Testicular sperm extraction-outpatient surgical procedure
Gonadal shielding during radiation therapy (S)	Use of shielding to reduce the dose of radiation delivered to the testicles	Case series	Only possible with selected radiation fields and anatomy Expertise is required to ensure shielding does not increase dose delivered to the reproductive organs
Testicular tissue cryopreservation Testis xenografting Spermatogonial isolation (I)	Freezing testicular tissue or germ cells and reimplantation after cancer treatment or maturation in animals	Has not been tested in humans; successful application in animal models	Outpatient surgical procedure
Testicular suppression with gonadotropin releasing hormone (GnRH) analogs or antagonists (I)	Use of hormonal therapies to protect testicular tissue during chemotherapy or radiation therapy	Studies do not support the effectiveness of this approach	

S Standard, *I* Investigational
Lee et al. [1]

References

1. Lee SJ, Schover LR, Partridge AH, Patrizio P, Wallace WH, Hagerty K, et al (2006) American Society of Clinical Oncology recommendations on fertility preservation in cancer patients. J Clin Oncol 24(18):2917

2. Parenthood Options: Women (2011) Fertile Hope. http://www.fertilehope.org/learn-more/cancer-andfertility-info/parenthood-options-women.cfm

3. Parenthood Options: Men (2011) Fertile Hope. http://www.fertilehope.org/learn-more/cancer-and-fertilityinfo/parenthood-options-men.cfm

4. Financial Assistance (2011) Fertile Hope. http://www.fertilehope.org/financial-assistance/index.cfm

Guides for Choosing a Fertility Provider and Service [1–3]

Fertility Resource Guide

Fertility Resource Guide is an online searchable database that includes reproductive endocrinologists, sperm banks, financial assistance, adoption agencies and legal services in the United States, Canada, and Puerto Rico. After selecting search criteria, the results will list the name of the centers and the services provided, given the opportunity to compare center and view their websites.

http://fertilehope.org/tool-bar/referral-guide.cfm

Choosing a Doctor or Service

This online guide assists in determining which doctor, agency, or professional is best for the patient or client. Information is provided on choosing a reproductive doctor or agency, and questions to consider with surrogacy and choosing a Preimplemantation Genetic Diagnosis (PGD) provider.

http://www.fertilehope.org/learn-more/cancer-and-fertility-info/how-to-choose-a-doctor.cfm

Male and Female Services

General Fertility/IVF services

Infertility is the inability to conceive after one year of unprotected intercourse in women under 35, or after 6 months in women over 35, or the inability to carry a pregnancy to term. In vitro fertilization (IVF) is the process in which unfertilized eggs are collected from a female partner, sperm is collected from a male partner, and the two are put together in a laboratory in order to achieve fertilization [1, 2].

Preimplanatation Genetic Diagnosis (PGD)

PGD is a process that allows the possibility to identify particular aspects of an embryo. A cell is removed from an embryo and is evaluated for some particular traits. About 500 genetically related diseases can be tested for such as cystic fibrosis, Huntington's disease, and fragile X syndrome. Cost varies around $15,000 for a single treatment [1, 2].

Male Services

Sperm Retrieval Services & Testicular Tissue Freezing

Testicular sperm extraction can be accomplished with several different techniques. The most effective approach uses an operating microscope to identify areas of the testicle with sperm production [2]. Extraction or retrieval of testicular tissue can be done to freeze testicular tissue prior to cancer treatment.

Sperm Banking

A chance for men who store their sperm and undergo cancer treatment to father a biological child has enhanced significantly. Quality of semen is usually best before any treatment has started. Patients should consider banking at least two specimen spaced 48–72 h apart [2]. Specimens are stored in liquid nitrogen tanks in sperm banking facilities.

Female Services

Egg Cryopreservation

Egg cryopreservation is the process by which human eggs are rapidly cooled in order to preserve them [1]. This technology is appropriate for women at risk of losing ovarian function or premature ovarian failure, including cancer patients who have to undergo radiation or chemotherapy.

In Vitro Maturation (IVM)

IVM can be offered to post puberty patients, preferably before the onset of cancer treatment, to reduce the risk of genetic damage to the oocytes [1]. Eggs are retrieved using a transvaginal ultrasound probe and then matured in a laboratory. The mature oocytes are either fertilized by patient's partner and then the resulting embryos are frozen or the mature oocytes can be frozen without fertilization. Cost vary from $2,400 to $5,000.

Ovarian Tissue Cryopreservation

Ovarian failure is correlated to chemotherapy and radiation. This option is when one ovary or a portion is removed surgically. The ovarian tissue containing immature primordial follicles is then frozen. The ovarian tissue can be thawed and undergo further development before fertilization, once the patient is cured of her disease [1].

Third Party Reproduction

Adoption

Different types of adoption [1, 2]:
- Private Placement – birth parent(s) place the child directly with the adoptive parent(s) without an agency as an intermediary. Cost varies from $10,000 to $15,000.
- Private Agency – an agency that has been authorized by the state to act as an intermediary between adoptive parents and birth parents. Cost varies from $15,000 to $30,000.
- Public Agency – state provides adoption services for children who are in its custody. There is little or no cost.
- International – through agencies with programs in foreign countries. Adoption requirements of the country of the child's origin and requirements of United States citizenship and Immigration Services must be satisfied. Cost varies from $7,000 to $30,000, not including travel expenses.

Egg and Embryo Donation

When a woman cannot produce eggs or has poor quality eggs, she can receive eggs from another woman. A woman can still experience pregnancy and if she has a male partner can have a genetic link to the child. Donor egg cycles use the same technology as IVF. Cost varies from $25,000 to $30, 000 [1].

Sperm Donation

Sperm donation is the use of donor sperm to become pregnant. The sperm is placed into the woman's uterus via a tiny tube during ovulation. Cost varies from $1,500 to $3,000 on average of 3–6 cycles [2].

Surrogacy

A traditional surrogacy arrangement is an option for a cancer patient who may not be able to carry a child because of a hysterectomy due to cancer, damage to her uterus because of radiation, or concerns about her health as result of cancer /or cancer treatment [1].

Financial Assistance Services

Although diagnostic tests for infertility are often covered by insurance, the cost of treatment usually is not. In the United States, about 15–20% of all high technology treatments are covered by insurance [3]. Without insurance coverage patients have to pay for treatments which can range from several thousands of dollars. Having a consult with a financial advisor at the infertility practice and discuss questions about insurance and service costs would be the first step to deciding about fertility treatment.

Non Profit Organizations

For more information on the aforementioned services refer to the following:

American Fertility Association (AFA)
- Free membership
- Online community where you receive access to AFA educational material via the web based program "No Barriers"
- Find expert advice from world renowned physicians during AFA-moderated online sessions

www.afa.org

American Society of Reproductive Medicine (ASRM)
- Provide information on infertility, menopause, contraception, reproductive surgery,

endometriosis, and other reproductive disorders.
- Online patient features include:
  - Find a doctor
  - Patient booklet
  - Patient fact sheet
  - FAQs
  - Topic index
  - Links to professional organizations

www.asrm.org

Cryogenic Laboratories, Inc. Priority Male: Sperm Banking by Mail Program
- First US sperm bank
- Donor sperm, sperm banking, and sperm and embryo storage services
- Accredited by American Association of Tissue Banks

www.cryolab.com

Extend Fertility, Inc.
- Provide women with information on medical solutions and reproductive health
- Connects women with Extended Fertility partner center with success in frozen eggs
- Team comprised of doctors, scientist, and business leaders that solely specialize in egg freezing

www.extendfertility.com

Fertile Hope
- A **LIVESTRONG** initiative, as a fertile resource for cancer patients, dedicated to providing reproductive information, support and hope to cancer patients and survivors whose medical treatments present the risk of infertility.

www.fertilehope.org

The ARC Fertility Program
- Nation's largest network of reproductive endocrinologists and premier fertility programs
- Unique treatment packages and financing programs to help overcome insurance coverage

www.arcfertility.com

The InterNational Council on Infertility Information Dissemination (INCIID)

- Helps individuals and couples explore their family-building options
- Provides current information and immediate support regarding the diagnosis, treatment, and prevention of infertility and pregnancy loss, and offers guidance to those considering adoption or childfree lifestyles
- "From INCIID The Heart" is a program designed to provide free IVF to those without insurance who have both financial and medical need for the procedure

www.inciid.org

Resolve: The National Infertility Association
Benefits of membership include:

- Medical call-in hours
- Member to member contact system
- Local Resolve support
- Physician referrals
- Annual Subscription to Family Building
- Savings on Publications
- Advocacy

www.resolve.org

References

1. Parenthood Options: Women (2011) Fertile Hope. http://www.fertilehope.org/learn-more/cancer-and-fertility-info/parenthood-options-women.cfm
2. Parenthood Options: Men (2011) Fertile Hope. http://www.fertilehope.org/learn-more/cancer-and-fertility-info/parenthood-options-men.cfm
3. Financial Assistance (2011) Fertile Hope. http://www.fertilehope.org/financial-assistance/index.cfm

Index

A

Adolescents, 33–34
Amenorrhea, 6, 9, 12, 41, 47–48, 66, 77, 80–81, 83–85, 92
Antineoplastic agents, 65
Assisted reproductive technologies, 15–19, 96, 104, 153, 169–170, 192–193, 205, 211–212
Azoospermia, 6, 30–32, 34–35, 38, 65–66, 151

B

Breast neoplasms, 64

C

Cancer
    fertility, 78–81
    predisposition, 19, 104–106, 111–112, 154
    survivorship, 156
    treatment (male/female), ix–x, 1–7, 11, 14–16, 18–20, 22, 30–31, 38, 42, 53, 61–63, 68–69, 72, 78, 82–83, 93, 100, 106, 116–117, 119–123, 126–127, 143, 151–153, 155, 157–161, 166–167, 171–172, 176–181, 183–184, 188, 190, 193–194, 212–213, 216–217
Chemotherapy, 2–3, 6, 10–18, 21–22, 31, 33–34, 36–37, 41–43, 45–49, 52–54, 63, 65–66, 78, 80–81, 83–85, 90–93, 98–100, 121, 123, 133, 135, 142, 151–152, 158, 176–178, 182, 213, 216
Childhood coping, 132
Communication, 22, 62, 68–69, 71, 100, 117, 131–139, 141, 143–144, 147, 152–154, 160, 175–184, 188
Contraception, 41–56, 72, 176–179, 183–184, 217

D

Decision making, 18, 117–118, 126, 133, 144, 153, 160, 169, 179, 194, 199

E

Embryo, 16–19, 21, 78–79, 93, 104, 108–110, 154, 182, 198–202, 206–208, 211–212, 216–217
Ethics, 119, 179–180, 187, 189, 192–194

F

Female infertility, 170
Fertility
    preservation, 10, 93, 166–167, 183–184, 193–194, 212–213
    infertility, 69

G

Gonadal toxicity, 6–7, 11, 13–14, 21, 31, 35, 77, 81, 85, 99

I

Infertility, male, 170
Institutional Approach, 165–173
Intestacy, 198, 204–206
Intimacy, 62–63, 67–71
In vitro fertilization, v, 3, 9–10, 14, 16, 29, 79, 93, 118, 127, 153–155, 182, 189, 206, 211–212, 215

L

Legacy, 144, 145, 148
Legal, 90, 96, 104, 119, 122–123, 125, 145–146, 190–191, 197–209, 215

M

Menopause, 6, 10–11, 14, 16, 20, 41, 63, 65–67, 71, 78, 80, 90, 92, 121, 152, 158, 170, 184, 217

O

Oncofertility, 9, 11, 22, 100
Oncology, 10, 30, 53, 55, 70, 72, 91–92, 94, 147–148, 151–161, 165–173, 177, 179–182, 188, 212
Ovarian reserve, 7, 10–11, 13, 80, 82–83, 91, 108

P

PACT, 131, 147–148
Parenthood after cancer, 166–168
Parenting history, 131, 133, 139
Parenting with cancer, 131–139, 141–148
Pediatric oncology, 151–161, 177, 180–181
Posthumous, 30, 119, 189–191, 198, 204–206
Pregnancy, 83–85, 89–100, 176–177, 184, 189–190
Preimplantation genetic diagnosis, x, 19, 104, 211
Program, x, 43, 69–72, 131, 135, 147, 166–169, 171–172, 180–181, 183, 189, 216–218
Providers, 7, 22, 38, 53, 55–56, 72, 85, 100, 112, 126, 139, 148, 160–161, 172, 175–184, 194–195, 206, 215

R

Radiotherapy, 3–5, 7
Reproduction, 1–7, 29–30, 33–34, 38, 61–62, 69–70, 80, 119, 152–155, 169, 179–180, 182–183, 189–192, 204, 216

Reproductive age, 22, 30–31, 90–93, 96, 98, 155, 168,
    190
Reproductive health, 42, 77, 91, 116, 118, 122, 151–160,
    166, 175–184, 217

S
Semen preservation, 30, 33–34, 36–37, 202, 204
Sexual assessment, 69–70
Sexuality, x, 61–63, 65, 67–72, 157, 176–177
Sperm retrieval, 34–38, 215–216
Stages of illness, 131, 141–148

Status, ix, 7, 10–11, 31, 49, 63, 65, 84, 93, 107, 124,
    154–157, 160–161, 183, 189, 191, 198–201, 203,
    206
Supporting children, 146–148
Survivorship, ix, 62, 78, 91, 131, 143, 147, 154, 156, 160,
    165–167, 172, 176, 179

Y
Young adults, 2, 6–7, 30, 41–43, 53, 55, 61–63, 66–72,
    77, 115–116, 118, 121, 126, 136, 153–154, 156,
    172, 176, 183

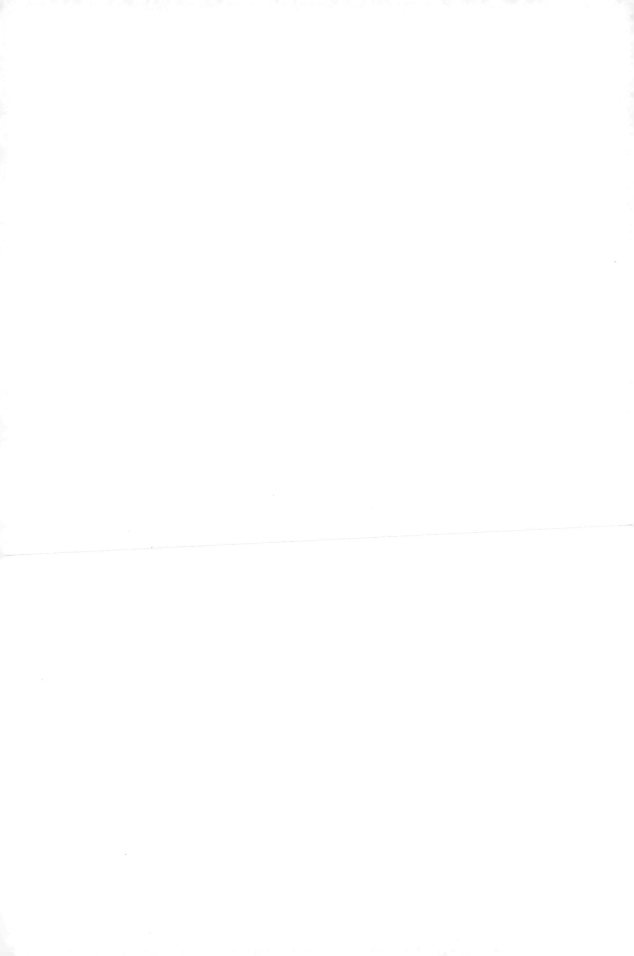

CPSIA information can be obtained at www.ICGtesting.com
Printed in the USA
LVOW112012250613

340187LV00003B/3/P